Avian Surgical Anatomy and Orthopedic Management

SECOND EDITION

Susan E. Orosz, PhD, DVM, DABVP(Av), DECZM(Av)

M. Scott Echols, DVM, DABVP(Av)

Patrick T. Redig, DVM, PhD

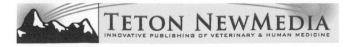

TETON NEWMEDIA
INNOVATIVE PUBLISHING OF VETERINARY & HUMAN MEDICINE

Executive Editor: Carroll C. Cann

Teton NewMedia
5286 Dunewood Dr,
Florence, OR 97439
541.991.3342
www.tetonnm.com

ISBN # 978-1-59161-052-6
Print number 5 4 3 2 1

Library of Congress Cataloging-in-Publication Data on file.

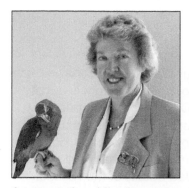

Dr. Orosz is an internationally known avian veterinarian and anatomist. She received her PhD in human neuroanatomy from the University of Cincinnati Medical Center in 1980 and her DVM degree from The Ohio State University in 1984. From 1986-2000, Dr. Orosz taught avian medicine and surgery at The University of Tennessee, College of Veterinary Medicine where she attained the rank of professor. During her tenure at the University, she advanced the Avian and Exotic Animal Medicine Service at the Teaching Hospital as Service Chief and developed the ABVP Avian Residency Program in Avian Medicine. She obtained board certification in Avian Medicine through the American Board of Veterinary Practitioners and the European College of Avian Medicine. Dr. Orosz authored the award-winning prede- cessor to this text, Avian Surgical Anatomy: Thoracic and Pelvic Limbs, and co-authored Manual of Avian Medicine with Dr. Glen Olsen. She has written on a variety of avian topics for research publications, including avian anatomy, fungal diseases and their treatment, and neurology. Dr Orosz is a past president of the Association of Avian Veterinarians (1995) and served as scientific editor for its journal, The Journal of Avian Medicine and Surgery, from 2000-2003. She received the Merck Award for Creative Achievement in 1994 and was the recipient of the Excellence in Avian Research from the AVMA in 1997. Dr Orosz was awarded the Dr. TJ Lafeber Avian Practi- tioner Award in 2007. Dr. Orosz has served as a committee member to the Secretary of Agriculture's Advisory Committee on Foreign Animal and Poultry Diseases and as a consultant for the Lafeber Company. Dr. Orosz is owner of the Bird and Exotic Pet Wellness Center in Toledo, OH.

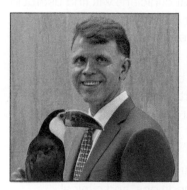

Dr. M. Scott Echols is a boarded avian specialist veterinarian living in Salt Lake City, Utah. Dr. Echols was the 2005 recipient of the T.J. Lafeber Avian Practitioner of the Year Award, 2007 Texas Veterinary Medical Association Non-Traditional Species Practi- tioner of the Year, 2007-2008 President of the Association of Avian Veterinarians and Texas A&M 2018 Distinguished Alumnus. He is also the creator of several educational DVDs including Captive Foraging and The Expert Companion Bird Care Series. Dr Echols founded the Grey Parrot Anatomy Project to better define bird anatomy and develop new diagnostic and therapeutic advances that apply to numerous branches of medicine. Additionally, he creates innovative imaging technology for use with animals and humans and is the founder of Scarlet Imaging where he works to help science achieve better answers that change the world. His animal and anatomy themed artworks have been featured on the cover of several journals, recognized for two Wellcome Image Awards and displayed in numerous museums and galleries across the world. Dr Echols is a frequent author, lecturer and visiting professor internationally covering topics relative to human and animal health. He lives with his wife Layle and daughter Alaina who also enjoy animals and nature.

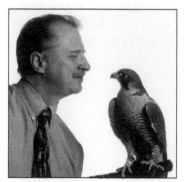

Dr. Patrick Redig DVM, PhD, is Professor Emeritus at the College of Veterinary Medicine, University of Minnesota and founder and former director of The Raptor Center, a world-renowned institution of raptor conservation and medicine. He obtained his DVM from the University of Minnesota in 1974 and his PhD in physiology at the same insti- tution in 1979. He assumed a position as an assistant professor in 1981 and rose to the level of Full Professor in the Department of Small Animal Clinical Sciences. A falconer since his early teens with a keen interest in raptor protection, he seized the opportunity to initiate and develop a program designed to promote conservation of birds of prey through the medium of veterinary medicine and public outreach. From this platform, he nurtured, through research and practice, the nascent art of avian medicine and the establishment of The Raptor Center. Responding to the need for an armamentarium of tools to treat the hundreds of traumatically injured raptors presented annually, he developed unique and affordable methods for orthopedic management that are a major component of this edition of the book. These methods have been taught to thousands of students around the globe through residencies and internships at The Raptor Center as well as workshops offered at many venues domestic and abroad. Dr. Redig is the author of numerous original research articles on topics ranging from anesthesia and orthopedic surgery to West Nile virus disease, avian influenza, asper- gillosis, and lead poisoning. In addition, he has authored numerous chapters in most contemporary avian medicine books and convened two international symposia on raptor biomedicine. Beyond veterinary medicine, he also served as the overall coordinator for restoration of the peregrine falcon in the Midwest United States and was appointed by the U.S. Fish & Wildlife Service to the California Condor Recovery Team where he served as coordinator of outreach on lead poisoning for 15 years. He served for six years on the Committee on the Environment of the American Veterinary Medical Association and as Treasurer for the AAV. He is a recipient of the T.J. Lafeber Avian Practitioner of the Year Award and the Minnesota Veterinary Medical Association's Veterinarian of the Year. He retired in 2018 after forty-five years of dedication to the cause of raptor conservation and continues to work on their behalf. The endowed Patrick T. Redig Chair in Avian Medicine and Conservation at The Raptor Center ensures his legacy will endure.

PREFACE

Avian Surgical Anatomy: Thoracic and Pelvic Limbs by Orosz, Ensley and Haynes, was published in 1992 and has served as a standard guide for those performing orthopedic surgery on birds. That foundational work is out of print but the need for a concise source of avian surgical anatomy has not changed. Our objective in this edition has been to recapture the musculoskeletal anatomy of the original work and to expand the scope to include comprehensive coverage for the clinical management of common fractures of the long bones of birds, primarily raptors. The procedures described have been honed over two decades of development and refinement by clinicians at the Raptor Center at the University of Minnesota. In addition, we have included details of the vascular anatomy of the limbs, further informing the surgeon and clinician.

The class Aves includes thousands of species with countless anatomic variations. Although it is impractical to represent every species, birds commonly encountered in private practice and rehabilitation medicine including poultry, pigeons, parrots and birds of prey were chosen for this book. Details of the vascular anatomy of the limbs were obtained by high resolution digital computed tomography imaging of the appendicular skeleton of several diverse bird species. These images provide a unique comparative aspect that clinicians will find useful in conducting surgical procedures. This new information is intended to help the reader better understand skeletal and vascular anatomy, and thus improve interpretation, reporting of findings, treatment and teaching.

This new information is intended to help the reader better understand relationships between musculoskeletal and vascular anatomy, helping the surgeon preserve vasculature during complex orthopedic procedures. It is our hope that it will enrich the interpretation, reporting of findings, development of treatment methods and the teaching of management procedures for orthopedic issues in birds.

Since publication of the first edition, numerous advances have been made and published relative to avian orthopedics. In this edition, you will find comprehensive discussion of orthopedic conditions, and clinical management that represents best treatment options and current practices. The title of the book has been changed to reflect inclusion of that information.

As our knowledge of avian anatomy, health and disease progresses, so does the need for improved resources that convey this valuable information. Over time the information contained herein will also need to be expanded and updated. The authors humbly submit this work to the veterinary and scientific community for review and scrutiny. We hope that it will contribute to the betterment of avian care.

Respectfully,

Drs. Susan E. Orosz, M. Scott Echols and Patrick T. Redig

ACKNOWLEDGEMENTS

PRIOR CONTRIBUTORS

We would like to acknowledge those individuals that made the first edition of Avian Surgical Anatomy: Thoracic and Pelvic Limbs possible. Two of the previous authors, Carol Haynes, our illustrator and Dr Phil Ensley were instrumental in providing illustrations of great quality and clarity and in getting the atlas off the ground. It started with a small grant provided by Dr Werner Heuschle and the Zoological Society of San Diego. I was a veterinary student at The Ohio State University seeking to better understand the surgical anatomy of the wings and legs, to facilitate improved surgical support to injured California condors that were then precariously close to extinction. The project morphed into a standalone surgical atlas that has been used around the world. Other individuals were also acknowledged in the first edition and all were integral in making it happen. These included Eric Bergman, who worked then, and now to help assemble and edit the work for production. My father, Julius Orosz, was my (SEO) guiding light and drew the original thumbnail sketches, showing how we could turn these drawings into a unique, practical, and beautiful atlas. The completed book won the book category at the highest level of recognition (Distinguished) and was runner up for the Best of Show award at the Society of Technical Communication's International Competition in 1993.

ANATOMICAL IMAGING ASSISTANCE

While we have included most of the original illustrations, new imaging technology has also been used to create the second edition. We wanted to demonstrate anatomic variability and advance our understanding of anatomy relative to commonly performed orthopedic procedures in birds. High resolution computed tomography (CT) was used to create the detailed digital skeletal and vascular images found throughout the book. The Grey Parrot Anatomy Project (www.avianstudios.com/the-grey-parrot-anatomy-project) has been established in part to discover and report anatomy of avian (and other) species. Funds made available through generous donations have been used to develop CT protocols and scanning time to create images in this book.

The images are standardized to include a minimum of four approximately orthogonal views per section: the distal wing, humerus and leg. The shoulder was divided into three main views (dorsal, ventral and cranial) with an additional dorsal oblique view. In some birds, these sections are further divided, and additional views are provided to show greater detail such as the hip of the military macaw.

Most of the CT scans were created using the Siemens Inveon Preclinical Micro-PET/CT unit at the Preclinical Imaging Facility, University of Utah HSC Cores in Salt Lake City, Utah (www.cores.utah.edu/preclinical-imaging). The scans were conducted under the direction of Dr Ed Hsu and his students, Samer Merchant and Gavin Yeip, at the University of Utah Department of Biomedical Engineering as a part of the Grey Parrot Anatomy Project. This scanner produces 'slices' 100 μm or less creating incredibly detailed images. Because the CT unit bore is small (about 5 inches), tissues that can be scanned are limited by their size. For many of the below listed birds, the entire leg or wing could be placed in the scanner. However, for the golden eagle, the shoulder girdle was simply too large to scan, which is why the shoulder girdle of that species is not included in this book. Because of the exceptional detail and relatively large size, the golden eagle and military macaw images were made as standard plus oblique views to create more 'three dimensional' views of the bones and joints than those done with the other birds.

The domestic chicken and African goose were scanned using the Epica Vimago CT at Parrish Creek Veterinary Hospital and Diagnostic Center in Centerville, Utah. The scans were conducted under the direction of Drs Scott Echols and Doug Folland and staff including Crystal Wilcox, LVT and Jason Benzing, LVT also as part of the Grey Parrot Anatomy Project. The Vimago's large gantry allowed for scans of whole animals and thick tissues such as the breast and shoulder girdle of the chicken that would otherwise not be suitable for the Inveon Preclinical Micro-PET/CT scanner. At 200 μm slice thickness, the Vimago also produced high quality images required for this book.

SKELETAL ANATOMY INFORMATION

Common Name	Scientific Name	CT Image Slice Size	Views
Budgerigar	*Melopsittacus undulatus*	50 μm	Standard
Domestic Chicken	*Gallus gallus domesticus*	200 μm	Standard
Golden Eagle	*Aquila chrysaetos*	100 μm	Standard plus obliques
Great Horned Owl	*Bubo virginianus*	100 μm	Standard
Military Macaw	*Ara militaris*	100 μm	Standard plus obliques
Orange Winged Amazon	*Amazona amazonica*	100 μm	Standard
Pigeon	*Columba livia*	100 μm	Standard
Red Tailed Hawk	*Buteo jamaicensis*	100 μm	Standard
Umbrella Cockatoo	*Cacatua alba*	100 μm	Standard

The vascular anatomy was created using a perfusion process and product (BriteVu®, www.ScarletImaging.com) developed by Dr Scott Echols. Once the vascular system was properly perfused, the regions of interest were then CT scanned. Drs Scott Echols and Nick Kirk and the Parrish Creek Veterinary Hospital staff (especially Crystal Wilcox, LVT and Jason Benzing, LVT) performed the BriteVu® perfusions.

The arteriovenogram images were standardized to include four approximately orthogonal views per section: the distal wing, proximal wing, hip and stifle, and foot. There are additional views of the pigeon and painted stork. There are no distal limb images in the barn owl due to physical trauma to all extremities.

Understanding the location of the vasculature can prove quite useful during wound management, surgery and other treatments. Vascular anatomy is complex and can be quite variable between breeds and individuals. The images provided are not comprehensive and cannot be representative of all birds. However, the arteriovenograms do provide a guide as some vascular features appear to be common to many studied bird species.

ARTERIOVENOGRAM INFORMATION

Common Name	Scientific Name	CT Image Slice Size	Views
African Goose	*Anser anser domesticus*	200 μm	Standard
Barn Owl	*Tyto alba*	100 μm	Proximal wing and hip and stifle only
Painted Stork	*Mycteria leucocephala*	100 μm	Standard plus additional views
Pigeon	*Columba livia*	100 μm	Standard plus additional view

None of these images would have been possible without the donations of terminally ill and deceased birds by their loving caretakers. In common to all donors was the desire to learn and advance our knowledge about these magnificent animals. Many birds were submitted through the Grey Parrot Anatomy Project while only a handful were selected for this book. Criteria included acceptable bone density, normal anatomy (except for the pigeon with a fractured coracoid), lack of vascular disease and more. Many of the birds listed above were family members and beloved collections animals. Out of respect for the caretakers and their birds, personal details have been omitted. Every effort has been made to respect the wishes of the caretakers and present the images in a manner that can benefit the scientific community and those who care for birds.

Additionally, we would like to thank those that provided photographs to help explain principles like with our Andean Condor and those that provided a similar feel to the wonder of birds as in the first edition. One of those individuals we want to thank posthumously and his family for allowing us to use his photos. Some of these exquisite photos were taken by Kevin Blaylock during several ecotours hosted by the Phoenix Landing Foundation. Kevin was enamored by the elegance, ingenuity, grace, and joyful nature of wild parrots. Kevin was also passionately dedicated to giving parrots better lives in captivity. He was on the Phoenix Landing Board of Directors and was one of its most treasured volunteers. He facilitated the rehoming of many birds, and he inspired people with his enthusiastic teaching skills. We lost Kevin at an early age, but his love for birds, as obvious through his photos, will last long into the future. It (SEO) is my joy to honor his life and work in this book. Kevin Wayne Blaylock, (October 8, 1972 - June 17, 2017)

The staff, board members and bird caretakers at Tracy Aviary in Salt Lake City assisted with coordinating and establishing photo sessions and by providing some of the images found throughout the book. These contributors include Darris Howe, Helen Dishaw, Lindsay Hooker, Michiko Berceau, Aron Smolley and Kate Lyngle-Cowand. Brian Smyer, a professional photographer also provided images taken of birds residing at Tracy Aviary. Andy, Tracy Aviary's beloved Andean condor, posed beautifully to help create the topographical anatomy images.

The golden eagle on page 293 was taken by Dawn Scalise Giffard. Cover art by Dr. Scott Echols and Manu Carrasco, artist, falconer and naturalist.

Finally, our families who have supported and endured our work must be recognized. Without their encouragement and tolerance of long hours pursuing this goal, this book would not be possible.

DEDICATION

We dedicate this text to our feathered patients and their health care.

FOREWORD

Paracelsus, a 16th century Swiss physician, was the first to describe medicine as both an art and a science. In this long-awaited book, Avian Surgical Anatomy and Orthopedic Management, readers will find both parts to this whole. While anatomy reflected in this book details important facts, the surgical section depicts decades of creative problem-solving to ensure better outcomes for avian patients.

For over two decades, I have had the privilege of knowing and working with the authors of this book. I learned the basics from Pat Redig, eventually taking over leadership of his brainchild, The Raptor Center at the University of Minnesota; I have taught workshops and been friends with Susan Orosz for almost two decades; and Scott Echols is a treasured colleague in the world of avian medicine. Each of these wonderful people is a brilliant, passionate teacher. Combined, they bring over 100 years of experience and expertise to create an incomparable team for writing this book.

The first edition of this book, Avian Surgical Anatomy, written by Dr. Orosz in 1992, has stood the test of time as an invaluable reference. Those of us who own dog-eared and worn copies have carefully protected them as they have become irreplaceable over the years. My own copy makes regular trips from its home on my bookshelf to the surgical suite, where it is a mainstay as students make sense out of the altered anatomy of trauma and sculpt a plan that gets a patient back on the wing.

In bringing the second edition to fruition, Dr. Orosz recruited the leading avian orthopedic surgeon in the world, Dr. Redig, and one of the most innovative clinicians in avian medicine, Dr. Echols, to curate and present the most up-to-date information available in avian orthopedics. Moving beyond the first book's sections on surgical approaches to avian bones, this edition has been expanded to include both surgical and non-surgical treatment options for orthopedic patients, as well as post-operative management and care. Advanced diagnostic imaging has also been included as new tools have built the knowledge base of anatomy far beyond the careful and detailed dissections that were the foundation of the original book.

From start to finish, this book provides accessible information that is practical for a clinical setting. It starts by presenting general principles and orthopedic techniques for avian orthopedic patients, then moves to detailed drawings and explanations of relevant anatomy and surgical approaches. Clinicians can turn to this book for step-by-step instructions on orthopedic methods, as well as the foundational information needed to extrapolate the information to the many varied presentations seen in avian practice. The depth of anatomical detail enclosed in this book is enhanced with cutting-edge diagnostic images that are both beautiful and revealing in ways not seen before in avian medicine.

Like its predecessor, this book will quickly become a "must have" text for all veterinarians working with feathered patients. I am certain that with its breadth of new information and presentation of tried-and-true methods, readers will find this book to be a treasured resource for their practice of avian medicine and surgery. With its superb illustrations, it is a masterpiece. And with its practical approach, clinicians have a definitive, scientific and evidence-based tool for managing avian orthopedic cases.

Julia B. Ponder, DVM, MPH
Executive Director, The Raptor Center
Associate Professor, Veterinary Population Medicine
College of Veterinary Medicine, University of Minnesota

Scope of this Book

This book – from text to pictures – is designed to provide information that enhances the surgical and medical care of the wings and legs of birds. It is based on the original text, Avian Surgical Anatomy: Thoracic and Pelvic Limbs, published over 25 years ago. Unfortunately, the atlas had a limited press run and is out of print, so it is not generally available for use. Realizing the book's purpose remains vital, the authors wanted to provide the information in an expanded manner and include the most tried and true surgical approaches developed by Dr. Patrick Redig at The Raptor Center, University of Minnesota.

While many of the drawings from Avian Surgical Anatomy: Thoracic and Pelvic Limbs have been used in this text, we have expanded our understanding of the anatomy by adding, for the first time, a large collection of CT images of the wings and legs of a variety of bird species. We chose to provide a diverse group of species, because avian veterinarians see a variety of birds in practice. This is an important distinction from dog and cat veterinarians that see a diversity of breeds. The species of birds range from frugivorous parrots to carnivorous condors. As you look at the CT images provided, it is important to remember that each is an individual bird of that species. There may be variations within the species but since this technology is so new – particularly the micro CT that was used on many of the smaller birds – the range of variations is not known at this time. However, as you can see from looking at the CT images from each portion of a limb, there is considerable variation between species.

The familiar anatomic drawings from the original book, in which we used the turkey vulture to document basic anatomy of the wings and legs are included. We also provide CT scans for the readers to develop their three-dimensional understanding of the same structures. CT scans are provided that first image the standard anatomic positions, followed by oblique views. This is done to encourage readers to develop their ability to visualize a three-dimensional image of the anatomic portion of the limb. Once they can visualize the basic anatomy of the wing or leg, the reader is challenged to use the obliques of the CT images to better understand that portion of the wing or leg by visualizing it in their head. Variations of the limbs among species can then be studied using a variety of CT images including oblique views from diverse species. The concept of building an anatomic image and being able to flip and see things in layers is important in understanding an individual surgical or medical avian patient. This is particularly vital with traumatic wounds where one must quickly determine anatomic landmarks.

We have provided arteriovenograms of portions of the limb or its entirety depending on the species and the size of the bird. These provide an idea of the interspecies variations in birds of the circulatory system. They also help the surgeon to know where important blood vessels lie, as well as gain an appreciation of the degree of perfusion in surrounding tissues.

After developing an understanding of the anatomy of the wings and legs, additional chapters are provided with information explaining concepts of avian orthopedics and post-operative patient management. This is critical as avian patients are extreme athletes and require different care from mammals. After the anatomic chapter of each limb, a chapter follows providing step-by-step information for repairing fractures relative to that region. These approaches have stood the test of time with raptors and other bird species with fractures that have been repaired by the veterinarians of The Raptor Center, University of Minnesota. The person that developed these approaches is one of the authors of this text, Dr Patrick Redig, and his work, drawings and thoughts on repair are well represented. These are the approaches that he and his colleagues at The Raptor Center have used to train other veterinarians and veterinary students around the world with the goal of returning birds to function.

A table of homologous terms is provided and will be useful for comparing terms from older textbooks since the names of the muscles have changed over time.

We are excited that this text provides under one cover the detailed anatomy and surgical protocols for fracture repair of the wings and legs of birds. Its new depth and breadth with the inclusion of CT images of the bones and joints and of arteriovenograms will allow those individuals working with a diverse group of species to have the knowledge to do what is necessary to properly surgically manage the legs and wings of their avian patients.

CHAPTER 2

Anatomic Form and Function

Terms of Orientation and Direction

The planes of the body, lines of direction and the points of relative position follow the terminology of the four-legged or quadruped animals. While confusing, birds are bipedal, yet their orientation is not that of a true biped. Depending on species, the back of a bird may be more horizontal than vertical. Based on this understanding, the back of the bird in this text is dorsal and the underside is ventral **(Figures 2-1 and 2-2)**.

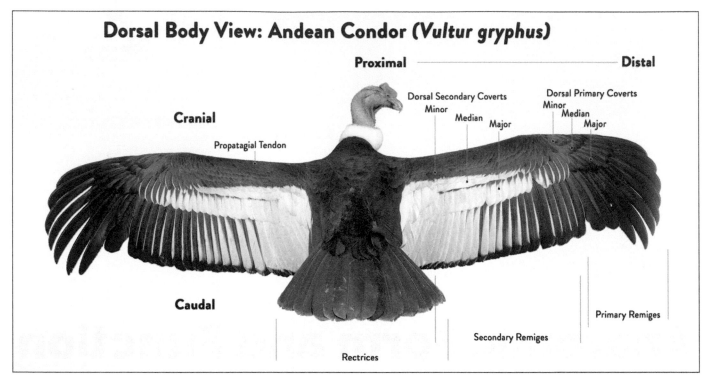

Figure 2-1. Dorsal body view: Andean condor *(Vultur gryphus)*.

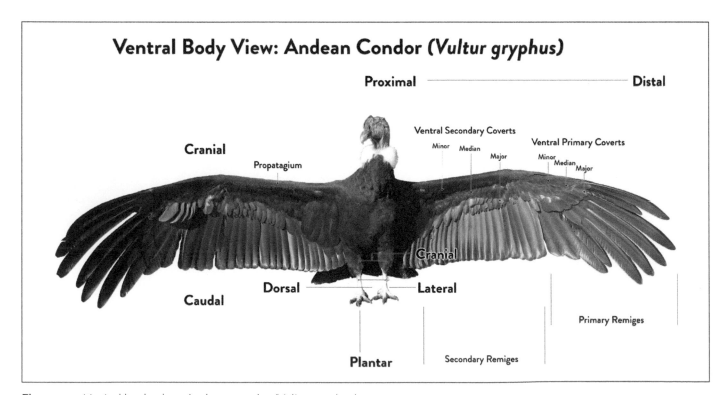

Figure 2-2. Ventral body view: Andean condor *(Vultur gryphus)*.

Lateral Body View

There are 2 lateral sides- the right and the left sides. The head-end is termed rostral, cranial or anterior; the tail-end is termed caudal or posterior **(Figure 2-3)**.

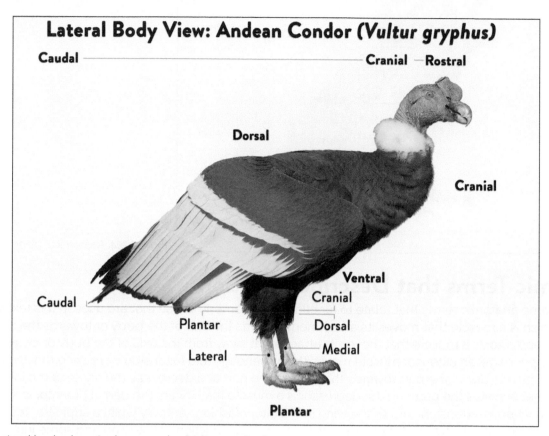

Figure 2-3. Lateral body view: Andean condor *(Vultur gryphus)*.

Anatomical Planes of the Body

A sagittal plane passes in a line through the body from dorsal to ventral and the midsagittal plane divides the body into right and left halves. The frontal (coronal) planes go through the body at a 90-degree angle to the sagittal planes. The frontal plane divides the body into dorsal and ventral parts. A transverse plane cuts the body at right angles to the sagittal and frontal planes **(Figure 2-4)**.

An organism can be divided into 3 main planes that describe body parts in relation to each other's axis. All planes are imaginary lines that act as boundaries of the body. The sagittal (median) plane runs parallel to the longitudinal axis of the bird dividing it into left and right sides. The coronal plane divides the body into dorsal and ventral portions. The transverse or axial plane runs perpendicular to the sagittal and coronal planes and divides the body into superior and inferior (or cranial and caudal) regions.

Medial refers to the placement of an object in relation to another object which is, by definition, laterally placed. Medial is also defined as toward the median plane (or middle) of the body. Conversely, lateral is also defined as moving away from the median plane or toward the side(s). These terms are often used with vessels and nerves and refer to their relation to the body.

Anatomic Terms Used for Comparison

There are many terms that are applied for purposes of comparison. These commonly include external *(externus)* and internal *(internus)*; superficial *(superficialis)* and deep *(profundus)*; distal *(distalis)* and proximal *(proximalis)*; ascending *(ascendens)* and descending *(descendens)*; major *(majorus)* and minor *(minorus)* and long *(longus)* and short *(brevis)*.

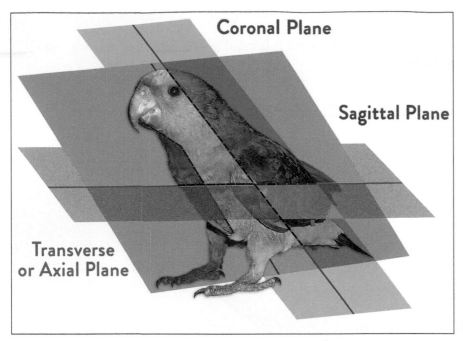

Coronal Plane

Sagittal Plane

Transverse
or Axial Plane

Figure 2-4. Anatomical planes of the body.

Anatomic Terms that Describe Function

There are some anatomic terms that relate to function or movement. Those that are used in this text include: adductor which is a muscle that moves its attachment towards the axis of the body or towards the axis of the appendage; abductor is a muscle that moves its attachment away from the axis of the body or away from the axis of the appendage; an extensor muscle moves the appendage into extension increasing the angle of the joint; a flexor muscle draws the part towards the body or the part and decreases the angle of the joint; a levator is a muscle that elevates the part and the depressor is a muscle that lowers the part; a pronator is a muscle that, with the wing when in extension, draws the wing in a rotatory fashion ventrally while a supinator rotates the extended wing dorsally. There are several muscles that indicate function of the wing and some include: pronator superficialis and profundus muscles; supinator muscles; similarly, for the leg, flexor hallicus longus and extensor hallicus longus muscles; and abductor pollicis and adductor pollicis muscles.

There are other muscles that are named to indicate their connections, positions or relationship to other structures. Examples include: Iliotibialis cranialis, femorotibialis externus; ischiofemoralis and the interosseous dorsalis and ventralis muscles.

From an anatomic perspective, the wing in lateral extension and outstretched, as when flying, is the anatomic position of the bird. In this position, there is a dorsal surface to the wing (See Figure 2-1) and a ventral surface (See Figure 2-2). The front, or leading edge, of the wing is cranial while the back, or trailing edge, is caudal. Most references in this text relate to the wing in this position.

However, in the literature the wing may be described in its resting position folded against the body wall. In this position, the dorsal surface becomes the lateral surface and the ventral surface becomes the medial surface. In this text, those terms are used more with bandaging and care of the wing at surgery.

For the leg in birds, the axis of the toes is at an angle to the axis of the leg with a line drawn through the middle or the midsaggital plane from proximal to distal. The portion of the leg containing the femur and tibiotarsus have 4 sides: cranial, caudal, medial and lateral, while the distal leg (distal to the 'hock joint') containing the tarsometatarsus and digits are labeled dorsal, plantar, medial and lateral. The upper surfaces of the toes while standing on the ground in anatomic position are dorsal; and the lower surfaces are plantar. Birds have a significant portion of the leg against the body wall, except when the legs are extended as in landing or seizing prey (as in raptors) or if you are a crane or a heron or similar.

The Feathers of the Wing

The feathers of the wing are composed of the long flight feathers or remiges (from Latin remus meaning oar) and their smaller covering covert feathers (tectrix). Covert feathers cover the flight feathers. In contrast, contour feathers cover the body. The flight feathers are divided into the primary flight feathers, secondary flight feathers and tertiary flight feathers (Figures 2-1 and 2-2 show primary and secondary flight feathers). Tertiary flight feathers arise from the caudal aspect of the humerus.

The primaries arise from the carpometacarpus also known as the bird's "hand" or manus. There are usually 10 primary flight feathers and they are numbered starting at the proximal carpus and advancing distally. Flighted birds have between 9 and 12 primary flight feathers. Some of the primary flight feathers insert onto the phalanges, while the other primary flight feathers insert on the caudodorsal aspect of the carpometacarpus. When there are 10 primary flight feathers, flight feather VII inserts on the minor digit, and flight feathers VIII-X insert on the major digit (see anatomy plates of the distal thoracic wing in Chapter 5). The fused bones of the carpometacarpus are also dorso-ventrally compressed to form a flattened surface to which the metacarpal primaries (primaries 1-6) attach.

The secondary flight feathers arise from the forewing and are attached to the caudal border of the ulna at the quill knobs. These can be observed in the photo of the skeleton of a California condor as the slight bumps on the caudal margin of the ulna **(Figure 2-5)**.

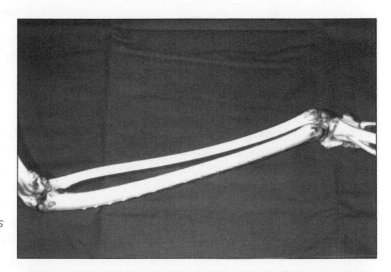

Figure 2-5. Dorsal view of a California condor *(Gymnogyps californianus)* showing the quill knobs on the caudal border of the ulna.

The length of the radius and ulna varies among species of birds and accordingly, there is a highly variable number of secondary flight feathers ranging, but not limited to, between 6 and 32. The secondary flight feathers are numbered starting at the carpometacarpal joint and the numbers advance proximally to the elbow. The alula consists of the alular digit, surrounding soft tissue and feathers. The alular digit is considered digit I or the pollex and has also been described as the bastard wing. The alula has between 2 and 7 flight feathers and these should be numbered from proximal to distal like the primary flight feathers.

Tertials, when present, arise from the region of the humerus. Not all birds possess tertials.

The shafts of each of the flight feathers are covered over by a covert feather. Those that cover over a primary flight feather are called primary coverts and those that cover over a secondary are secondary coverts. On the dorsal surface of the wing the coverts tend to be arranged in overlapping rows and the major coverts are the ones closest to the flight feathers, followed by the median coverts. The coverts that are smaller and more craniad are the minor coverts with marginal coverts on the area of the propatagium *(See Figures 2-1 and 2-2)*. These feathers form the elegantly crafted aerodynamic surface of the wing. The coverts on the ventral surface of the wing follow the same pattern but tend not to be arranged as uniformly in rows as those on the dorsal surface. Additionally, there is group of covert feathers that are found between the shoulder and the scapula that form the scapular coverts.

The trailing edge of primary feather 10 is covered by the leading edge of primary feather 9, and so on. Each feather is composed of a central shaft or rachis **(Figure 2-6)** with barbs coming off at about a 45-degree angle **(Figure 2-7)**. These barbs are slender but stiff filaments and form an external and internal vane of each feather.

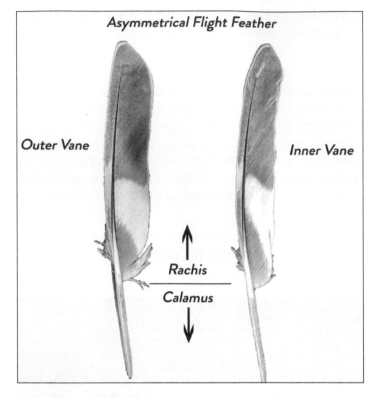

Figure 2-6. Structure of a flight feather. Flight feathers are highly organized and stiff enough to counteract wind resistance and ultimately produce lift. All feathers have a central shaft composed of the calamus (portion without barbs that inserts under the skin) and rachis (the portion of the feather shaft with barbs) (more commonly referred to as the "shaft'" that is visible).

Additionally, the width and shape of the barbs differ as the barbs on the leading edge or outer vane are shorter and stiffer than those on the trailing edge or inner vane *(See Figure 2-6)*. Anatomically, this produces a feather that is asymmetric about its long axis. Aerodynamically, the result is that a downward movement of the wing imparts a forward twisting motion to the feather shaft as the rear of the feather is elevated relative to the anterior edge. This produces the forward movement of the propulsive downward stroke of the wing. In **Figure 2-8**, you can observe this leading edge and the trailing edge and the differences in the length of the barbs. In this king vulture, the flight feathers are black, and the coverts are white.

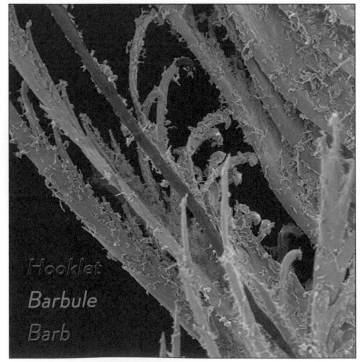

Figure 2-7. Microanatomy of the feather. The rachis gives rise to barbs angled away from the skin. Especially with flight feathers, the barbs give rise distally to regularly spaced barbules containing hooklets. However, the regularly spaced barbules on the proximal side (towards the body) of the barb do not contain hooklets. These hooklets attach to barbules arising from the proximal side of barbs linking each barb together. With each successive barb connected, the smaller outer and larger inner vanes of the asymmetrical flight feather are formed.

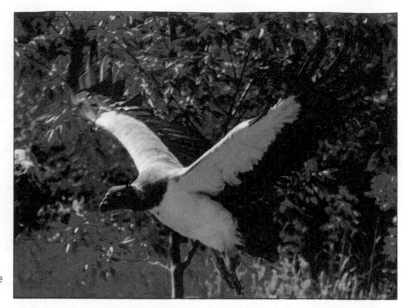

Figure 2-8. View of a king vulture *(Sarcoramphus papa)* in flight showing the primary, secondary, and covert feathers - the flight feathers are black and the covert feathers are white.

The arrangement of the flight feathers and that of the ligaments and muscles and the spreading of the remiges help to provide the shape to the wing for flight. The primary and secondary flight feathers are connected by the interremigial ligament **(Figure 2-9)**. While the spreading of the flight feathers is a consequence of extension of the wing, the interremigial ligament serves as a check ligament to hold each feather so that they overlap appropriately to form a continuous flying surface. The muscles that attach to the interremigial ligament provide voluntary control of these feathers as a response to applied flight loads.

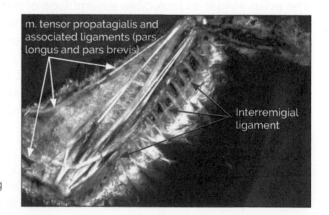

Figure 2-9. Dorsal view of a dissection of a turkey vulture demonstrating the structures of the propatagium and the interremigial ligament.

The triangular fold of feathered skin between the shoulder on the cranial margin of the wing that runs to and inserts onto the carpal joint is the propatagium. The tensor propatagialis longus tendon forms the support for the leading edge of the wing and the skin wraps around it dorsally and ventrally to be continuous with the coverts and the flight feathers. In addition to the tensor propatagialis longus tendon, there are elastic tissue fibers that run in several directions to support the propatagium to keep this structure taut and from vibrating as the wing moves through the air. The propatagium and associated structures form the cambered surface of the wing that generates lift. With forward motion of the wing, air is separated and accelerated over its dorsal convex surface creating an area of low pressure that generates lift (Bernoulli effect). The post patagium is the fold of skin that runs between the caudal surface of the ulna and the carpus or manus. The alular patagium is a fold of skin with feathers between the alula and the major digit **(Figure 2-10A & B)**.

The patagium is the feathered membranous tissue that spans the joints of the wing. There are four patagial membranes: propatagium, metapatagium, postpatagium, and alular patagium (or patagium alulae). All act to create a smooth contoured airfoil when the wing is in extension while allowing the wing to be freely flexed as the patagia are folded. The propatagium is the fold of skin spanning the shoulder to the carpus forming the cranial (leading) edge of the wing. The postpatagium is the thickened skin on the caudal aspect of the elbow extending distally to the wing tip. The calami of the primary and secondary remiges are embedded in the postpatagium. The metapatagium is the triangular skin fold spanning the lateral body wall to the caudal margin of the proximal

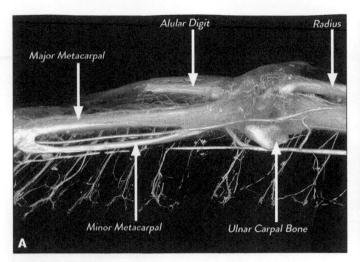
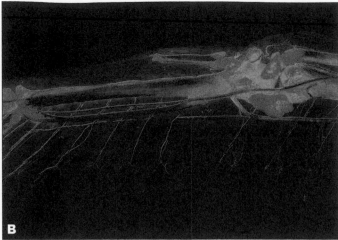

Figure 2-10A. Ventral view of the distal forewing, carpus and major and minor metacarpals.
Figure 2-10B. Using false color, the alular patagium is highlighted as blue tissue between the alula and major metacarpal bones.

wing or brachium. The alular patagium connects the alula to the cranial border of the major digit. The images **(Figures 2-10A & B)** show a ventral view of the distal forewing, carpus and major and minor metacarpals and their associated vasculature.

Aerodynamics and Their Clinical Implications

The avian wing is an incredible assemblage of bone, muscle, tendons, ligaments, elastic fibers, nerves, blood vessels, skin and keratin derivatives (feathers) that, despite what appears to range widely in shape and conformation, has been molded by the principles of aerodynamics and corresponding selection forces within the ecological niche occupied by a given bird. Much about aerodynamics has been learned from study of birds and the results applied to many types of aircraft. Conversely, an understanding of the aerodynamics of airplane wings contributes to understanding how bird's wings function. Such knowledge provides a useful conceptual framework in which to conduct restoration of birds that have sustained wing injuries and is therefore of importance to avian orthopedic surgeons.

The avian wing combines both the means of propulsion and the means of lift generation in its configuration. In flapping flight, the portion of the wing distal to the wrist joint, the carpus, in concert with the asymmetric form of the primary feathers, results in generation of forward propulsive forces (thrust). In gliding or soaring flight, where the wing is in fixed extended position, the carpus in concert with the forearm, the portion between the elbow and the wrist that gives rise to the secondary feathers, forms a fixed wing to which many of the considerations of conventional aircraft aerodynamics can be applied. These include the basic aerodynamic forces acting on a flying body which are thrust, lift, drag, and gravity. These forces are entrained by several aspects of the wing and include the overall shape or planform, camber, chord, span, aspect ratio, wing-loading, as well as drag-reducing elements such as turbulators, slotting, and speed and stall sensors (filoplumes). These aspects interact or combine to generate the forces of thrust, lift, and drag along with their control that are inherent to flying bodies. And while the fixed wing mode comparison with aircraft generates many similarities in principle, the fact that the avian wing does not have constant camber from root to tip even in its fixed mode, that the functional aspect ratio can vary tremendously depending on whether the wing is fully extended or partially retracted, and that the camber of the wing as formed by the patagium varies by the degree of wing extension as well as dynamic positioning during the flapping cycle, limits exact comparisons. Regardless, the ability to fly and the manner in which various birds fly is defined by aerodynamic principles and places constraints on the overall planform of the avian body including body weight, weight distribution, and muscle arrangement.

Detailed description and analysis of these aerodynamics parameters are outside the scope of this work, but much can be learned from detailed avian aerodynamics studies that have been conducted (Savile 1957, Tabalske 2001, Tucker 1993, Withers 1981, Drovetski 1996). A detailed on-line presentation of many aspects of avian aerodynamics is available at: http://people.eku.edu/ritchisong/554notes2.html. Another excellent reference, and delightful read, is the book Birds in Flight by Carrol Henderson (Voyager Press 2008). As will be noted, many of the photographs of birds and illustrations were taken from this book with permission, for which these authors are most grateful.

The basic components of the avian forelimb that function aerodynamically are detailed in **Figure 2-11A**. Aspects of these are detailed in the discussion below.

The leading edge of the wing – the point at which the air meets the wing and is deflected over and under the wing is an important component of wing function. In birds, this structure is formed by the propatagial tendon and

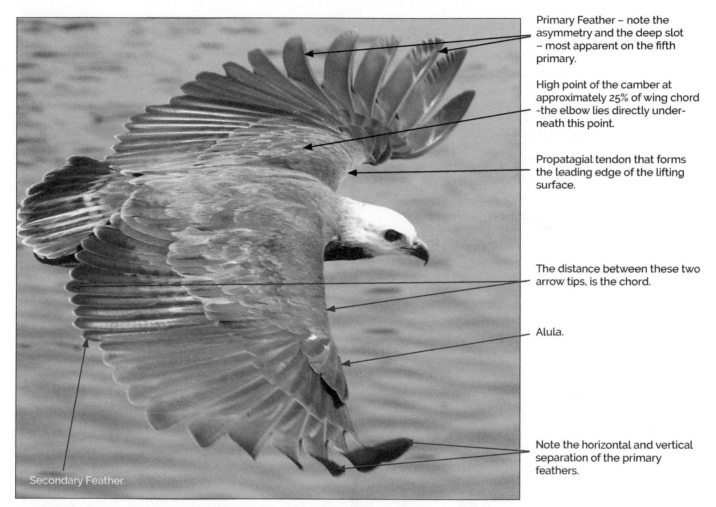

Primary Feather – note the asymmetry and the deep slot – most apparent on the fifth primary.

High point of the camber at approximately 25% of wing chord -the elbow lies directly underneath this point.

Propatagial tendon that forms the leading edge of the lifting surface.

The distance between these two arrow tips, is the chord.

Alula.

Note the horizontal and vertical separation of the primary feathers.

Secondary Feather.

Figure 2-11A. Dorsal view of the distal forewing, carpus and major and minor metacarpals.

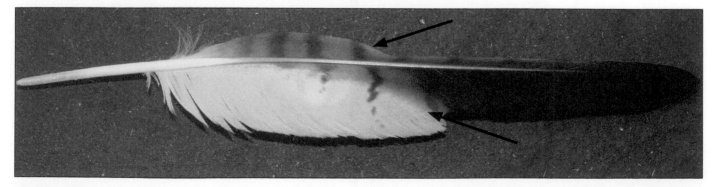

Figure 2-11B. Primary feather from a red-tailed hawk (*Buteo jamaicensis*) showing the abrupt changes (*arrows*) in the contour of the leading and trailing edges of the distal vane that forms a slot with an adjacent overlapping feather in the spread wing. (From Henderson 2008)

associated skin and feather structures **(Figure 2-11A)**. This structure – part tendon, part elastic fibers – extends from the shoulder to the carpus and is covered with small, tightly overlapping covert feathers that comprise the smooth, cambered upper surface of the wing. The angle of deflection of air molecules striking the leading edge and their subsequent behavior is significantly affected by the shape of the leading edge and its relation to the remainder of the wing. Maintenance of its integrity during management of wing injuries is paramount to return to normal flight capacity. Also, given the range of conformations that it can acquire during different stages or types of flight at any moment, loss of elasticity by scarring following injury can impact the function of the wing.

Other important and notable aerodynamic features of the avian wing include wing-type, aspect ratio, wing loading, and camber along with structural features including the alula, asymmetric flight feathers, and wing slots.

Wing Type

There are various classifications of wing-types for birds, generally splitting them into passive and active soaring, high lift, high maneuverability, high speed and combinations of these features **(Figure 2-12)**.

The most common wing shape is a semi-ellipse that provides a large envelope of flight capacity including rapid, short take-off and high maneuverability. It is found in passerines and ground dwelling birds and psittacines.

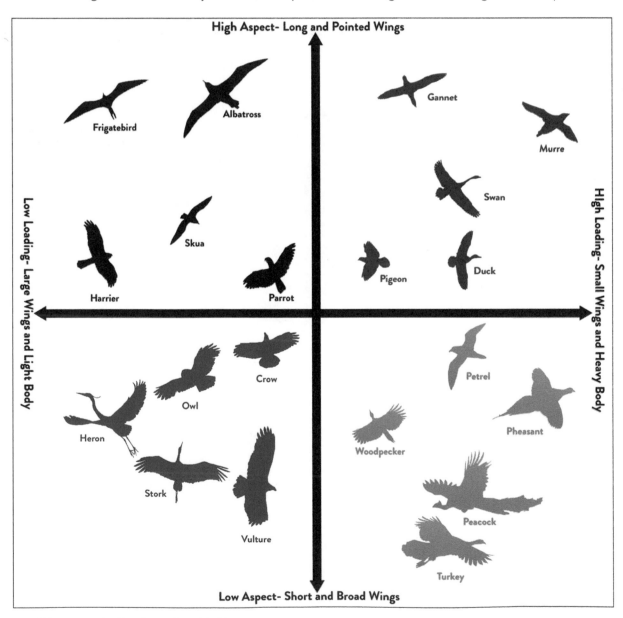

Figure 2-12. Wing aspect ratios for various bird types.

Modifications of this basic wing form such as increasing the length or slotting the primaries to afford capacity for soaring or long-distance migration are seen in many species of birds including many raptors. High lift wings are found in slow-flying birds such as herons and other marsh birds that take-off and land nearly vertically. Their wings are of a broad planform with a large curvature or camber. The highspeed wings are found in falcons, terns, nighthawks and swifts. They tend to be longer and narrow with sharp points and shallow cambers. Slotted wings are those where the outer 5-6 primary feathers separate into finger-like projections that reduce drag **(Figure 2-13)**. Slots are found in wings of terrestrial soaring birds such as eagles, hawks and vultures, as well as in some high maneuvering ground dwelling birds where slots function to prevent stalling with abrupt maneuvers. Within all these categories, the aerodynamic property of aspect ratio is the major determining factor of wing shape and is a major factor in wing performance **(Figures 2-14A & B)**.

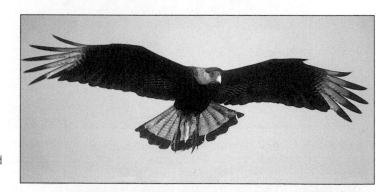

Figure 2-13. Slotted wingtips in a soaring northern crested caracara (*Caracara cheriway*). (Photo: C. Henderson).

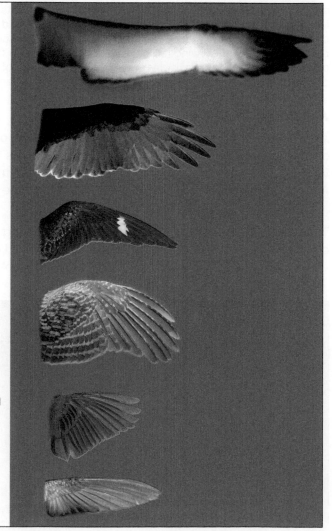

Long, narrow, high aspect ratio wing suited for dynamic soaring (sp. - white capped albatross, *Thalassarche steadi*)

Long, broad moderate aspect ratio wing with slotted tips suited for combined overland soaring and flapping flight (sp. turkey vulture, *Cathartes aura*).

Long, angular and pointed high-speed wing (sp. common nighthawk, *Chordeiles minor*). Similar wing types found in falcons.

Short, broad, midrange aspect ratio and usually highly cambered wing suited for explosive take-offs and maneuvering (sp. greater prairie chicken, *Tympanuchus cupido*).

Short and broad, low aspect ratio wing suited for abrupt maneuvers in heavy cover – common in song birds (sp. indigo bunting, *Passerina cyanea*). Note slight degree of slotting.

Long, slender, straight oar-like wing suited for specialized flight modes (sp. green hermit hummingbird, *Phaethornis guy*).

Figure 2-14A. Variations on avian wing plan form (modified from Henderson 2008).

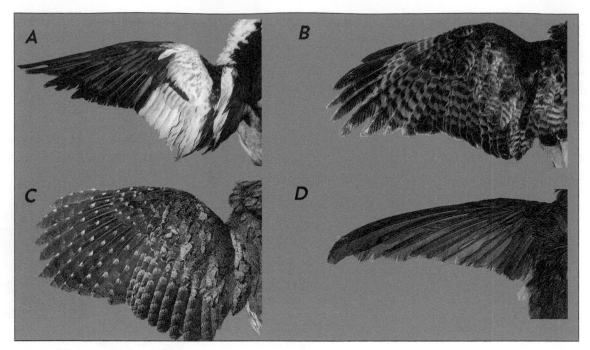

Figure 2-14B. Further information on variations on avian wing plan form. Bird wings come in many types of shapes and sizes, all to serve different functions. This diagram depicts adult left wings in partial extension as viewed from their dorsal surface; *(A)* common merganser *(Mergus merganser)*, *(B)* red-tailed hawk *(Buteo jamaicensis)*, *(C)* tawny frogmouth *(Podargus strigoides)* and *(D)* black-chinned hummingbird *(Archilochus alexandri)*. High speed wings *(A)* are medium to long and relatively narrow. Birds with high speed wings can sustain fast flight. The passive soaring wing *(B)* is common among land soaring birds. Also called the slotted high lift wing due to the wide gaps (or slots) between the primary feathers (in full extension), this wing type takes advantage of rising columns of hot air allowing the bird to soar. The elliptical wing type *(C)* is designed for short bursts of controlled flight and maneuvering through tight spaces such as in highly wooded areas for catching food and avoiding predators. The elliptical wing requires sustained flapping for flight and results in relatively slow speed. The hovering wing *(D)*, classic with hummingbirds, is designed for tight flight control and hovering. In hummingbirds, articulation and movement are principally at the shoulder (instead of the wrist) and wings tend to be small relative to body size.

Aspect Ratio

Aspect ratio is the ratio of wing length to wing width or chord. It is calculated as the square of wing-length divided by its surface area – it fundamentally defines how the wing flies in terms of lift, speed, and maneuverability and there is a rough correlation to the habitat and ecological niche of the bird to which it is adapted. Aspect ratios range from approximately 2 in quail-like birds to 16 in albatrosses **(Table 2-1)**.

The functional aspect of a high aspect ratio wing (long and narrow) is to compensate for loss of lifting surface created by wing-tip vortices that swirl up over the end of the wing and destroy lift by having a longer and narrower wing. High aspect ratio wings are found in dynamic soaring birds such as gulls and albatrosses **(Figure 2-15)**.

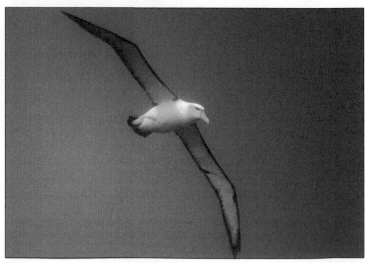

Figure 2-15. High aspect ratio of the white-capped albatross *(Thalassarche steadi)*. (Photo: C. Henderson).

Table 2-1. ASPECT RATIOS OF SELECTED SPECIES OF BIRDS

WING SHAPE GROUP	COMMON NAME	SPECIES	ASPECT RATIO	REFERENCE
Elliptical	American Crow	*Corvus brachyrhynchos*	6.1	Savile 1957
Elliptical	House Sparrow	*Passer domesticus*	5.5	Savile 1957
Elliptical	Quail	*Not specified*	1.8	Withers 1981
Elliptical	Pheasant	*Phasianus colchicus*	5.5	Henderson 2008
Elliptical	Magpie	*Pica hudsonia*	5	Hedrik et al. 2003 Lees et al. 2016
Elliptical	Blue Jay	*Cyanocitta cristata*	4.83	Lees et al. 2016
Elliptical	Blue and Gold Macaw	*Ara ararauna*	4.6	Bhargavi1 et al 2017
High Speed	Peregrine Falcon	*Falco peregrinus*	6.5	Savile 1957
High Speed	Wood Pigeon	*Columba palumbus*	6.36	Lees et al. 2016
High Speed	American Black Duck	*Anas rubripes*	7.0	Savile 1957
High Speed	Chimney Swift	*Chaetura pelagica*	8.6	Savile 1957
High Speed	Cockatiel	*Nymphicus hollandicus*	6.7	Hedrick 2003
High Speed	Teal	Genus *Anas*	6.15	Lees et al. 2016
High Speed	Wigeon	*Mareca americana*	7.46	Lees et al. 2016
High Speed	Mallard	*Anas platyrhynchos*	5.64	Lees et al. 2016
High Speed	Common Loon	*Gavia immer*	10	Savile 1957
High Aspect Ratio	Tundra Swan	*Cygnus columbianus*	8.5	Savile 1957
High Aspect Ratio	Herring Gull	*Larus argentatus*	8.1	Savile 1957
High Aspect Ratio	Wandering Albatross	*Diomedea exulans*	15.6	Warham 1977 – Savile 1956
High Aspect Ratio, slotted	Osprey	*Pandion haliaetus*	10	Henderson 2008
Slotted High Lift	Golden Eagle	*Aquila chrysaetos*	7.4	Savile 1957
Slotted High Lift	Red-tailed Hawk	*Buteo jamaicensis*	5.8	Savile 1957
Slotted High Lift	Northern Harrier	*Circus cyaneus*	7.1	Savile 1957
Slotted High Lift	Screech Owl	*Otus asio*	5.5	Savile 1957
Slotted High Lift	Andean Condor	*Vultur gryphus*	7.9	McGahan 1973
Slotted High Lift	Turkey Vulture	*Cathartes aura*	7	McGahan 1973

A low aspect ratio wing affords explosive take-off capacity and high maneuverability as found in many gallinaceous birds, including ring neck pheasants *(Phasianus colchicus)* **(Figure 2-16)**. Low aspect ratio and elliptiform wings are found in forest dwelling and ground birds where their inherent features are essential for survival. Aspect ratios of most birds are in the range of 4-8.

Wings may also be categorized as high speed and low lift or low speed and high lift – the former being thin (low cambered) and tapered, such as found in falcons and swifts while the latter are deeper and broad such as found in herons and egrets.

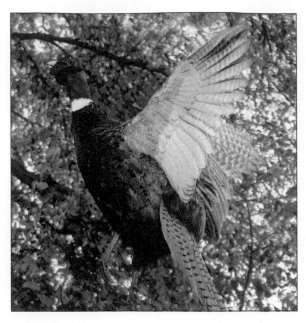

Figure 2-16. Low aspect ratio wing of the ring neck pheasant *(Phasianus colchicus).* (Photo: C. Henderson).

Camber

Camber is the front to back curvature of the wing over its dorsal surface that forms the airfoil. This shape serves to split the oncoming air at the leading edge with the air passing over the upper surface being accelerated in a manner that generates lift **(Figures 2-17 and 2-18)**. Some birds such as herons have a deep camber that generates a high lift wing **(Figures 2-19 and 2-20)**. Such birds are also slow flyers. Falcons and waterfowl fly at high speeds and the camber of their wings is much reduced. With an ability to alter the camber of the wing through flexion and extension to match different flying circumstances, the avian wing is the envy of aerodynamic engineers.

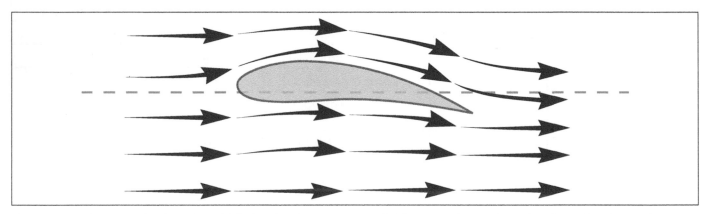

Figure 2-17. Schematic drawing of an airfoil showing the separation of airflow over the cambered surface. The air over the upper surface is accelerated generating a region of lowered pressure compared to the bottom surface (Bernoulli's principle) which, along with angle of attack (below), generates lift. (From Henderson 2008).

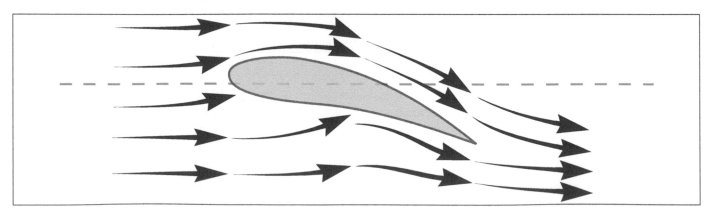

Figure 2-18. Angle of attack and attached airflow – generates more lift, but it has not reached the point of stalling. Compare to figure 2-22. (From Henderson 2008).

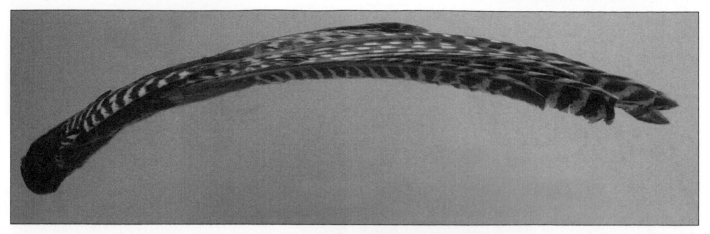

Figure 2-19. High cambered, high-lift wing of a turkey (*Meleagris* sp.). (From Henderson 2008).

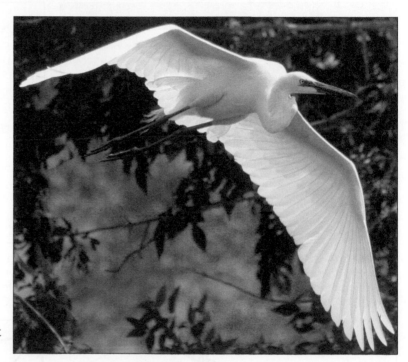

Figure 2-20. Highly cambered wing of the great egret (*Ardea alba*) – a high lift wing. (Photo: C. Henderson)

Features of Avian Wing that Reduce Drag and Prevent Wing Stalling
Slotting

Wing tip slots are drag reducing devices created by varying degrees of foreshortening of the anterior and posterior webs of the outer 5-6 primaries, so-called emargination, that results in gaps or slots being present between the primaries when the wing is in full extension **(Figure 2-21A-D)**. This slotting, which results in gaps between the feathers in both horizontal and vertical planes, reduces the magnitude of turbulent drag-inducing vortices that shed off the wing tip and destroy lift. They function to create vertical and horizontal separation of the wing tip vortices thereby reducing the production of a wake which has a high drag component (Tucker 1993).

Slots are particularly evident in thermal soaring birds, the characteristic flight seen in eagles, buteo hawks, vultures, pelicans **(Figure 2-21A-D)** and other birds that utilize rising overland air thermals.

Many aspects of avian flight, especially landing and taking off as well as gliding, involve maneuvering at low airspeeds and high angles of attack of the wing. In such circumstances, the wing, or portions of it, will stall leading to a loss of lift. In a stall the normally bound flow of air over the wing becomes disrupted and a chaotic mass of swirling air known as a burble traverses its way cranially from the trailing edge **(Figure 2-22)**. This can be observed in images of birds in landing configuration at high angles of attack **(Figure 2-23A, B)**.

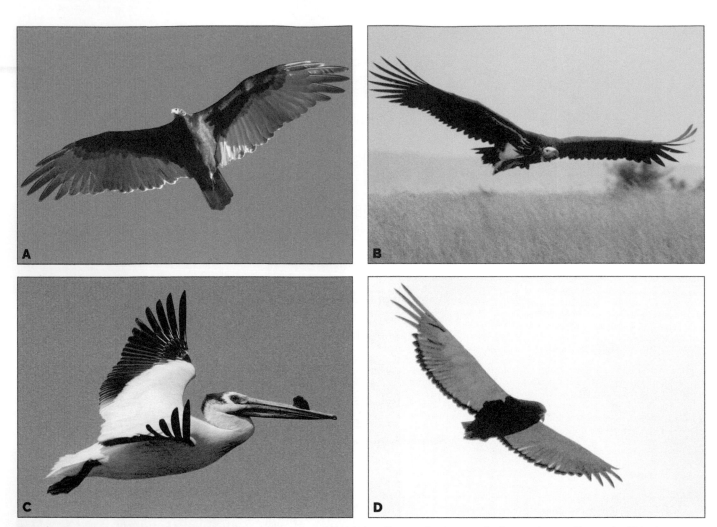

Figure 2-21A-D. These images demonstrate various terrestrial birds with excellent capacity for soaring on thermals. **A)** turkey vulture *(Cathartes aura)*, **B)** lappet-faced vulture *(Torgos tracheliotos)*, **C)** white pelican *(Pelecanus erythrorhynchos)*, **D)** Bateleur eagle *(Terathopius ecaudatus)*. The latter, an extremely aerial bird of the African savannah, demonstrates wing-slotting taken to the extreme to maximize drag reduction and enhance gliding ability. (Photos: C. Henderson).

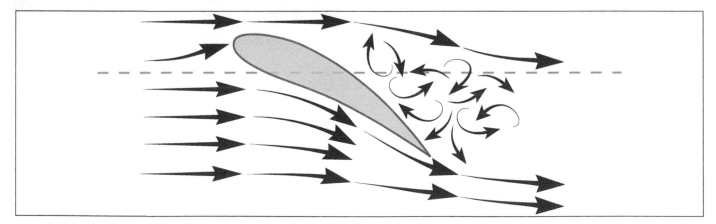

Figure 2-22. The formation of a burble in a stalled wing at a high angle of attack is illustrated. (From Henderson 2008).

Alula

The alula **(Figure 2-24)** is a single feather or group of feathers, depending on species, attached to the first digit at the carpus. When deployed at slow speed and high angles of attack such as occur in gliding flight, take-off or landing, serves to energize the boundary layer over a portion of the wing thereby preventing airflow separation from the cambered surface and limiting the tendency of the wing to stall **(Figure 2-24)**. It can be seen deployed in soaring birds that attain the best glide ratio at airspeeds just above the stalling speed, and in most birds as they are taking off or landing, both maneuvers occurring at low airspeeds **(Figure 2-25)** and high angles of attack **(Figure 2-26)**.

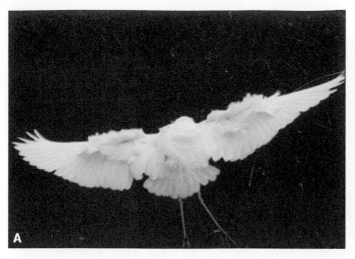

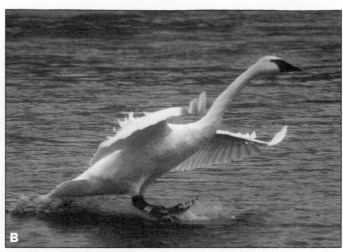

Figure 2-23A & B. These images demonstrate ruffled feathers on the back of **A)** a snowy egret *(Egretta thula)* and **B)** a trumpeter swan *(Cygnus buccinator)* due to turbulence generated by a stalled wing during landing. (Photos: C. Henderson).

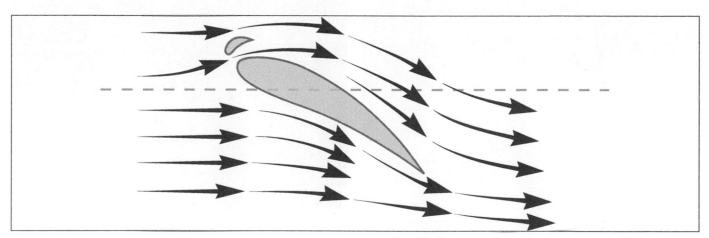

Figure 2-24. This is an illustration of how the alula, when deployed, alters the airflow over a portion of the wing immediately downstream such that it remains attached to the airfoil. (From Henderson 2008).

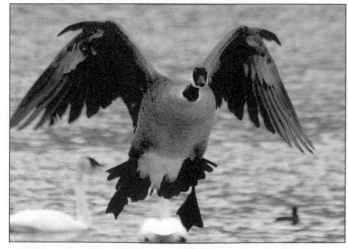

Figure 2-25. In this image, the extended alula of a Canada goose *(Branta canadensis)* in landing configuration can be observed. (Photos: C. Henderson)

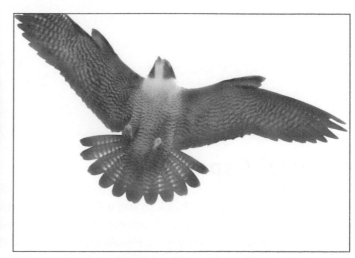

Figure 2-26. In this image, a peregrine falcon *(Falco peregrinus)* in an abrupt high angle of attack turn extends its alulas. (Photo: C. Henderson).

Pointed Wings

Narrowing of the wings at the tips is found in high speed flyers and serves to reduce the flat plate area that is responsible for producing wing-tip vortices that contribute to drag **(Figure 2-27A-C)**.

Among different groups and species of birds, these structural features have been extensively molded through natural selection. These molded modifications enable characteristic modes of take-off and landing, flight style, lifting capacity, gliding, soaring, diving, abrupt maneuvering, and hovering that we associate with different species.

This brief consideration of aerodynamics of avian wings and its correlations to lifestyle and ecological niche only partially explains the relationships of the overall flight apparatus (wings, tail, muscles, bones, cardiovascular and respiratory systems) that combine to give a bird its characteristic flight style and capacity. A full explanation necessarily requires examination of not only aerodynamics of the fixed wing, but also the kinematics of flapping flight, muscle anatomy and physiology (Tobalske 2001), details of flight feather structure (Pap et. al., 2015), metabolism and energy production/delivery and ecological positioning, much of which remains uninvestigated and correlated, to fully grasp the complexities of avian flight (Alerstam et. AL, 2007).

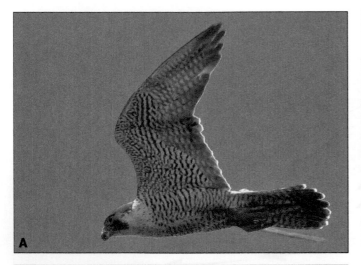

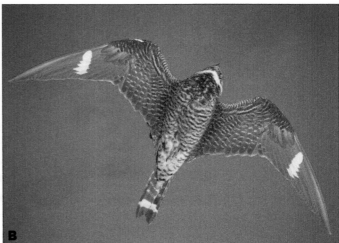

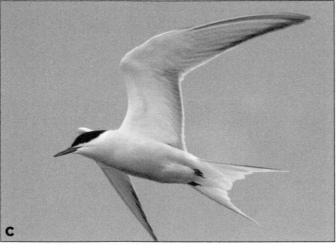

Figure 2-27A, B & C. Pointed, high speed wings of: **A)** peregrine falcon (*Falco peregrinus*), **B)** common nighthawk (*Chordeiles minor*), **C)** common tern (*Sterna hirundo*). Note slight degree of slotting in the wing tips of the falcon. (Photos: C. Henderson).

Clinical Aspects

With minimum reflection, it should be clear that in effecting repair of an injured wing or otherwise managing birds intended for release back to the wild where they have to fly for survival, it is of utmost importance that the integrity of all the various structures of the wing be restored and/or maintained in order to maximize the capacity of the patient to fly well. Presently, one can do no better than to thoroughly comprehend the article "A Review of Biomechanics and Aerodynamic Considerations of the Avian Thoracic Limb" (Beaufrere, 2009). The essential aspects of this article are summarized below and accompanied by the authors' personal observations.

Deviations or compromise of the elasto-tendinous propatagium that forms the leading edge of the wing between the shoulder and the wrist due to deep lacerations, improper bandaging methods or traumatic scarring will severely interfere with airflow over the dorsal wing. Repairs of lacerations require tension relief over the affected area while the sutured tissues are healing (see Redig in Samour's *Avian Medicine*, 3rd edition, p. 350 for method). The patagium also tends to scar and contract in the aftermath of humeral fractures especially if a figure-of-8 bandage is used for support after surgery. Physical therapy is vital to maintaining its integrity during recovery from orthopedic procedures involving the humerus or radius/ulna.

Impaired use of or damage to the alula may interfere with the bird's ability to redirect airflow over the wing at high angles of attack and result in unintentional stalling of the wing as the bird maneuvers. There is an inherited condition in captive-bred peregrine falcons where the alula folds forward of the wing and certainly impairs ability to control airflow over the wing. Correction of this problem involves tying the alula back into an over correct position for 2-3 weeks causing the feathers to re-orient in the feather follicles.

Improperly aligned bones, particularly in rotational planes, will interfere with the angular presentation of the wing in various flight attitudes and portions of the flapping cycle. Clearly, great attention to this detail must be attended to when conducting orthopedic procedures on any of the long bones of the wing. Fractures of the coracoid bone appear to be enigmatic. Analysis from a structural and kinematic point of view would suggest that its integrity is a requirement for function of the pectoral muscles. Yet, there are thousands of birds now rehabilitated and released where the coracoid was managed conservatively, and post-healing alignment was lacking – The majority of cases successfully regained flight capacity with physical therapy and exercise. Conversely, attempts to surgically repair the coracoid, while achieving successful union, often fail owing to the added morbidity associated with surgery.

Damage to joints, whether arising from the original injury or from iatrogenic causes may severely compromise the complex movements of the wing at the shoulder, elbow and carpus. Such events must be avoided or mitigated at all costs. The orthopedic procedures detailed in other parts of this book strive to provide methods of pin placement that avoid joint compromise. Following recovery, careful evaluation of joint range of motion is essential in determining a rehabilitated bird's ability to fly normally. This can be conducted by direct physical examination and passive range of motion exercises. Evaluation of flight as a bird is observed flying away from the observer on a creance provides a means of noting compensatory shifts in body rotation, leg positioning, or dissimilarity in wing beats as a means of detecting deficiencies in wing function. Where these occur, one can only strive to restore normalcy with continued vigorous exercise.

Improper feather management – whether through breakage, loss, or inadequate repair (imping) - will negatively impact wing efficiency through increased drag, loss of lift, and impaired maneuverability. Missing feathers, whether from viral infections such as circovirus or West Nile virus or loss of primary and tail feathers that have been pulled are problematic. Large flight feathers should be preserved throughout the process and never be pulled from their follicles; pulling them often results in follicular damage and replacement by distorted feathers. Secondary feathers and coverts tolerate removal. When feathers are repaired by imping, it is important to replace a broken feather by imping at its base (so that the normal flexibility of the rachis is maintained) and to use a feather that is as close to an exact match as possible with regard to species, gender and feather position. Birds should not be released to the wild without a full complement of intact feathers.

Lastly, the patient's weight should be controlled during recovery. Wing loading, the ratio of the bird's weight to its wing area, is a factor in flight efficiency. Overweight birds, in addition to being poorly athletically conditioned, are also going to be less agile and have reduced flight efficiency due to the excess weight.

An understanding of aerodynamics and wing mechanics of the bird focuses the attention of the veterinary orthopedic surgeon toward conducting restorations in a way that maintains the integrity and structure of all the various components of the wing that contribute to flight. Such attention is vital for wild birds that are released and important for the psittacine or other companion bird that is intended to live a long, pain free and mobility capable life in its domestic environment.

Tail Region

The tail consists of free caudal vertebrae that end with 4-6 fused vertebrae that form the pygostyle. The flight feathers of the tail are termed the rectrices from the Latin word, rector (retrix f.) meaning governor. These feathers are asymmetrical, but symmetrically paired. The first pair, feather 1, is the central most feather (1a) and its pair (1b) are attached to the middle point of the pygostyle. The remaining rectrices are attached into dense fibro-adipose tissue, the rectrical bulb, that sits dorsally on the pygostyle. Most commonly there are 6 pairs of rectrices. The tail spreads by lateral movement of these overlapping pairs of feathers. As with the remiges, there are coverts that cover these rectrices both dorsally and ventrally **(Figure 2-28)**.

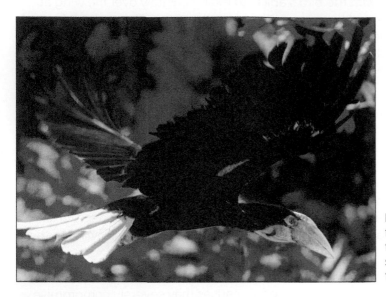

Figure 2-28. Hornbill flying. Note the white rectrices fanning out to show the overlap pattern. The shaft of the feather is centered with both vanes relatively the same size. This is different from the aysmetrical arrangement of flight feathers. (Photo: Kevin Blaylock).

Pelvic Limb or Leg

In this text, the entire hind or pelvic limb will be referred to simply as the leg. The hip joint is where the leg articulates with the trunk via the ilium. The ilium is partially fused to the remainder of the pelvic bones — the pubis and ischium and the synsacrum. The synsacrum is a bony plate of fused vertebrae incorporating the caudal thoracic vertebrae and most of the lumbar vertebrae.

There are typically three long bones comprising the avian leg, the femur, the tibiotarsus and the tarsometatarsus. The femur is the most proximal bone of the leg and is tucked against the body wall. This bone along with associated musculature is also referred to as the thigh. The joint between the femur and the next portion of the leg is the femorotibiotarsal joint which in mammals is the stifle joint **(Figure 2-29)** and is similarly referred to in birds. The tibiotarsus is the bone distal to the femur and is also called the leg, lower leg, or the crus in some anatomic texts. The proximal row of tarsal bones fuse to the distal end of the tibia in birds, thereby rendering it more accurately described as the tibiotarsus. Lateral to the tibiotarsus is the shortened fibula. Since it is greatly reduced in birds, they have a limited ability to rotate their distal leg. The distal row of tarsal bones fuse to the proximal metatarsus thereby changing it anatomically to the tarsometatarsus. The intervening joint is a true intertarsal joint in birds. The true, and lengthy, name of this is the tibiotarsal-tarsometatarsal joint, but it is generally referred to as the hock given its anatomic and functional similarity to the tibiotarsal joint in mammals. The next joint is between the tarsometatarsus and the toes. The toes form the final component of the anatomical pes and most avian texts use the term foot to describe the toes. A perched bird at rest exhibits a moderate amount of flexion in both the stifle and hock joints so that the femur, stifle and the proximal portion of the tibiotarsus are hidden under the feathers.

The length of the leg varies with the locomotion specific to the species of the bird. Long-legged birds **(Figure 2-30)** spend a significant amount of time running or walking. Short legs are found in birds that are hoppers, those that spend time clinging to surfaces and dabbling ducks. Loons (also cormorants, penguins, and other highly specialized diving birds) are unique in that their legs are set far back on the body, an adaptation for underwater swimming, that also renders ground locomotion difficult. In most ground-dwelling birds, the center of gravity is mid-body. This arrangement allows them to walk well on land, but compromises flight ability.

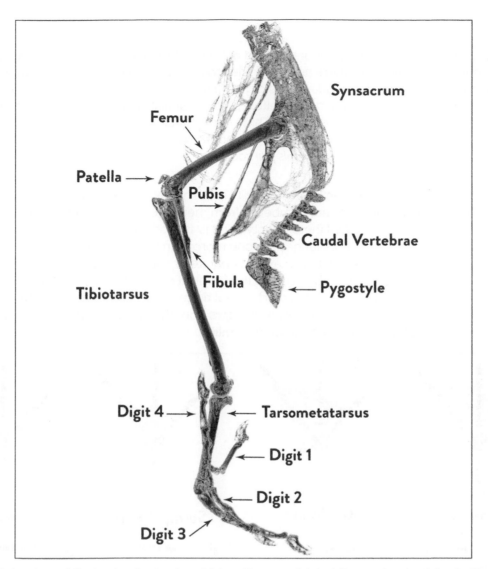

Figure 2-29. Skeletal structure of the leg in a budgerigar *(Melopsittacus undulatus).* See anatomic plates in Chapter 7 for further elaboration on the bony anatomy of the leg.

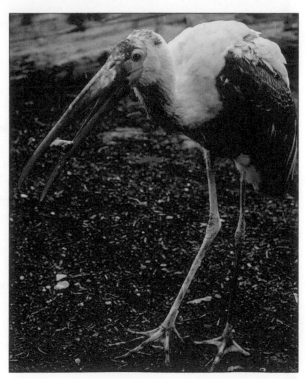

Figure 2-30. Painted stork *(Mycteria leucocephala)* showing the long legs of this species.

Foot

All birds are digitigrade (i.e., they walk on their toes and not the entire foot). The foot of a typical bird has 4 toes and except for polydactyl individuals, there are no species that have more than 4 toes but there are some that have fewer. Only the ostrich has 2 toes (didactyl) as digits I and II are absent. There are several bird species that have 3 toes (tridactyl) and usually it is the digit I (hallux) that is vestigial or absent. Tridactylism is associated with species that are runners, waders, or climbers. Three-toed species include the ratites except the ostrich (emu, cassowary and rhea), diving petrels, many of the waders, some of the woodpeckers and one species of passerine, the three-toed parrot bill (*Paradoxornis paradoxus*).

Following the conventions of mammalian anatomy, digit I is the hallux and, although rearward projecting, it is regarded as the most medial digit; digits are numbered from medial to lateral. Digit I can be directed forward or backward in some species as can digits II (heterodactyl) and IV (zygodactyl). The phalanges are the bones of the toes and in most birds the numbers of phalanges are one more than the digit number. For example, digit I has 2 and digit II has 3 phalanges **(Figure 2-31)**. Toes may be separate or connected with webbing **(Figures 2-31 and 2-32)**. The claws are the horny epithelium that covers the terminal digit of each of the toes. It consists of a harder dorsal plate that makes up the lateral sides, the hard, dorsal ridge, and a softer ventral plate. This difference in firmness accounts for the curvature of the claw as it grows from the base. In general, the claw tends to be straighter in those species that are larger and ground dwelling.

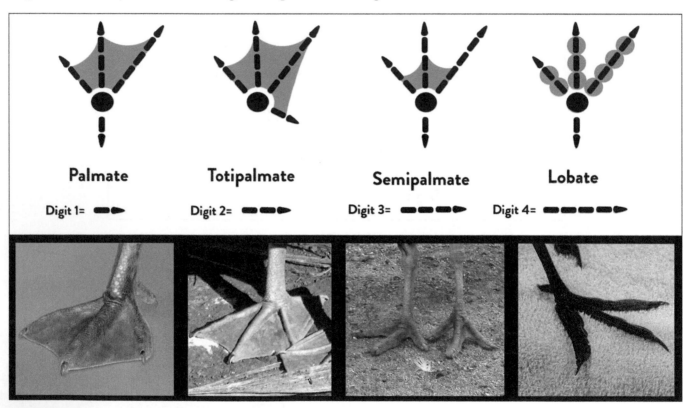

Figure 2-31. Types of webbed feet used in swimming or walking in mud. The palmate example is represented by the domestic goose (*Anser domesticus*), the totipalmate by the great white pelican (*Pelecanus onocrotalus*), the semipalmate by the African black oyster catcher (*Haemotopus moquini*), and the lobate by the American coot (*Fulica americana*).

The arrangement of the 4 toes depends on function. Many of the species have 3 toes pointing forward and one pointed back (digit I), the anisodactylous foot. The other common form is to have 2 toes pointed forward (digits II and III) and 2 pointed back (digits I and IV) or the zygodactylous foot. This type of foot is suited for climbing and grasping. The zygodactylous foot is commonly found in woodpeckers, parrots, toucans, cuckoos, and owls. The pamprodactylous foot has the ability to point all 4 toes forward. The syndactylous foot is one where digits III and IV are partially united by a bony fusion as in some of the kingfishers **(Figure 2-32)**.

The types of toe arrangements are:
• Anisodactyl: three toes forward (2,3,4) and one toe back (1). Illustrated by purple martin (*Progne subis*).
• Didactyl: two toes forward (3,4). Illustrated by ostrich (*Struthio camelus*).

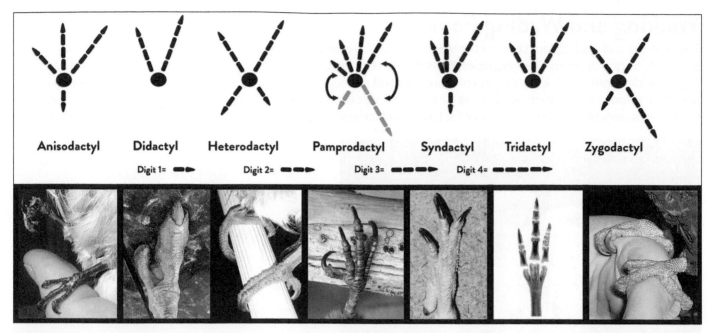

Figure 2-32. Arrangement of toes.

• Heterodactyl: two toes in front (3,4) and two toes in back (2,1). Digit 2 is caudal and medial. Illustrated by a green backed trogon *(Trogon viridis)* courtesy of Dr Andreas Frei.

• Pamprodactyl: the two inner toes are in front (2,3) and the other toes (1,4) can rotate forward and backward. Illustrated by speckled mousebird *(Colius striatus)* courtesy of Dr Erika Crook.

• Syndactyl: three toes in front (2,3,4) and one behind (1). Illustrated by laughing kookaburra *(Dacelo novae-guineae)*.

• Tridactyl: three toes in front (2,3,4). Illustrated by southern cassowary *(Casuarius casuarius)*.

• Zygodactyl: two toes in front (2,3) and two behind (1,4). Illustrated by rainbow lory *(Trichoglossus moluccanus)*.

Grasping Foot

The grasping type of foot is designed for grasping as well as perching and may be of two forms. The aniso-dactylous foot of passerines and raptors has toes that are freely moveable along the axis of each digit, and the hind or caudal toe (hallux) is opposable allowing excellent perching. The zygodactylous foot is conducive for grasping. Parrots can perch with one foot and eat their food with the other one **(Figure 2-33)**.

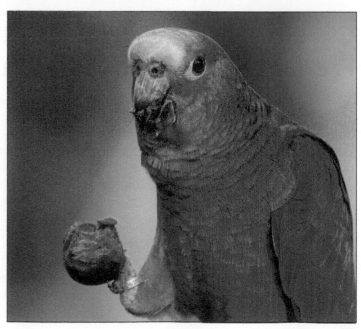

Figure 2-33. An example of the zygodactylous foot of a parrot eating a bocaiúva fruit *(Acrocomia aculeata)*.

Walking and Wading Foot

The walking and wading foot spreads the weight out on the plantar surface of the toes **(Figure 2-34)**. This foot lacks the ability to grip or grasp. The wading foot has partial webbing between the toes or hyper-developed digital pads (e.g., lobes) to spread the weight of the bird out over soft surfaces. The webbing of the toes provides a greater surface area for the foot. In birds such as rails and jacanas, the digital lobes are greatly elongated to enable these species to walk across vegetation. With this type of foot, digit I, which points backward, is often reduced, vestigial, or absent.

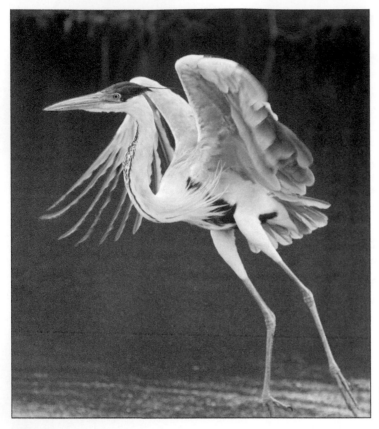

Figure 2-34. Cocoi heron (*Ardea cocoi*) on the Pantanal in Brazil possesses wading-type feet

Swimming Foot

The swimming foot has webbing between all 4 digits or the 3 toes that point forward. In those species that have the 3 toes with webbing, digit I is free and small. Some may spend most of their time swimming while the style and movements of the foot varies depending on the species.

Classification of Waterfowl Based on Modes of Locomotion, Feeding Habits, and Environmental Needs

Waterfowl can be classified via genetics, taxonomy and feeding and movement styles. How a bird feeds and moves around relates to anatomic adaptions that have evolved for its ecological niche **(Figure 2-35A, B, C, D)**. For example, most domestic ducks are mallards (*Anas platyryhnchos*) and are dabblers that walk on land and feed and spend time on water. However, not all ducks are dabblers nor are all well suited for terrestrial walking. Other classifications of waterfowl include divers, perchers and grazers. Understanding these differences helps one to create environments for captive animals that best suit their anatomy, thereby improving their welfare. This information can also be important when considering pre- and post-operative care for leg injuries in waterfowl.

Dabblers are those waterfowl that feed primarily on the surface of water or graze under shallow water. Traditionally this group is assigned to ducks in the subfamily Anatinae. These birds rarely dive and tend to have their legs placed more centrally on their body, walk well on land and even feed terrestrially. Examples of dabbling ducks include mallards, shovelers, pintails, teals, widgeons and gadwalls (all *Anas* genus). Most swans are also dabblers. Dabblers live in a combination of soft (grassy) land and shallow ponds, creeks or other water sources.

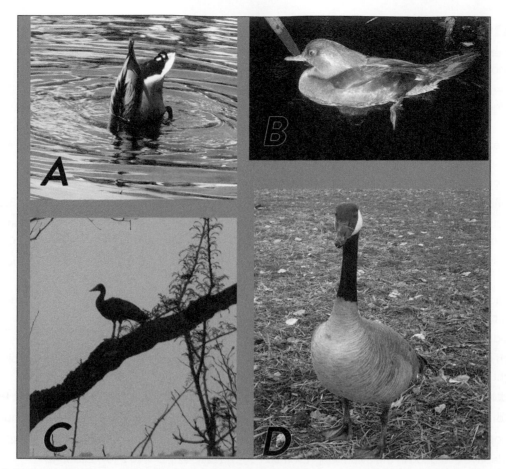

Figure 2-35A, B, C, D. Waterfowl types. This diagram shows examples of the 4 waterfowl types based on basic feeding and locomotion categorization. **A:** The mallard *(Anas platyrhynchos)* is the classic dabbler. Dabbling (depicted here) is the process of shallow feeding were the head and feet are submerged and the caudal half of the body visibly sticks out of water. **B:** Divers, such as this hooded merganser *(Lophodytes cucullatus)* feed only when submerged. Their caudally placed legs allow for forward propulsion while underwater however walking on land is difficult. **C.** Perchers, such as this silhouetted spur-winged goose *(Plectropterus gambensis)*, can frequently be found sitting on logs and trees. **D.** Grazers such as this Canada goose *(Branta canadensis)* spend most of their time walking on land and are primarily herbivorous.

Divers are those waterfowl that feed primarily under water. Ducks of this group belong to the subfamily Aythyinae. Compared to dabblers, divers have legs placed more caudally on their bodies to propel them underwater. However, divers tend to walk poorly on land, if at all. Examples of divers include bufflehead *(Bucephala albeola)*, *Aythya* genus birds such as pochard, scaup, canvasback and redhead, and ruddy *(Oxyura jamaicensis)* ducks. Other divers include mergansers, loons, and cormorants. Divers require water deep and wide enough for them to completely submerge their body and swim underwater. Further, many cannot take-off from land and require a run across water to become airborne.

Perchers perch in trees, on top of logs or other raised surfaces. Examples of perchers include Mandarin *(Aix galericulata)*, wood *(Aix sponsa)*, torrent *(Merganetta armata)*, maned *(Chenonetta jubata)*, muscovy *(Cairina moschata)* and some whistling ducks *(Dendrocygna* genus) and the pygmy *(Nettapus* genus) and spur-winged geese *(Plectropterus gambensis)*. Although not true of all, perchers tend to have longer legs and necks than dabblers and certainly divers. This group benefits from access to a combination of land, air (perched in trees, etc.) and water.

Grazers are primarily limited to herbivorous geese that eat terrestrial grasses, grains, and other plants. Grazers are good walkers and spend a significant amount of time foraging on land. The Canada goose *(Branta canadensis)* is a grazer. These waterfowl generally feed over large areas and benefit from dips in water, the frequency varying by species.

All waterfowl require water deep enough to completely submerge their head as needed to clear their nares. This is considered a basic welfare need.

Recommended Reading

1. Alerstam T, Rosen M, Baeckman J, et. al. Flight speeds among bird species: allometric and phylogenetic effects. *PLoS Biol.* 2007;5(8): e197. 2007 Jul 17.doi: 10.1371/journal.pbio.0050197.

2. Bhargavi S, S Venkatasen, Gramesh, TA Kannan. Morphometrical analysis of the wing of the blue-and-yellow macaw *(Ara ararauna)* with reference to the aerodynamics. *Int J Curr Microbiol App Sci.* 2017;6(8):2707-2710. http: doi.org/10.20546ijcmas.2017.608.3244.

3. Beaufrere H. A review of biomechanic and aerodynamic considerations of the avian thoracic limb. *J Avian Med Surg.* 2009;23(3):73-185.

4. Cornell Laboratory of Ornithology. www.birds.cornell.edu.

5. Drovetski SV. Influence of the trailing-edge notch on flight performance in galliforms. *Auk.* 1996;113,802-810.

6. Hedrick TL, Tobalske BW, Biewener AA. Estimates of circulation and gait change based on a three-dimensional kinematic analysis of flight in cockatiels *(Nymphicus hollandicus)* and ringed turtle doves *(Streptopelia risoria). J Exp Biol.* 2002; 205:1389-1409.

7. Henderson CL. *Birds in Flight: The Art and Science of How Birds Fly.* Minneapolis: Voyageur Press, MBI Publishing Company; 2008. 160pp.

8. Lees JJ, Dimitriadis G, Nudds RL. The influence of flight style on the aerodynamic properties of avian wings as fixed lifting surfaces. PeerJ 4cc2495; DOI 10.771/peerj.2495. 2016. Accessed March, 2022.

9. McGahan J. Gliding flight of the Andean condor in nature. *J Exp Biol.* 1973; 58:225-337.

10. Pap PL, Osvath G, Sandor K, et al. Interspecific variation in the structural properties of flight feathers in birds indicates adaptation to flight requirements and habitat. *Funct Ecol.* 2015; 29:746–757.

11. Pennycuick CJ. Mechanics of flight. In: Farner DS, King JR, eds. *Avian Biology.* Vol. 5. New York: Academic Press; 1975:1–75.

12. Rayner JMV. Form and function in avian flight. In: Johnston RF, ed. *Current Ornithol.* Vol. 5. New York: Plenum Press; 1988.

13. Redig PT. Orthopedic surgery. In: Samour J, ed. *Avian Medicine.* 3rd edition. St. Louis: Elsevier; 2016:312-358.

14. Savile DBO. Adaptive evolution in the avian wing. *Evolution.* 1957; 11:212-224. DOI 10.2307/2406051.

15. Tobalske B. Morphology, velocity, and intermittent flight in birds. *Amer Zool.* 2001; 41:177-187.

16. Tucker VA. Gliding birds – reduction of induced drag by wing tip slots between the primary feathers. *J Exp Biol.* 1993; 180:285-310.

17. Warham J. Wing loadings, wing shapes and flight capabilities of Procellariiformes. *N.Z. J Zool.* 1977.;4(1):73-83. https://doi.org/10.1080/03014223.1977.9517938.

18. Withers PC. An aerodynamic analysis of bird wings as fixed aerofoils. *J Exp Biol.* 1981; 90:143–162.

CHAPTER 3

Overview of Fracture Management

Pre- and Post-Operative Management of the Orthopedic Patient

Attention to pre- and post-operative management of the patient as well as fracture fixation is crucial for success in avian orthopedics. While companion birds typically have low energy fractures (e.g., closed transverse fracture of the tibiotarsus), many are nutritionally and/or structurally compromised and have poor bone quality and less than optimal body condition that will complicate management attempts. Wild birds typically have good bone quality and adequate levels of conditioning and fitness. However, wild birds are often severely compromised by some form of significant trauma that causes a given bone to be fractured along with attendant soft tissue injury. It can also result in damage to internal organs **(Figure 3-1)** and other parts of the body. Head injuries and accompanying ophthalmologic damage often occur concurrently with long bone fractures necessitating a superficial and fundic ophthalmic exam as part of the admission process to inform triage decisions. A few days of stabilization prior to surgery can mitigate the impact of many of these factors and contribute to the overall success of the repair process.

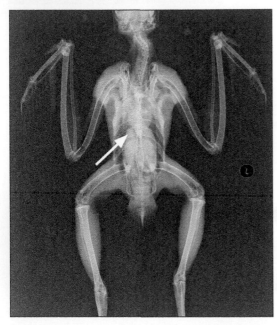

Figure 3-1. White *arrow* shows gas displacement of heart and liver suggesting internal organ damage.

Post-operatively, physiological impacts of prolonged anesthesia that often accompany orthopedic procedures, wound management, pain, and adaptation to externally applied splints, bandages, and fixation devices require a period of careful management and monitoring. Appropriate post-operative care is needed to maintain the health of the patient and respond to problems associated with their adaptation to the fixation hardware and bandages. Throughout, the underlying principle is to reduce additive morbidity at every opportunity, whether from tissue handling, hardware and bandage fit and comfort, housing, handling while providing infection prevention and maintenance of fitness. For these reasons, it is recommended that orthopedic patients be hospitalized for several days post-operatively so that trained hospital staff can properly monitor and manage circumstances that require immediate attention.

Readers are encouraged to consult material on these subjects in the regularly updated avian texts, such as *Current Therapy in Avian Medicine and Surgery* (Speer, ed. Elsevier 2016) or *Avian Medicine*, 3rd edition (Samour J, ed. Elsevier, 2016), and peer-reviewed journals for updated information on these topics on an ongoing basis, particularly regarding pain management. However, many of the basics are relatively immutable and will be covered here.

Examination and Assessment of the Orthopedic Patient

Optimizing the probability of success in an orthopedic case begins with attention to the patient first, and the fracture second. No fracture needs to be repaired immediately and there are advantages in delaying the undertaking for a few days, even up to a week, to stabilize the patient and give the soft tissues in the vicinity of the fracture some time to recover from the injury.

The basic elements of patient stabilization, hydration, warmth, ventilation (oxygen box if necessary) and protection from additional stress, need to be attended to as first order items. While attending to these or shortly after, when the patient has gained some strength, a thorough physical examination is conducted. It is recommended for any surgical procedures that the patient be treated with current anesthetic and analgesic protocols. For example, consider presurgical analgesic and anesthetic combinations combined with inhalant anesthesia. Multi-modal pain management should also be considered for all painful procedures. The sedated or anesthetized bird is generally safer for the animal and clinical staff. It makes collection of samples for a minimum database (CBC, chemistry panel, wound cultures, etc.) easier, and allows the patient to be easily positioned for imaging (x-rays or CT) in several planes to obtain needed information about overall condition (e.g., internal trauma) and assessment of the fracture(s). Procedures such as cleaning and debridement of soft tissue wounds, application of temporary fixation or coaptation, and initial antibiosis can also be undertaken without undue patient stress or causing additional injury through uncontrolled movements.

Radiological assessment is imperative for adequate pre-operative assessment. Obtain orthogonal view radiographs of long bone fractures along with a whole-body radiograph in at least the VD view or consider regional imaging or more advanced CT scans. Parameters to assess include fracture character and location, relative density, and bone condition. Proximity to joints and type of fracture (transverse, comminuted, oblique) determine load-sharing capacity and impact the choice of fixation. Factors influencing bone condition include the presence of pre-existing and possibly contributory issues such as avian tuberculosis, bone tumors, medullary bone, osteomyelitis and osteoporosis. The presence of abundant medullary bone if the patient is a female in laying condition will interfere with the ability to insert an intramedullary pin.

Broken bones need to be stabilized to prevent overriding of the fractured bone ends or projection of fragments through the skin. If the fracture is closed, stabilization is needed to prevent further trauma to the fracture site. Open fractures are more prone to osteomyelitis, so thorough cleaning, antibiosis, and bandaging are especially important in addition to stabilization. The use of a temporary, rapidly installed, partial external skeletal fixator is recommended for long bones as part of the physical examination process. Soft tissues may require debridement, treatment of infection, and protection from desiccation. It is often necessary and desirable to stage these procedures as a severely traumatized patient may not be able to withstand the handling and manipulation associated with the simultaneous conduct of all these items.

In most cases, the initial examination will conclude with the application of bandaging to protect soft tissue wounds and prevent the affected limb from moving until the definitive fixation is applied.

Management of Wounds Associated with a Fracture

External evaluation of long bone fractures involves careful handling of all tissues; gentle debridement, often best accomplished with a warm-saline soaked cotton-tipped applicator to probe the wound; trimming of sharp, exposed bone spikes; and careful removal of feathers and debris from around the injury site. If the patient is sufficiently stable, it may be useful to remove feathers from the anticipated locations of surgical approach and insertion of fixation hardware. Plucking can be used for feather removal so long as the skin is not torn. Feathers may need to be cut to avoid skin damage in some areas. Large, deep wounds should be irrigated with warm saline or other isotonic fluids. While there is a general caveat typically issued about inadvertently flowing saline into an open humeral fracture, the authors have never found this to be problematic. Wounds may be partially closed with suture or staples and a dependent area left open into which a sterile gauze seton is inserted to allow for drainage. This will be in direct contact with a wet-to-dry bandage that is applied in a later step to wick fluids away from the wound site.

Fractures of the ulna are often accompanied by a large hematoma that fills the space between adjacent secondary feathers **(Figure 3-2)**. The pressure on the skin can lead to ischemic necrosis, rupture and the formation of a large open wound. Hematomas should be resected and the clotted blood removed as part of the pre-surgical examination.

Open wounds are, by their nature, infected by or at the time of examination and mandate systemic antibiotics. While best practices dictate the acquisition of a culture and sensitivity determination, there is a critical need for immediate antibiosis. Until determined otherwise, the presence of anaerobic as well as aerobic organisms can be assumed. Skin organisms are commonly gram-positive while bite wounds often introduce gram-negative bacteria. Broad based antibiotics that cover anaerobic and aerobic organisms should be considered. A combination of clindamycin (Antirobe, Zoetis Inc., Kalamazoo, MI, USA) and augmented penicillin (Clavamox [amoxicillin and clavulanate potassium], Zoetis, Kalamazoo, MI, USA)) is a good first-line therapy to begin the process, subject to change if the sensitivity indicates otherwise when it becomes available.

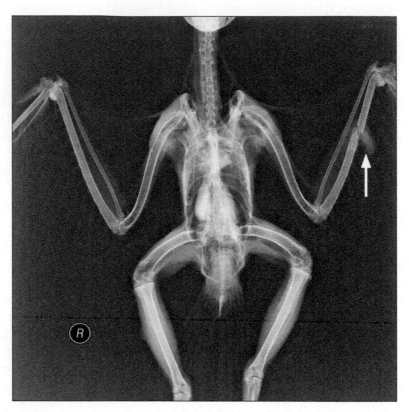

Figure 3-2. Radiographic view of the hematoma that often accompanies a fracture of the ulna. These contain a mass of clotted blood that needs to be removed during the admission process.

Summary

Careful attention to pre-operative conditions sets the stage for planning and performing the needed orthopedic procedure with a stabilized patient as well as informs triage decisions. Maximizing the potential for success depends heavily on appropriate attention to careful examination and stabilization of the patient at the outset.

Recommended Reading

1. Speer B.L., ed. *Current Therapy in Avian Medicine and Surgery.* St. Louis: Elsevier; 2016.

2. Samour *J. Avian Medicine.* 3rd ed. St. Louis: Elsevier; 2016.

CHAPTER 4

General Considerations for Management of Fractures: Methods and Materials

General Approaches to Management of the Avian Orthopedic Patient

The goals in fracture management, whether in avian or mammalian applications, include establishing early and rigid stability of the bone fragments while maintaining normal longitudinal and axial alignment of the bone; ensuring opposition of applied forces; and promoting load-sharing when possible (transverse fractures). If possible, fracture management will permit limited return to function. Additionally, whether using a surgically applied fixation device or external coaptation, the preservation of soft tissues is paramount for maintaining bone integrity. Exact anatomic alignment of comminuted fragments is not necessary and moreover their manipulation runs a high risk of detaching them from scant soft tissue vasculature attachments.

Where possible, fixation devices should promote load sharing with the bone, which contributes to the stability of the fixation construct. The use of fixation that will allow return of the limb to normal function or at least allows range of motion movement as soon as possible, will shorten healing times and minimize secondary complications. It will also promote patient mobility and comfort. In cases of periarticular fractures, the use of a trans-articular fixator that fixes the joint in place becomes an exception to allowing range of motion movement. Throughout, the clinician must make every effort to reduce morbidity by applying sound treatment techniques.

In general, bone healing rates in birds are approximately twice that of a comparable mammalian bone (Tully 2002). Well managed humeral fractures will heal in as little as 3 weeks; forelimb fractures require about 4 weeks and metacarpal fractures heal in 5-6 weeks. Healing times are longer in fractures of more distally located bones on a given limb, as well as in cases with comminuted or open fractures, or more distal diaphyseal fractures. Open fractures and those that are or become infected as well as those occurring in patients that are metabolically or nutritionally compromised will take longer to heal, have a higher complication rate and an overall lower rate of success.

Materials and Procedures for Coaptation

Coaptation (bandages and splints) is useful as an adjunct to surgical management of fractures for additional stabilization, for patient comfort and for wound protection. In a few instances, especially for wing fractures, it is a useful mode of stabilization for bone healing because the wing is not load-bearing during the healing period. An inviolate principle of coaptation is that the device must immobilize the joints above and below the fracture site. The use of coaptation as a primary mode of fracture immobilization in all but a few situations will have a higher rate of complication and poorer outcome than use of a hardware device. The various cases presented below include some where coaptation was the method of choice and the rationale for that choice is also provided.

For fractures of the pectoral limb, there are 3 modes of coaptation that are used: the simple body wrap, the figure-of-eight bandage and the metacarpal curved edge splint. For the pelvic limb, there are two: the Altman tape splint and the modified Schroeder-Thomas splint. There are notable limitations to the use of each and coaptation is seldom a satisfactory choice for leg fractures. In select cases, cage rest may be a viable option **(Figure 4-1)**.

The simple body or tape wrap consists of a piece of non-stretchy adhesive tape that is wrapped around the body and incorporates a wing affected by a fracture; the unaffected wing is left free. The tape is applied directly to the feathers for good adhesion; some feathers will necessarily be stripped off when the tape is removed, but they will regrow readily. The simple body wrap is an effective way to immobilize a wing, and it does not have any inherent characteristics that cause permanent damage. It is used pre-operatively to stabilize a wing prior to surgery, post-operatively for patient comfort for the first 3-5 days post-op and as an adjunct to wings restrained in a figure-of-eight bandage or a curved edge splint in the case of metacarpal fractures. Simple body or tape wraps, or sometimes no bandaging with cage rest alone, are also the preferred choice of management for coracoid fractures.

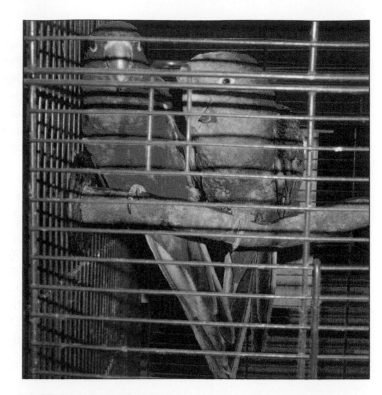

Figure 4-1. This pair of conures was attacked by a raccoon the previous day. With both birds, there was moderate bruising scattered over the wings and legs from thrashing about the cage. However, there were no fractures or penetrating wounds. The birds recovered uneventfully by taking a hands-off approach and letting the birds quietly recover in their cage and re-arranging their environment to prevent a repeat attack.

The figure-of-eight bandage, as its name suggests, is a multi-layer bandage configured in a figure-of-eight wrapping that effectively immobilizes the elbow and the metacarpal joint. It is marginally useful for stabilizing fractures between the elbow and the carpus; however, bone alignment may be poor. If both the radius and ulna are fractured, management with a bandage often results in the formation of a synostosis, a bony bridge between the two. Wings confined in this bandage are also typically bandaged to the body with a tape wrap. This bandage is not suitable for immobilizing fractures of the humerus unless the wing is also taped to the body. In all its uses, this bandage can cause stretching and deformity of the propatagium, the tendino-elastic tissue that forms the leading edge of the wing. For this reason, it needs to be applied in a manner that does not overly impinge on the propatagium, and it must be removed every few days so that physical therapy can be applied.

The curved-edge splint is used exclusively for the immobilization of fractures of the metacarpus. It is made from a flat piece of a thermoplastic material that extends from the wrist joint to the end of the phalanges on the ventral surface. It is molded to fit the contours of the joints between the bone elements of the metacarpus and held in place with adhesive tape. In addition, the entire wing is taped to the body for the duration of time that the splint is in place.

Legs present more challenges for coaptation because a) they cannot be simply bandaged to the body, and b) birds will invariably try to bear weight on them which applies distractive forces to the fracture site.

The tape splint, historically referred to as the Altman tape splint, is limited to stabilization of leg fractures in small patients – typically those weighing less than 100 g. Tape splints attempt to sandwich the affected area of a limb between several layers of adhesive tape applied face-to-face on either side of the leg and crimped tightly. Some clinicians choose to further strengthen the splint by applying super glue to the bandage material which hardens upon drying. Others incorporate small wood splints in the bandage as an alternative means to provide rigidity (Hatt J-M). Its best application is for tarsometatarsal fractures that cannot be otherwise managed surgically. A tape splint is likely to be unsuccessful in stabilizing a non-load-sharing fracture of the tibiotarsus as the surrounding muscle prevents crimping the splint tightly enough to immobilize the fracture. In either application, this splint does not achieve the principle objective of immobilizing joints on either side of the fracture. It may have use in some instances where other options are unavailable, but the complication rate is high.

The modified Schroeder-Thomas splint, though bulky, can be an effective mode of primary stabilization in select circumstances. It is suitable for leg fractures occurring in the tibiotarsus and tarsometatarsus; it is not suitable for femoral fractures. It is composed of a malleable wire frame that has a ring at the top that fits around the leg and lays up against the body wall, and two struts that descend along the cranial and caudal aspect of the leg, bent to follow the contours of the leg so that the bird can reasonably and comfortably hold the leg in a near normal perching position. By sizing the wire to the bird, clinicians can tailor this device to a wide range of avian patients. It can be fashioned from appropriately sized (in the judgment of the clinician), malleable wire. Standard coat hanger wire (3/32-in diameter) is near perfect for birds weighing 500-1200 g. Soft wire used in taxidermy is available at craft stores and various online sources in a variety of sizes that can accommodate smaller birds. Bigger birds, requiring larger wires, will require imagination and resourcefulness. One author (P. T. R.) has used it on birds ranging from cockatiels to macaws to mid-size raptors (e.g., red-tailed hawks).

Methods of Application
Body Wrap
The goal in the application of this bandage is to fix the wing against the body as it would be held in normal perching position without a) constricting the respiratory movements of the bird, and b) not trapping the legs under the bandage. Materials needed consist only of white adhesive tape (do not use stretch bandage such as Vetrap™ [3M, Maplewood, MN, USA]) of a width proportional to the size of the patient. This may range from one-quarter inch in 100-g birds, to half-inch for 300-500 g birds, 1 inch for birds around 1 kg and 2 inches for 4-kg patients. Use of sedation or anesthesia will greatly facilitate handling of the bird for its application. Bandaging steps are shown below **(Figure 4-2A-J)**.

One to two repeated wraps are generally sufficient. Check to ensure the tape is sufficiently loose so the bird can breathe in an uninhibited fashion. Fold the opposite wing back into a resting position and ensure that the tips of the primaries cross in symmetrical fashion over the tail. Ensure that the stifle joints are free to extend so that the bird can perch normally.

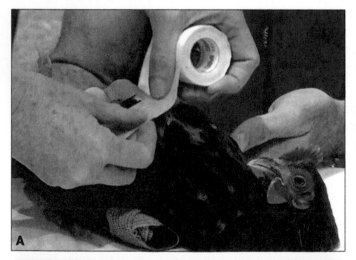

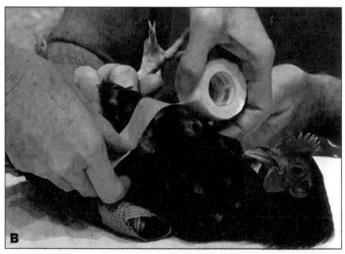

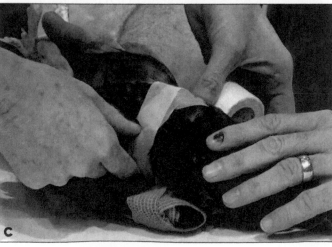

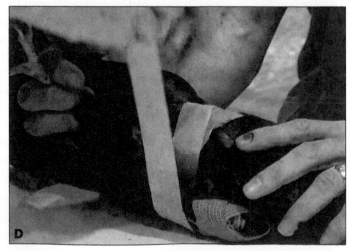

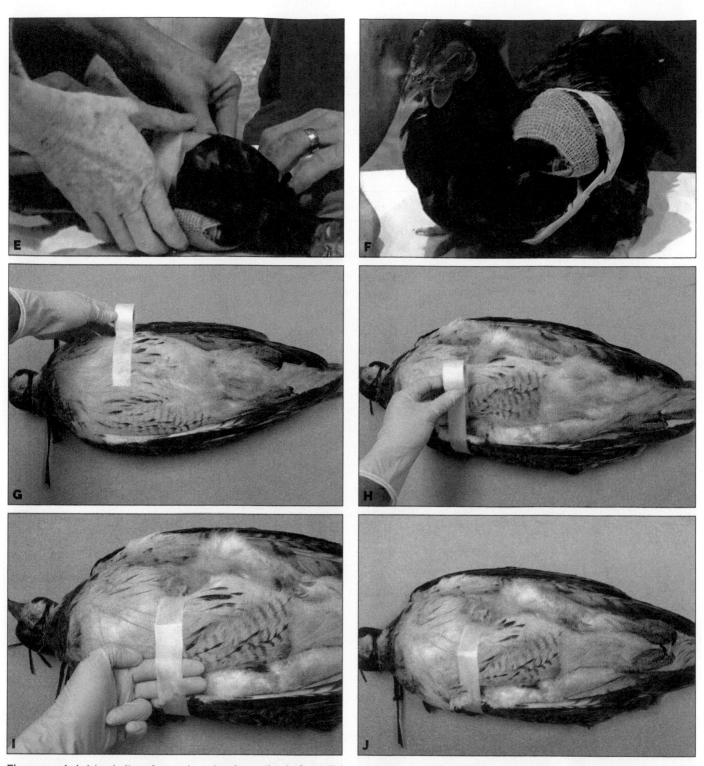

Figure 4-2A-J. A body "tape" wrap is a simple method of stabilizing an injured wing leaving the unaffected limb free. Use appropriately sized tape (1" tape for this small chicken-*Gallus domesticus domesticus*) applied directly to the feathers. Image G is that of a red-tailed hawk *(Buteo jamaicensis)* with a simple body wrap applied; the clinician is checking the bandage for appropriate tension. **A)** With the bird in dorsal recumbency, position the tape over the central portion of the keel. **B)** Press the tape on the feathers making the tape flat and even and hugging the body snuggly although not so tight as to affect respirations. **C)** Pass the tape around the body laterally in the caudal portion of the axillary spaces. When placing tape, ensure the feathers are laying in a normal position and are not disrupted as a result of the tape. Make at least one pass around the body such that the tape is now sticking upon itself. Subsequent passes may include the cranial portion of the axillary space of the unaffected wing. **D)** Incorporate the affected dorsal (lateral) portion of the wing with the next pass. **E)** After incorporating the affected limb, either complete the bandage by taping the tape to itself such that it is stable or provide one more pass over the injured wing. **F)** The bandage should be light and comfortable for the bird. Notice how the wing (even with a figure of 8 bandage in addition to the body wrap) is in normal resting position on this chicken. Excess, tight, poorly positioned and heavy bandages contribute to patient discomfort and may further complicate the injury. **G-I)** The body wrap is also demonstrated in a red-tailed hawk *(Buteo jamaicensis)*. When complete **(I)**, the body wrap should be snug across the body and loose enough to allow two fingers to slip under the bandage across the lateral pectoral region.

Figure-of-8

The figure-of-8 wing bandage is one of the more challenging to properly place on birds and has the greatest potential to cause damage if incorrectly performed. The goal is to restrain the wing in its normal anatomic position and allow bones to heal in their proper configuration **(Figure 4-3A-R)**.

When completed, the bandage should stabilize the elbow and carpal joints without over-flexing the carpus. The leading edge of the primary feathers should lie parallel to the secondary feathers.

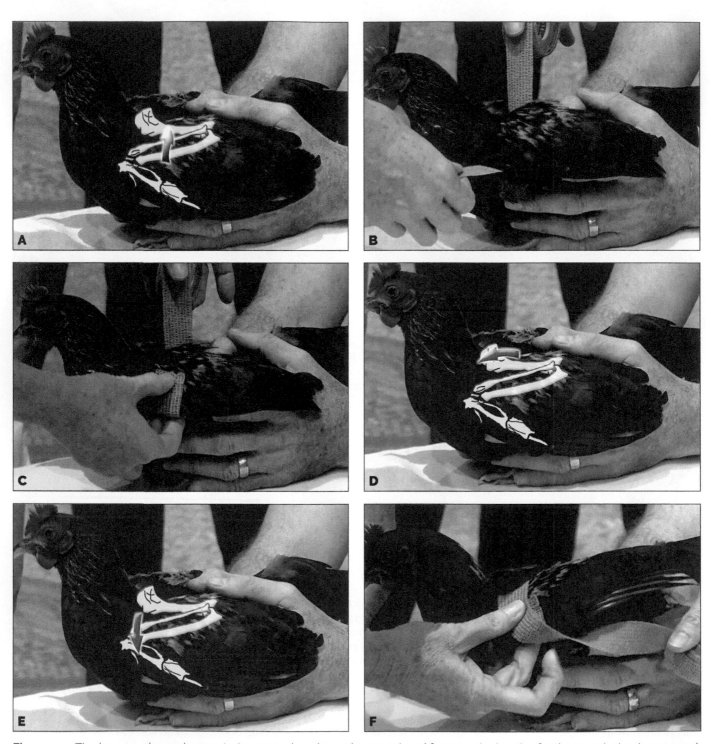

Figure 4-3. The images above demonstrate proper bandage placement and focus on laying the feathers and wing in a normal "folded" resting position against the body. The "lateral" aspect of the resting wing is the dorsal side when outstretched for flying. The "medial" aspect of the resting wing is the ventral side when flying. Black arrows indicate that the bandage is passing along the medial side of the wing. Green arrows indicate that the bandage is on the lateral side.

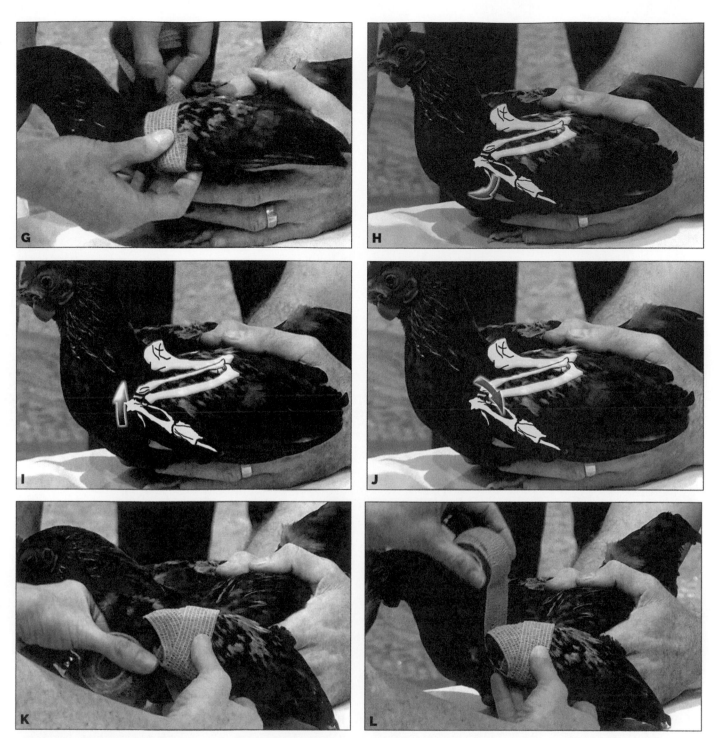

Figure 4-3. *(continued)* **A.** A bandage of appropriate width (1-in [~2.5 cm] in the small chicken *[Gallus domesticus domesticus]* used in the example) starts at the leading edge of the carpus and travels along the medial side of the wing exiting at the caudal aspect of the axillary space. **B.** The bandaging material is positioned on the medial side of the wing resting in the cranial portion of the axilla. **C.** The bandage starts at the leading (cranial) edge slightly draped over the lateral (dorsal) carpus. **D-E.** The bandage then travels over the dorsal portion of the wing connecting to the starting edge (slightly draped over the lateral carpus). **F.** The bandage has traveled over the dorsal surface of the wing meeting the starting point. **G.** Another pass is made along the ventral portion of the wing essentially creating another starting layer and ending again at step F. The example shown here is typically reserved for larger birds as a single pass may be enough for smaller species. **H-J.** Once the bandaging has returned to the starting point (as a first or second pass), the material is wrapped along the cranial to medial aspect of the carpus. The bandage is then returned across the lateral aspect of the carpus back to the starting point. **K-M.** The bandage is continued to wrap the carpus. This step is critical in that the bandaging material is kept as close to the carpus (without slipping) as possible. More proximally placed bandages (those toward the elbow) risk damaging the propatagium. As a rule, keep the bandaging material away from the elbow.

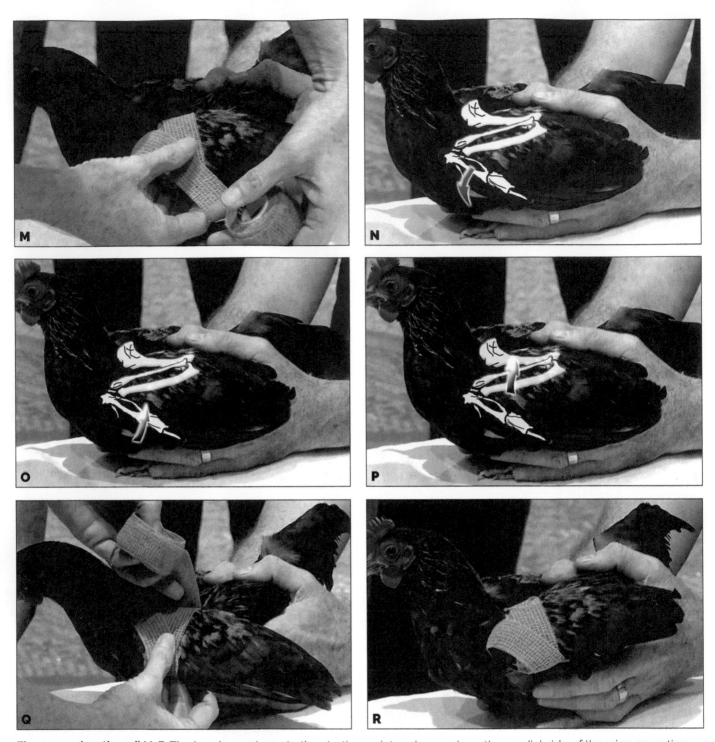

Figure 4-3. *(continued)* **N-P.** The bandage returns to the starting point and goes along the medial side of the wing repeating the pattern. **Q.** The second pass of the figure of 8 bandage repeats. Depending on the species, 1-3 passes of the bandage may be needed. If too bulky or tight, the bandage will be uncomfortable. In very small birds (<200 g), only one layer is used to avoid excessive bulk. **R.** When complete, the wing should rest against the body in a normal position.

Application of a figure-of-eight bandage using a red-tailed hawk *(Buteo jamaicensis)* **(Figures 4-4A-I)**. (Credits: Hugo Lopez, intern at The Raptor Center, St. Paul, Minnesota, USA).

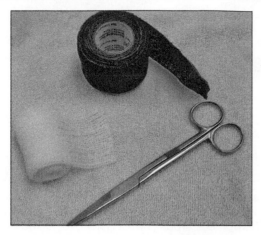

Figure 4-4A. Materials required. 2-inch wide (5 cm x 5 cm) conforming gauze (e.g., Kling Gauze™ Johnson and Johnson Products, Inc, New Brunswick, NJ, USA). 2-inch wide self adherant bandage such as Vetrap (e.g., Vetrap™, 3M) or similar bandaging material, Scissors.

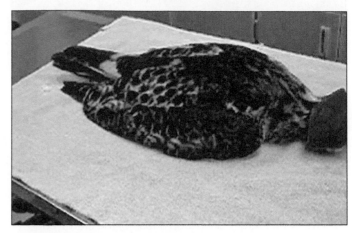

Figure 4-4B. Patient positioning and preparation for bandage application. The bandage may be applied with the bird in either dorsal or ventral recumbency per operator preference. Anesthesia or sedation facilitates, but is not necessary, for application. Important Steps: Place patient on its keel with the injured wing closest to you. Gently extend the wing. Gather primary, secondary and tertiary covert feathers together.

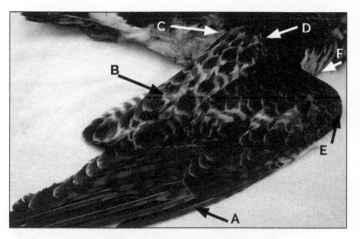

Figure 4-4C. Important landmarks for bandage application include: *A* # 10 primary flight feather, *B.* elbow, *C.* axilla, *D.* scapular or tertiary coverts, *E.* carpometacarpus or wrist, and *F.* propatagium.

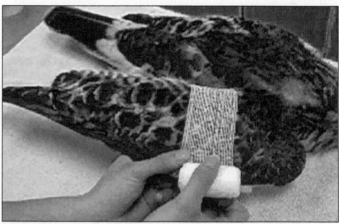

Figure 4-4D. Initiating the placement of the conforming gauze on the wing. Orient the gauze roll so that, as gauze is being applied, your tension tightens the gauze on the roll as opposed to having it unwind ahead of you. Slide the free end of the gauze from dorsal to ventral into the axilla. Pull the free end of the gauze under the ventral surface of the wing to the outer wing margin (last primary) and pinch the free end with thumb and index finger. Draw the gauze roll over the dorsal aspect of the wing toward the leading edge and the # 10 primary flight feather.

Figure 4-4E. Continuing the application of the conforming gauze wrap. Wrap the gauze around the leading edge, under the wing and bring the roll from ventral to dorsal through the axilla. Again, pinch the free end now overlapped with more gauze, where it overlays the last primary (#10). Continue wrapping the gauze in this manner until four complete rounds have been applied. (The number of wraps will vary in different species, with fewer wraps for smaller species because of weight limitations and the bulk of the bandaging). Keep the gauze placed as high into the axilla as possible and do not allow it to slide distal to the elbow.

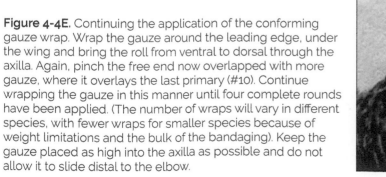
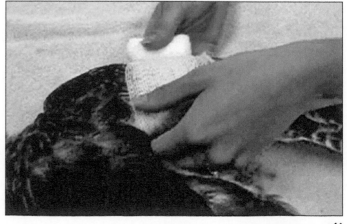

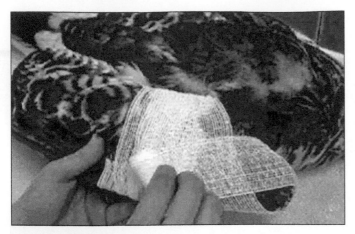

Figure 4-4F. Initiating the figure-of-8 pattern. After the 4 rounds of gauze, on the next lap, instead of bringing the roll over the wing margin, bring it up ahead of the cranial edge of the carpometacarpus and wrap it over the propatagium. After coming around the carpometacarpus, come across the dorsal aspect of the wing, angling caudad. Come over the cranial edge of the #10 primary flight feather, under the wing, and back up through the axilla (as before). Continue this figure of 8 pattern until a multi-layered firm bandage has been applied. Two points are critical: 1) do not over flex the elbow or the carpometacarpus—the outer-edge of the # 10 primary flight feather should lie flush with the edge of the outmost secondary feather, and 2) the propatagium must not be compressed. This bandage immobilizes with its bulk, not its tightness.

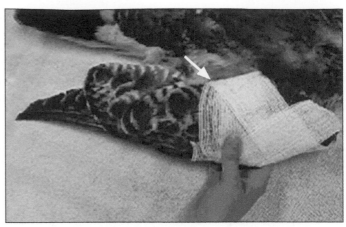

Figure 4-4G. Caveats and checkpoints before proceeding further. Propatagium is not compressed or deformed by gauze. Carpometacarpus or wrist is not over flexed – the edge of the #10 primary flight feather should be aligned with the cranial edge of the outermost secondary flight feather. The gauze should extend no more than half a width distal to the elbow *(arrow)*. Scapular coverts are included in the bandage. Wing should lie against the body in a manner nearly symmetrical to the unbandaged wing.

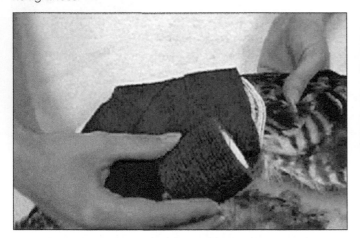

Figure 4-4H. Application of the Vetrap overwrap. Begin the application of Vetrap in the same manner as the gauze. Wrap it once around the wing, then begin the figure-of- 8 by bringing it up over the carpometacarpus and propatagium for one or two rounds. Continue the figure-of-8 pattern until the gauze is completely covered. Fold loose edges over the wrist and compress the layers with your fingers. Be certain that all loose edges of gauze are tucked under the Vetrap. Check again to ensure that the carpometacarpus or wrist is not over flexed and that the propatagium has not been compressed.

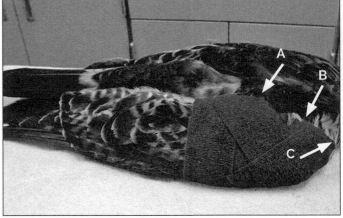

Figure 4-4I. The completed figure-of-eight bandage. Note that: Tertiary coverts *(A)* are included within the wrap. Propatagium *(B)* is not compressed. Carpometacarpus or wrist *(C)* is not over flexed and the primary flight feathers are aligned. All gauze tufts are covered (to prevent the bird from pulling at them). Wing lies comfortably along the body.

Curved Edge Splint

Materials required for this splint include a rectangular piece of 1.2-mm (small patients) or 2.4-mm (large patients) thick thermoplastic bandaging material, warm water (160° F/ 71° C) in a suitable container (beaker or open pan), white adhesive tape, and overwrapping material such as Vetrap™ (3M). The thermoplastic is cut to a length that extends from the proximal edge of the carpometacarpus to the end of the last digit. Immerse the plastic in the hot water bath until it becomes soft and malleable. Apply it to the ventral side of the wing. Fold the outside edge up to ninety degrees so it runs along the leading edge of the wing – it should not be wrapped around the edge of the wing. Now mold the material so that it conforms to the contours of the underside of the wing along the length of the metacarpus and carpometacarpus. Allow the plastic to cool and harden. If desired results are not attained, replace the material in hot water and repeat the process. Take an appropriately wide piece of white adhesive tape, one on the dorsal surface and one on the ventral surface and sandwich the splint material between the two adhesive surfaces **(Figure 4-5A-D)**. Complete the process by taping the wing to the body.

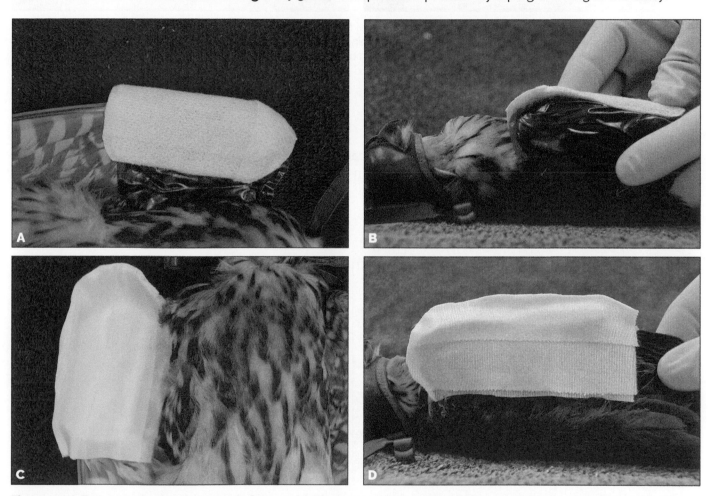

Figure 4-5A-D. A curved-edge splint made from moldable thermoplastic. A piece of thermoplastic is cut to the length of the metacarpus and molded to the ventral aspect of the bone **(A)** with a right-angle bend covering the leading edge of the bone **(B)**. The splint is sandwiched in place using overlapping pieces of adhesive tape applied ventrally **(C)** and dorsally **(D)**. Used with permission from Speer B, ed. *Current Therapy in Avian Medicine and Surgery*. 1st ed. St. Louis: Elsevier; 2016.

Altman Tape Splint

This splint has moderate utility for temporary immobilization of midshaft and distal diaphyseal fractures of the tibiotarsus and for definitive immobilization of metatarsal fractures in small birds. Both the stifle and tibiotarsal-tarsometatarsal joints must be immobilized for this splint to function **(Figure 4-6A & B)**. To begin, wrap the leg in 1-3 layers of conforming gauze or elastic material (Vet Wrap™, 3M) to contain the feathers. Then, with the leg flexed in an approximate perching position, apply 2 pieces of white adhesive tape, opposing adhesive surfaces facing each other, on either side of the leg, extending from the stifle as far as possible to the digits. Pinch it down tightly on either side of the leg (a hemostat is useful). Two or three layers of tape may be used to achieve a desired level of stiffness followed by hardening with cyanoacrylate adhesive (Vetbond™ – 3M, Maplewood, MN, USA). Avoid use of cyanoacrylate adhesive such as used in modeling as the exothermic curing process may cause tissue damage.

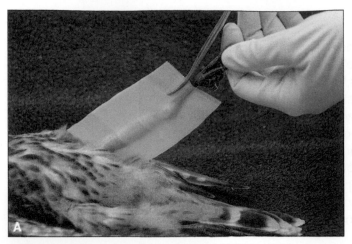
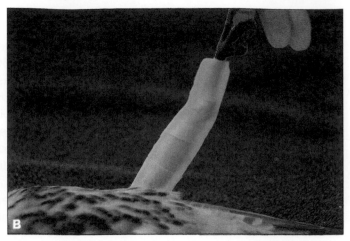

Figure 4-6A&B. Application of a tape splint to a distal tibiotarsal fracture in a merlin (Falco columbarius). After fracture reduction, the leg is lightly wrapped in a few layers of conforming gauze. Then, two layers of tape sandwiching the leg between the adhesive surfaces are applied and cinched down using a hemostat or other instrument as shown **(A)**. The splint edges are trimmed and hardened with cyanoacrylate **(B)**. (Used with permission from Speer B, ed. *Current Therapy in Avian Medicine and Surgery.* 1st ed. St. Louis: Elsevier; 2016)

Schroeder-Thomas splint

The modified Schroeder-Thomas splint, though bulky, can be an effective mode of primary stabilization in select circumstances. It is suitable for leg fractures occurring in the tibiotarsus and tarsometatarsus; it is not suitable for femoral fractures **(Figures 4-7A-K)**.

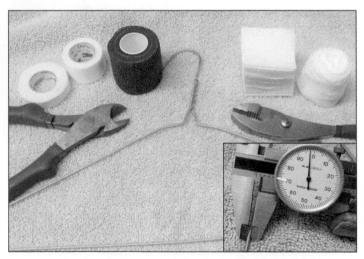

Figure 4-7A. Supplies needed: A piece of 3/32" (0.094-in, 2.4-mm) soft wire (e. g., coat hanger), wire cutters, pliers, 2-in x 2-in (5-cm x 5-cm) gauze sponges or equivalent, white adhesive tape, and Vetrap™ (3M). Inset shows wire diameter measured with calipers.

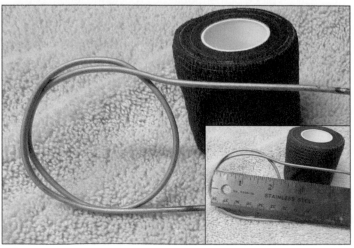

Figure 4-7B. Bending a ring in the wire. Anchor an appropriately sized mandrel (a round object such as a rod, piece of pipe or a can) of appropriate size in a vice; place the middle of the wire against the mandrel and bring the two free ends around 180 degrees to form the ring as shown. A 1-7/8-in diameter mandrel was used in this demonstration case and produced a 2-1/4-in diameter ring owing to spring-back in the wire.

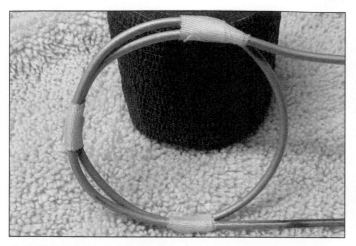

Figure 4-7C The ring is stabilized by placing adhesive tape stays at three locations.

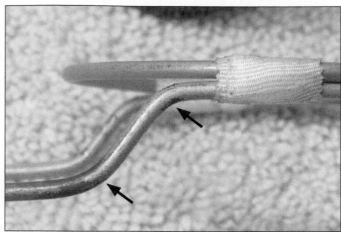

Figure 4-7D. In this step a two-bend jog *(arrows)* is formed in each of the struts to align the fixture with the bones of the limb and to angle the ring so that it will lie against the side of the patient's body.

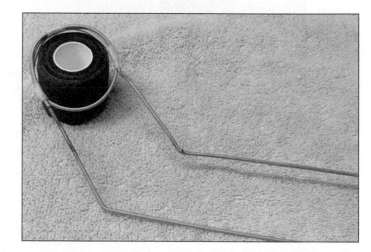

Figure 4-7E. The struts are bent at the appropriate distance from the ring to accommodate the natural flexion of the bird's leg at the hock (tibiotarsal-tarsometatarsal) joint – this step is best performed using the patient's leg as a guide for placement of the flexures.

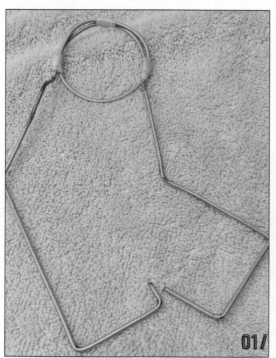

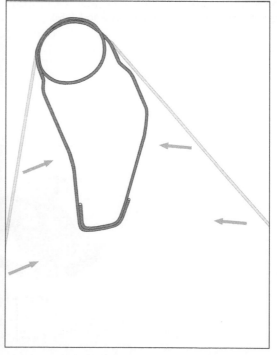

Figure 4-7F. The struts are now extended the length of the leg distal to the hock and trimmed to the appropriate length as determined by trial fitting. Once trimmed, the ends are bent toward each other at right angles to form the lower end of the splint.

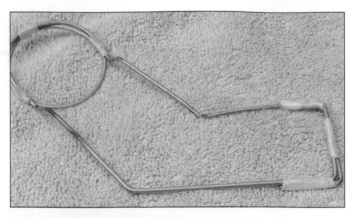

Figure 4-7G. The ends are now overlapped and taped together with white adhesive tape.

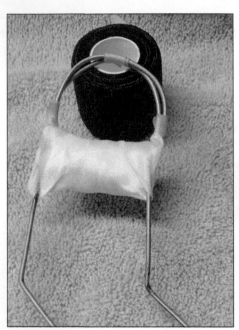

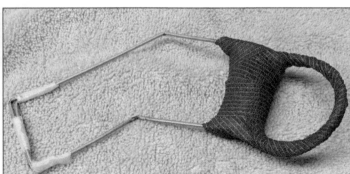

Figure 4-7H. The last steps in making the splint consist of padding the ring in the areas that are going to be in contact with the bird's body. Most of the padding (2-in x 2-in [5-cm x 5-cm] gauze sponges) is applied to the ventral part of the ring and then overwrapped with white tape and finally Vetrap™ (3M).

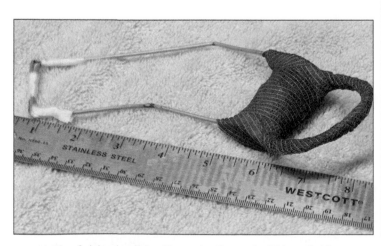

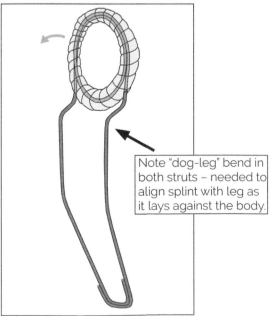

Note "dog-leg" bend in both struts – needed to align splint with leg as it lays against the body.

Figure 4-7I. The finished splint with a ruler for scale. This splint is appropriately sized for a 300-600 g bird such as an Amazon parrot, broad-winged hawk, or male peregrine falcon.

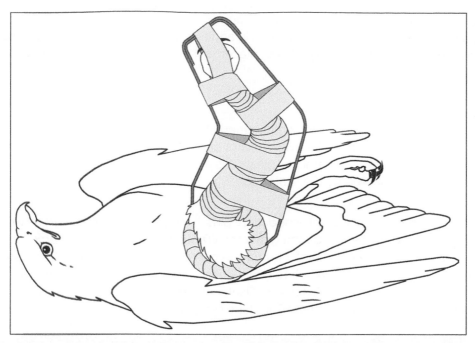

Figure 4-7J. The splint is applied as detailed in this sketch. The fracture is reduced and the leg of the patient is wrapped in conforming gauze. The leg is suspended between the struts using alternating white adhesive tape stays. With the leg suitably suspended, the entire splint is overwrapped with Vetrap™ (3M). Duct tape is a useful overwrap for patients that are inclined to chew at the splint. (Image by Frank Taylor). Birds adapt remarkably well to this device and this author has had it well tolerated by such notable chewers as macaws along with many species of raptors.

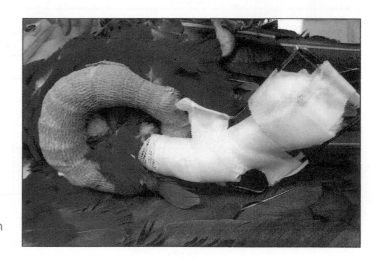

Figure 4-7K. Modified Schroeder-Thomas Splint mid-application on a blue and gold macaw (*Ara ararauna*). Completion involves overwrapping the entire construct with Vetrap™.

Surgical Fracture Management

Surgical management of avian fractures is typically accomplished with one of three options; intramedullary pinning, some variant of an external skeletal fixator (ESF) or a combination of the two known as a hybrid or tie-in fixator.

Equipment

Orthopedic work in most birds (< 2 kg) can be readily conducted with a minimum of specialized equipment. Beyond basic dissection equipment suitable for use in handling soft tissues in birds, the orthopedic gear required consists of a small 4-jaw pin driver (e.g., Mini pin driver – IMEX® Veterinary, Inc, Longview, TX, USA), a regular pin driver with a Jacobs chuck, and an assortment of bone handling tools (bone holders, thumb forceps, periosteal elevators, osteotome, rongeurs), and an assortment of needle-nose and locking-jaw pliers for handling the intramedullary pins and Kirschner-wire components of the fixator.

Radiology is an essential component of successful orthopedic management and it should be available in the immediate vicinity of the surgical proceedings so that, in addition to pre- and post-operative radiographs, intra-operative views may also be taken to guide pin placement and bone alignment when necessary.

Materials

The primary fixation methods used in birds include intramedullary pins, external skeletal fixators, and most importantly a combination of the two known as the hybrid fixator or external-skeletal-fixator-intramedullary-pin-tie-in (ESFIMPTI) or simply tie-in fixator. As the name suggests it is a combination of intramedullary pin and external skeletal fixator pins that are connected by the fixator bar.

The materials for these devices consist of intramedullary pins, both Steinmann pins and K-wires (Kirschner wires between 0.028 in [0.7-mm] and 0.078-in [2.0 mm] diameter) **(Table 4-1)**. English and Metric sizes for common pin sizes. Materials also include external skeletal fixator elements (ESFs) using conventional stainless-steel connecting bars and clamps, methylmethacrylate connecting bars (horse-hoof repair acrylic or similar) and more complex devices such as the F.E.S.S.A. system (Fixateur Externe du Service de Sante des Armees, Jorgensen Labs, Loveland, CO, USA) a.k.a. Fessa Tubulaire system.

Table 4-1. ENGLISH TO METRIC CONVERSION TABLE FOR COMMON PIN SIZES. THE MEASUREMENTS IN THIS TABLE ARE REFERENCED TO PIN SIZES AVAILABLE FROM IMEX VETERINARY, INC	
ENGLISH DIA. (INCHES)	METRIC DIA. (MM)
0.028	0.7
0.035	0.9
0.045	1.1
0.054	1.4
0.062 (1/16)	1.6
0.078 (5/64)	2.0
3/32	2.4
7/64	2.8
1/8	3.2
9/64	3.6
5/32	4.0
3/16	4.8
1/4	6.4

Intramedullary Pin

The hollow medullary cavity of most avian bones readily accommodates intramedullary pins. Generally, a pin is selected that fills approximately 50%-60% of the medullary cavity as determined by measurements taken from a radiograph pre-operatively. The singular useful attribute of the IM pin is that it strongly opposes bending forces; conversely, it has no ability to oppose torsional, compressive, or tensile forces that may be applied to bones. It must be used in conjunction with some other mode of stabilization – either coaptive bandaging or as a component in a hybrid fixator. The pin(s) must be secured in some manner to prevent removal by the patient.

Insertion of intramedullary pins can be done either in a retrograde or normograde manner. The former, which involves inserting the pin at a fracture site and driving it initially away from the fracture, seems the easiest and sometimes the most intuitive. However, it is also the most likely to cause iatrogenic injury or morbidity since a) if the fracture site is closed, it must be opened to gain access to the fracture end, and b) the pin is likely to exit the end of the bone through a joint. As will be noted in the case of the tibiotarsus, there are occasions when this is unavoidable. However, forcing a pin through a joint should generally be avoided. Under no circumstances should an IM pin be retrograded into either the radius, ulna or the humerus in a manner that causes it to exit at the elbow joint **(Figures 4-8A1, B1)**.

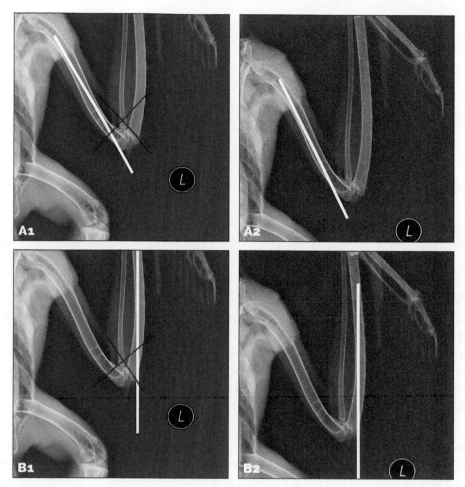

Figures 4-8A & B. These two figures demonstrate improper & proper placement of intramedullary pins in the humerus **(A1,2)** and the ulna **(B1, 2)**. Retrograde placement is to be avoided **(A1 and B1)**. In both instances, damage occurs to the triceps tendon and the elbow that inevitably results in degenerative joint disease. Normograde placement **(A2 and B2)**, where the IM pin is introduced at the apex of the distal curvature in the humerus and the ulna, avoids injury to the joint element. In the case of normograde placement in the humerus, the triceps tendon must be displaced medially so that the pin does not penetrate it.

Note that retrograde pin placement is acceptable for humeral fractures as long as the pin is introduced into the proximal fragment and exits at the proximal end.

Normograde placement involves inserting the pin at or near the proximal or distal end of the affected bone, away from the fracture site, and driving it toward the fracture. The principle long bones of the wing, the humerus and ulna, both have strong curvatures at the distal and proximal ends, respectively. This allows insertion of the IM pin at the apex of that curvature, and away from the elbow joint *(See Figure 4-8C and Figure 6-15C)*.

IM pinning of the radius is accomplished by insertion of the pin at the distal end near the metacarpal joint and driving it normograde. The femur is pinned by insertion at the fracture site and driving the pin retrograde, exiting at the hip. The tibiotarsus is pinned by inserting the IM pin on the tibiotarsal plateau and driving it normograde. There is some finesse involved in this method in that it requires approaching on the medial side of the stifle and, by percutaneous puncture, inserting the pin perpendicular to the leg (i.e., from medial to lateral) and underneath the patellar tendon. When halfway across the joint, the pin is directed into longitudinal alignment with the long axis of the bone, displacing the patellar tendon laterally; it is then advanced into the medullary cavity. While this pin is literally in the stifle joint, owing to the partially flexed position of the stifle in a perched bird, there is generally no appreciable long-term morbidity associated with placing the pin in this manner.

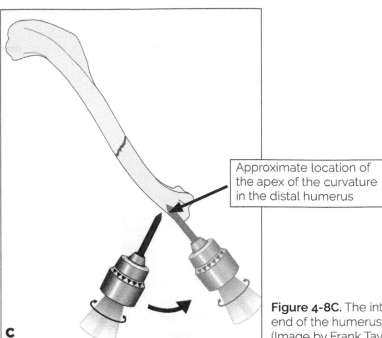

Figure 4-8C. The intramedullary pin is shown being inserted at the distal end of the humerus at the apex of its curvature for normograde placement. (Image by Frank Taylor).

External Skeletal Fixator

While various constructs involving Type I, II, and III external skeletal fixators (ESF) (Piermattei, Flo, and DeCamp 2006) may be used in birds, the Type II fixator is commonly utilized. Type I fixators, especially when applied to fractures of the pelvic limb distal to the stifle are prone to failure; however, they are useful for the ulna and metacarpus. They are generally good at resisting rotational movement as well as compressive or tensile forces. They also have a moderate capacity to oppose bending if they are comprised of sufficiently robust materials and are properly applied.

Important elements in placement include the use of appropriately sized, partially threaded, positive-profile ESF half-pins (IMEX Veterinary, Inc), designed for birds, ensuring that both trans and cis cortices of the bone are engaged by the threads, and that the pin is inserted at a 90-degree angle to the long axis of the bone. Pins should be approximately 25% of the bone diameter. Typical sizes would be 0.035-in (0.9-mm) pins for birds under 200 g, 0.045-in (1.1-mm) pins for birds weighing in the range of to 200-500 g, 0.062-in (1.6 mm) pins for birds 500-1200 +/- g, and 0.078-in (2.0-mm) pins for 1500-2500-g birds **(Figure 4-9A)**. "Center-threaded" pins with positive profile threads are also available in larger sizes **(Figure 4-9B)**.

For large waterfowl (swans, geese) and eagles, 1/8-in diameter Steinman pins (unfortunately, non-positive profile threads are the only options currently available) are used. Pin sizes are sometimes mixed within a construct at the surgeon's discretion to accommodate varying circumstances.

To complete the fixator, materials for making a connecting bar are needed. A length of soft latex tubing (e.g., Penrose drain, plastic drinking straw or tubing designed specifically for external fixators) filled with acrylic such as that used for repairing horse hooves (Technovit TM Horse Hoof Repair Acrylic, Jorgensen Laboratories, Inc., Loveland, CO, USA) has been found effective (van Wettere et al 2009). As well, dental acrylic (Caulk Dental AcrylicTM, Denstply International, Inc., Hork, PA, USA) or other products specifically engineered for this purpose (AcrylixTM ESF Acrylic. IMEX® Veterinary, Inc, Longview, TX, USA) may be found suitable. The acrylic is loaded in a syringe during the liquid stage of curing and injected into the mold. Alternatively, products such as the Acrylx™ ESF Acrylic system (IMEX® Veterinary, Inc) come complete with an applicator gun that mixes resin components during application and tube-filling which simplifies ESF construction. Acrylics are inexpensive and can be shaped to accommodate the contours of avian bones as well as small-to-modest misalignments of ESF pins.

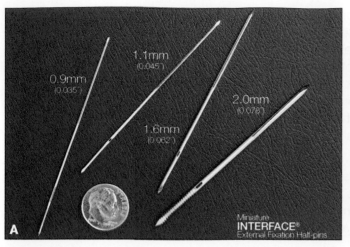
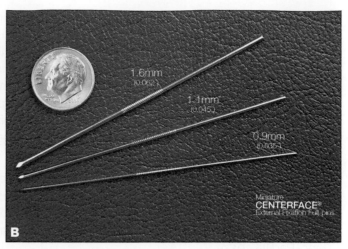

Figure 4-9A & B. Photograph of external-skeletal-fixator pins designed for use with acrylic connector bars. The threaded portion of the pin is larger than the diameter of the remainder of the shaft which obviates the necessity of pre-drilling holes in the bone and provides more surface area for gaining purchase on the bone cortex. The opposite end of the pin has a grooved surface that forms a mechanical lock with the acrylic material (photo courtesy of IMEX Veterinary, Inc). End-threaded pins **(A)** and center-threaded pins **(B)**.

The connector bar should be placed close to the skin to shorten the working distance of the pins (close placement of the bar will not be a problem because there is little swelling of avian skin wounds post-operatively). If using acrylic materials for the connector, biomechanical testing has shown that a bar of roughly the same diameter as the bone under repair is sufficiently strong **(Figure 4-10)**.

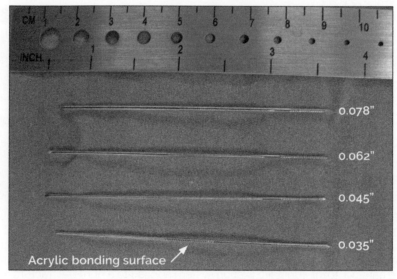

Figure 4-10. Roughened surface on acrylic interface pins. Refer to Table 1 for metric measurements of these pins.

A sufficient number of pins must be used when designing a robust construct. Generally, a minimum of two ESF pins must be placed in each fracture segment to assure fixator integrity. The strength of the construct increases exponentially with the addition of more pins and this should be given consideration, especially for Type II constructs applied to the tibiotarsus. Trans-articular configurations may be used to stabilize periarticular fractures and luxations of the elbow and stifle.

Other hardware possibilities include conventional Kirschner-Ehmer (KE) clamps and bars and the F.E.S.S.A. system (Jorgensen Labs) **Figure 4-11A & B**. In place of an acrylic bar, a stainless-steel tube drilled with holes for the ESF pins and orthogonally drilled holes that contain locking setscrews is provided. Its utility in repair of tibiotarsal fractures in falcons and many other avian species and cases has been demonstrated (Hatt J-M 2016, Mueller & Nafeez 2009). An advantage of this device is that it can be readily disassembled and reattached if problems develop in the post-operative period. On the other hand, it is less amenable to following the curvatures of bones such as the humerus or ulna, is limited in size availability, and is expensive.

External skeletal fixators are considered when IM pins cannot be used due to lack of an intramedullary cavity (e.g., tarsometatarsus), or where fractures are highly comminuted with significant soft tissue compromise. Type I fixators are suitable on the ulna where a hybrid fixator (below) is less suited and is the preferred method of fixation for metacarpal fractures. A Type II fixator can be used for tibiotarsal and metatarsal fractures in raptors and other large birds. (Note: A Type I fixator is not a sufficiently robust construct for either of these bones.) Application of a Type II fixator to the tibiotarsus requires placement of the most proximal ESF pin at a declining angle, lateral to medial, to avoid conflict with the body wall. Since the standard interface pins are only end threaded, in Type II applications, it is recommended that center-threaded pins be used to gain adequate purchase on the bone cortices.

Ring fixators may be used effectively to lengthen fractures where there has been significant bone loss and potential for foreshortening of the limb. The device allows periodic lengthening of the limb as new bone forms in a process referred to as bone transport osteogenesis. Transport osteogenesis has also been used to re-establish limb length in two raptor cases in the absence of bone graft options (Johnston et al, 2008; Ponder, Anderson, and Bueno-Padilla 2012).

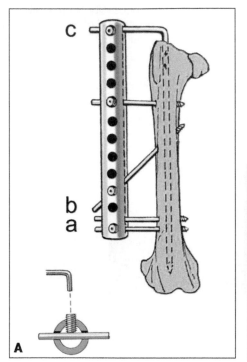

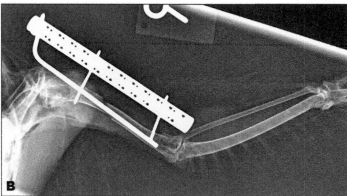

Figure 4-11A & B. A F.E.S.S.A. Tubular system 6/8-mm starter kit **(A)** (Jorgensen Labs). The 6-mm tube accepts pins of varying diameter 0.9 mm (0.035 in) to 1.8 mm (0.071 in) and the 8-mm tube accepts pins of 1.6 mm (0.063 in) to 3.2 mm (0.126 in). Design allows a placement of multiple pins close together in small fragments. Pins can be placed at an angle to the tube or straight through adjacent holes. Pins are locked into position by simple hex-head locking screws tightened by an Allen wrench (from Jorgensen Labs online catalog 2019). Tubulaire fixation system applied to a humeral fracture in a falcon **(B)** (from *Avian Medicine,* 3rd edition [Samour J, ed. Elsevier, 2016]

Tie-in Fixators

Tie-in fixators, presented in detail below, have proven to be an effective means of stabilizing long bone fractures in a variety of avian species (Bueno-Padilla et al 2015). As the name suggests they combine external skeletal fixator elements with an intramedullary pin. They are tied together with the external bar. As with Type II fixators, the bars may consist of conventional K-E bars and clamps, molded acrylic materials, or the F.E.S.S.A. (Jorgensen Labs) system.

Plates and Nails

Fixation modalities beyond those detailed above have been applied with varying degrees of success in a small number of cases; available information derives from individual case reports. Such cases include the use of an externally applied locking compression plate as an ESF connector bar on a tarsometatarsal fracture in an eagle (Montgomery et al 2011), an interlocking nail on a tibiotarsal fracture in a bald eagle (Hollamby et al 2004) and controlled studies to evaluate the utility of various miniplate systems for fracture management in pigeons (*Columba livia*) (Christen et al 2005; Gull et al 2012). Most of these approaches must be regarded as works in progress limited by a small range of suitably sized plates and nails, insufficient strength of plates, additional morbidity inherent in their placement, and expense (J. Ponder, P. Redig 2016).

Experience has shown that use of full-circumference cerclage to align and stabilize fragments in oblique fractures is contraindicated in avian orthopedics. Cerclage wire is inherently incapable of contributing to the robustness of fixation and the morbidity associated with wrapping it around the bone fragments leads to separation of the bone from its vital soft tissue attachment. This in turn results in loss of bone viability and formation of sequestra.

Coaptation methods tailored for use in birds can be used for temporary stabilization, as an adjunct to fixation, or as a sole means of stabilization in limited circumstances. Available coaptation methods for wings include body wraps, figure-of-8 bandages and curved edge splints. Coaptation for management of legs is rarely a suitable option for definitive stabilization; however, methods used include tape splints, modified Robert Jones type bandages and modified Schroeder-Thomas splints. Readers are referred to more comprehensive coverage of these topics (J Ponder, P Redig 2016) or Avian Medicine, 3rd edition (Samour J, ed. Elsevier, 2016).

Management Decisions: Summary

The decision whether to use surgical or nonsurgical fracture management techniques in any given case is based on the ability to meet orthopedic objectives, as well as on the resources and expertise available. In wild birds, restoration of full function to a point indistinguishable from a bird with no history of injury is the goal and overall management decisions are driven not only by an understanding of the orthopedic considerations outlined above but also comorbidities (especially eye and other injuries that affect release potential for wild species), age of the bird (e.g., pre-fledging age birds are likely to imprint while in captivity and cannot be released), and ability to re-assimilate when released. In companion birds, less than full function may be acceptable so long as the patient can be expected to have a pain-free life. Regardless, not all stabilization methods are created equal and there is not an equivalency between implantation of fixators and coaptive bandaging for many fractures, especially those of the pelvic limb. A poorly chosen or inadequately applied stabilization device, lacking adequate robustness, has a high likelihood of failing. Compromising orthopedic principals due to lack of experience or resources should not be a driver in choosing the mode of fixation. Approaching decision making in a fracture case with an understanding of orthopedic principles and how they apply to specific situations is paramount in producing satisfactory clinical outcomes, reducing patient stress, and avoiding costly and often less satisfactory "do-overs".

Surgical Fracture Management: The Tie-in Fixator

A most versatile and effective system for long-bone fixation in birds is the external skeletal fixator-intramedullary (ESF-IM) pin tie-in or hybrid fixator. This system is inexpensive, adaptable, easily learned, and effective. This fixator construct consists of an intramedullary pin, two or more ESF pins, and an external connecting bar that joins these components in a so-called tie-in configuration. This fixator completely stabilizes a fracture against all applied forces, firmly anchors the intramedullary pin, allows near complete freedom of movement of the limb (i.e., no coaptation is required for additional support), and permits easy access to any wounds for post-operative management. It has been the ideal management choice for most fractures of the humerus, ulna, femur, and tibiotarsus in birds. In its application it resembles an I beam with two parallel members (the IM pin and the fixator bar) linked via a shear web (the ESF pins and the bent-up end of the IM pin so as to be in the same plane as the ESF pins), which results in a very strong structural entity **(Figure 4-12)**. It also has other advantages. While conventionally, only two ESF pins are used, placement of additional pins on either side of the fracture significantly increases its robustness, a consideration in the management of fractures in long bones (Van Wettere 2009). Further, it can be sequentially dismantled during bone healing, a process referred to as dynamization, which transfers load to the bone as it starts to heal, a process that speeds the rate of healing and contributes to the strength of the callus (Egger 1993). Lastly, when fracture healing is complete, the fixator is removed in its entirety, leaving no hardware attached to the bird, an important consideration for birds that are released to the wild.

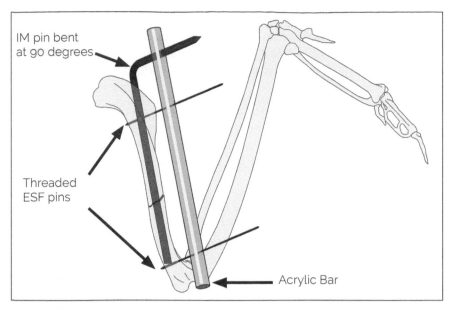

IM pin bent
at 90 degrees

Threaded
ESF pins

Acrylic Bar

Figure 4-12. This diagram illustrates the main elements of a hybrid fixator on an avian humerus. Note the exit of the IM pin, which was introduced at the fracture site and driven retrograde, exiting at the proximal end of the humerus. Note also that owing to curvatures in the proximal and distal ends of the humerus, the ESF pins do not share medullary cavity space with the IM pin. The combination of intramedullary pin tied to the acrylic bar by the ESF pins and the bent end of the IM pin effectively forms an I-beam. (Image by Frank Taylor)

The ESF-IM tie-in is effective for most diaphyseal long-bone fractures in birds where the medullary cavity is not large enough and the fracture location and character permit insertion of an IM pin. With modification, it can be adapted for more proximal or distal fractures in proximity to a joint using cross-pinning techniques.

There are two significant aspects of the application of the tie-in fixator at any location that are common to all placements: 1) bending the intramedullary pin and 2) application of the acrylic fixator bar. Both are described at this point and should be referred to in subsequent sections of the book where application of various fixators is presented.

It is essential that the intramedullary pin be stabilized with locking jaw pliers (e.g., Vice-Grip™, Irwin Tools, Huntersville, NC, USA) when it is bent in order to prevent transfer of bending forces to the bone leading to bone breakage. The IM pin is typically bent after the ESF pins have been inserted. Stabilization of the pin is accomplished by grasping the IM pin with the pliers at its exit point and locking it, then slip a Jacob's chuck over the pin to a point very near the pliers, leaving a little space for a bending radius **(Figure 4-13)**. With a firm grasp on the pliers, use the chuck to bend the pin into a 90-degree angle. Remove the pliers and chuck and rotate the pin as necessary to align it with the other pins in the fixator.

The installment of the acrylic connector bar and method of applying an acrylic fixator bar to a tie-in fixator using a latex rubber mold (Penrose drain) **(Figures 4-14A-I)**.

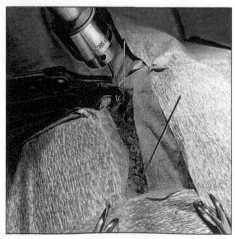

Figure 4-13. Clamping the IM pin with a locking jaw pliers to absorb the bending forces and preventing fracture of the bone. The pin should be bent at a right angle to the long axis of the pin in order to avoid torqueing forces in the fixator.

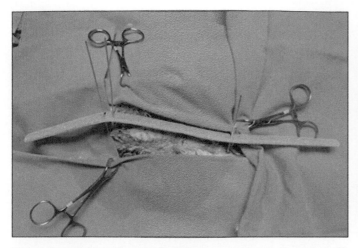

Figure 4-14A. Placement of a Penrose drain as a mold for the fixator bar. The tubing is first slightly stretched and placed alongside the pins; the sites for the pins are marked with an ink pen. The tubing is then forced onto the pins beginning with the longest pin – usually the bent IM pin – at each of the marked locations. Lubrication of the pins with saline will lessen the formation of ragged holes that would otherwise leak acrylic during its cure process.

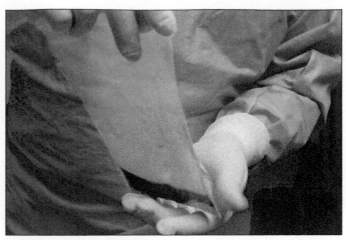

Figure 4-14B. Mixing of hoof acrylic reagents in zip lock bag: Mix Technovit® (Jorgensen Laboratories, Loveland, CO, USA) in a plastic sandwich bag. Estimate the amount of material needed and decant two parts of dry powder to one part of liquid monomer into the sandwich bag. For a starting point, place about 20 ml of powder and 10 ml of monomer into the bag – this is enough to fill a ½" x 7" latex tube. Seal the bag and knead the material to mix it. The mixture starts to thicken after 2-3 minutes. Have two 12-ml irrigation syringes immediately available to decant this mixture into. Technovit® is a hoof repair acrylic material. Alternatively, pre-packaged tubes of methacrylate resin in a mixing applicator gun (Acrylx™ IMEX Veterinary Inc., Longview, TX, USA) can be used.

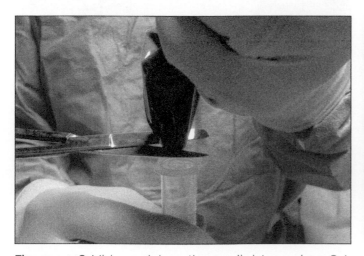

Figure 4-14C. Mixing and decanting acrylic into a syringe. Cut the corner from the baggie and express the acrylic material into a 12-ml irrigation syringe.

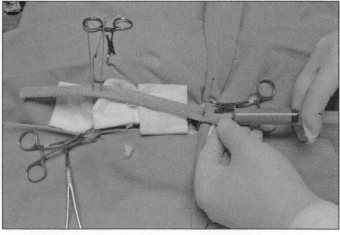

Figure 4-14D. Filling Penrose drain: Cut the small tip of the irrigation syringe back so a large bore is available. Insert it into the open end of the latex tubing and eject with moderate force. There may be some leakage around the pin holes, but if the latex is not stretched excessively, it should be minimal. Squeeze the tubing around the hub of the syringe so that as the tubing fills, it can be slightly expanded with excess acrylic. Leave syringe tip in the latex tube and continue to apply slight pressure on the plunger to keep the tube full until the material becomes viscous enough to not leak around any of the pins. It will take about 5-8 minutes for the acrylic to cure. An exothermic reaction occurs in the final stages of cure; however, the ESF pins radiate heat sufficiently to the exterior so that tissues are not affected. If desired, sterile cool fluids can be flowed onto the curing acrylic and pins to absorb heat. Alternatively, soaking the 2-in x 2-in (5-cm x 5-cm) gauze sponges placed around the construct with saline will control heat.

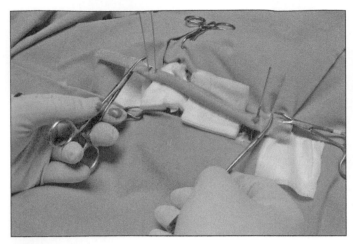

Figure 4-14E. Holding the latex mold with clamps while acrylic cures. It is important to keep the mold straight (i.e., avoid sagging in the unsupported mid-section). This can be done by inserting 2-in x 2-in (5-cm x 5-cm) gauze sponges to support that section as shown.

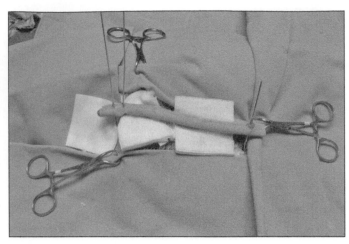

Figure 4-14F. Connector bar after the acrylic has cured and the excess Penrose drain has been trimmed.

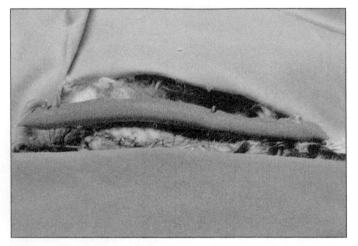

Figure 4-14G. Photo and illustration of the completed tie-in fixator. After the acrylic has cured, excess materials are trimmed. At this point, the area is dried by dabbing with sponges. After the drapes are removed, further drying of skin and feathers should be done with a warm-air dryer (e.g., hair dryer) before further bandaging. Triple antibiotic ointment can be placed over any suture lines and around pin tracts.

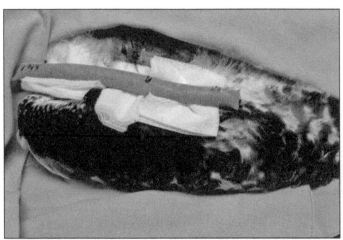

Figure 4-14H. Fluffing" - sterile 2-in x 2-in (5-cm x 5-cm) gauze pads - was placed between the fixator and the skin to absorb exuded fluids and provide mild compression of soft tissues. This material is replaced 18–24 hours post-operatively.

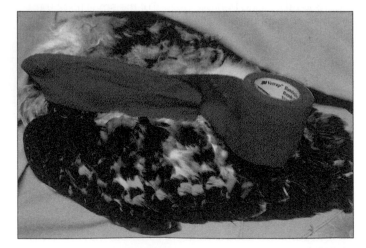

Figure 4-14I. Completed fixator with elastic bandage applied to cover fixator and fluffing. (Red-tailed hawk [Buteo jamaicensis])

Recommended Reading

1. Bueno-Padilla I, Arent LR, Ponder JB. Tips for raptor bandaging. *Exotic DVM.* 2011;12(3):29–47.

2. Bueno I, Redig PT, Rendahl AK. External skeletal fixator intramedullary pin tie-in for the repair of tibiotarsal fractures in raptors: 37 cases (1995-2011). *J Am Vet Med Assoc.* 2015;247(10):1154-60.

3. Christen C, Fischer I, von Rechenberg B, et al. Evaluation of a maxillofacial miniplate 1.0 for stabilization of the ulna in experimentally induced ulnar and radial fractures in pigeons *(Columba livia). J Avian Med Surg.* 2005;19(3):185–190.

4. Egger EL, Gottsauner-Wolf F, Palmer J et al. Effects of axial dynamization on bone healing. *J Trauma.* 1993 Feb,34(2):185-192.

5. Gull JM, Saveraid TC, Szabo D, et al. Evaluation of three miniplate systems for fracture stabilization in pigeons *(Columba livia). J Avian Med Surg.* 2012;26(4):203–212.

6. Hatt J-M. In Samour J, ed. *Avian Medicine.* 3rd ed. Philadelphia: Elsevier; 2016;354. Fig. 12-36.

7. Hatt JM, Christen C, Sandmeier P. Clinical application of an external fixator in the repair of bone fractures in 28 birds. *Vet Rec.* 2007; 160:188–194.

8. Hollamby S, Dejardin LM, Sikarskie JG, et al. Tibiotarsal fracture repair in a bald eagle *(Haliaeetus leucocephalus)* using an interlocking nail. *J Zoo Wildl Med.* 2004;35(1):77–81.

9. Johnston MS, Thode HO, Ehrhart NP. Bone transport osteogenesis for reconstruction of a bone defect in the tibiotarsus of a yellow-naped Amazon parrot *(Amazona ochrocephala auropalliata). J Avian Med Surg.* 2008;22(1):47–56.

10. Montgomery RD, Crandall E, Bellah JR. Use of a locking compression plate as an external fixator for repair of a tarsometatarsal fracture in a bald eagle *(Haliaeetus leucocephalus). J Avian Med Surg.* 2011; 25:119–125.

11. Muller M, Nafeez JM. Use of the FixEx Tubulaire Type F.E.S.S.A System for tibiotarsal fractures in falcons. *Falco.* 2007; 29:25–29.

12. Murray M. Management of metacarpal fractures in free-living raptors. *Proc Annu Conf Assoc Avian Vet.* 2012;283–284.

13. Piermattei DL, Flo GL, DeCamp CE. *Brinker, Piermattei, and Flo's Handbook of Small Animal Orthopedics and Fracture Repair.* 4th ed. St. Louis: Elsevier; 2006.

14. Ponder JB, Anderson GM, Bueno-Padilla IB. Distraction osteogenesis in two wild raptor species. *Proc Annu Conf Assoc Avian Vet.* 2012;43–44.

15. Ponder JB, Redig P. Orthopaedics. In: Speer B, ed. *Current Therapy in Avian Medicine and Surgery.* St Louis: Elsevier; 2016:657–667.

16. Redig PT, Cruz L. The avian skeleton and fracture management, a sub-section in trauma-related medical conditions. In: Samour J, ed. *Avian Medicine.* 2nd ed. London: Elsevier; 2008:215–248.

17. Redig PT. Evaluation and non-surgical management of avian fractures. In: Harrison JG, Harrison LR, eds. *Clinical Avian Medicine and Surgery.* Philadelphia: Saunders; 1986:380–394.

18. Redig PT. The use of an external skeletal fixator-intramedullary pin tie-in fixator for treatment of long bone fractures in raptors. In: Lumeij JT, Poffers J, eds. *Raptor Biomedicine III.* Lake Worth, Fl: Zoological Education Network; 2000:239–254.

19. Tully TN. Basic avian bone growth and healing. *Vet Clin North Am Exot Anim Pract.* 2002; 5:23–30.

20. Van Wettere AJ, Redig PT, Wallace LJ, et al. Mechanical evaluation of external skeletal fixator-intramedullary pin tie-in configurations applied to cadaveral humeri from red-tailed hawks *(Buteo jamaicensis). J Avian Med Surg.* 2009;23(4):277–285.

Anatomy of the Shoulder Girdle and Wing

Shoulder Girdle and Skeleton

Shoulder Girdle

The shoulder girdle is composed of the coracoid and the scapular bones with the fused clavicles. The two clavicles, or furcula, are fused medially at the hypocleidium. This is often given the term "wishbone" in the vernacular. This bony plate where the clavicles fuse is connected to the sternum by the hypocleidial ligament. The coracoid bones act as supporting struts for the pectoral limbs by connecting them to the sternum. The clavicles along with the coracoid bones act in concert to counteract the forces produced by the contraction of the pectoral muscles during the downstroke of the wing.

Each scapula lies against the ribs and articulates with the coracoid and clavicle cranially. The length of each scapula varies by species with increased length associated with birds that spend more time gliding. The triosseal canal [canal triosseus], or foramen triosseum, is formed by the articulation of the coracoid, scapula, and clavicle. In some species, the canal is bounded by only two bones, the coracoid and scapula (Getty 1975). The triosseal canal is an important structure for flight as the tendon of the supracoracoideus muscle passes through it. This allows the change of direction for elevation of the wing. The bones that comprise the shoulder girdle may be pneumatized by the clavicular air sac. Pneumaticity of the bones of the shoulder varies among species.

Sternum

The breastbone or sternum of birds covers a large surface of the ventral thorax. In most birds, there is a central keel or carina that projects from the sternum for attachment of the powerful pectoral and supracoracoideus muscles. Some of the flightless birds le.g. ratites L. rati - raft) do not have this ventral projection or keel. These include ostriches, cassowaries, emus, rheas, and kiwis (Baumel 1983). The ventral segment of each of the sternal ribs articulates with the sternocostal processes of the sternum. The sternum may also have extensions of the clavicular air sac.

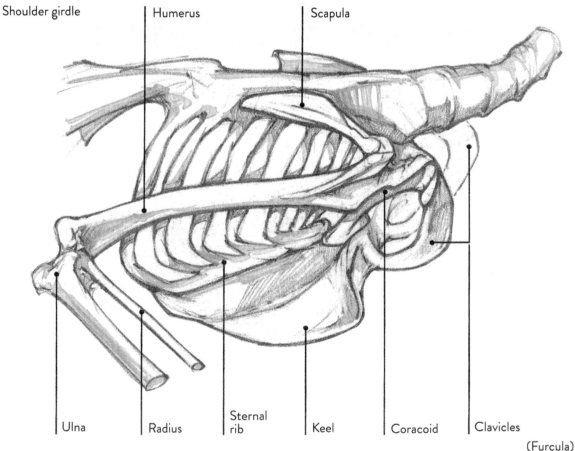

Shoulder girdle   Humerus   Scapula

Ulna   Radius   Sternal rib   Keel   Coracoid   Clavicles (Furcula)

Shoulder Girdle: CT Images

As described in Chapter 1, familiar anatomic drawings from the original book have been used to document basic anatomy of the wings and legs. In this Chapter, we provide computed tomography images of the shoulder girdle and other anatomical features for the readers to develop their three-dimensional understanding.

In this section, CT scans are provided that first image the standard anatomic positions of the shoulder girdle, followed by oblique views. Ready visualization of these features is especially important when quickly assessing traumatic injuries.

Computed tomography images of the shoulder girdle are presented for the orange-winged Amazon (*Amazona amazonica*), umbrella cockatoo (*Cacatua alba*), military macaw (*Ara militaris*), budgerigar (*Melopsittacus undulatus*), pigeon (*Columba livia*), domestic chicken (*Gallus gallus domesticus*), red-tailed hawk (*Buteo jamaicensis*), and great horned owl (*Bubo virginianus*). Structures are color-coded, allowing easy recognition and ready comparison across species. The shoulder girdle of the golden eagle was not imaged because it was too large for the scanner to capture the image in its entirety.

Orange-winged Amazon (*Amazona amazonica*)
Dorsal and Dorsal Oblique Shoulder Girdle

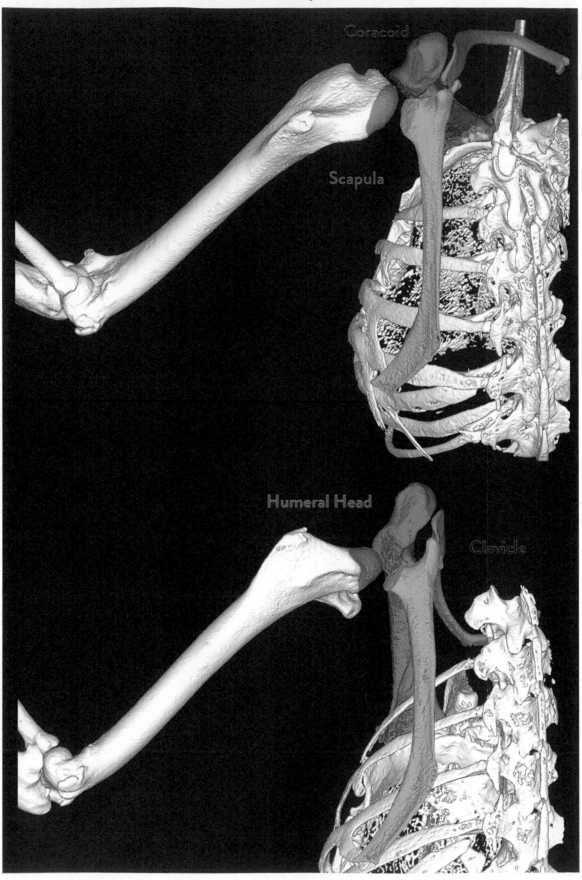

Orange-winged Amazon (*Amazona amazonica*)
Ventral and Cranial Shoulder Girdle

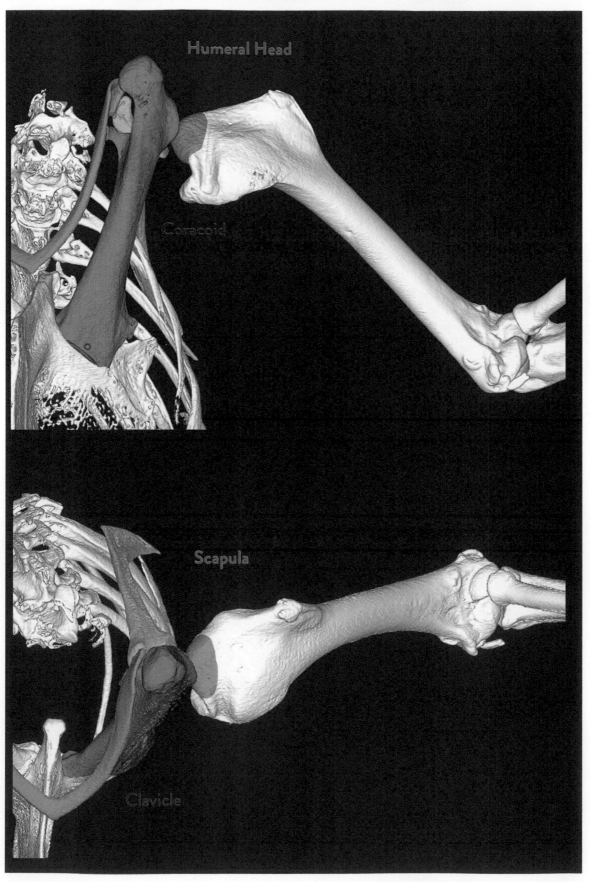

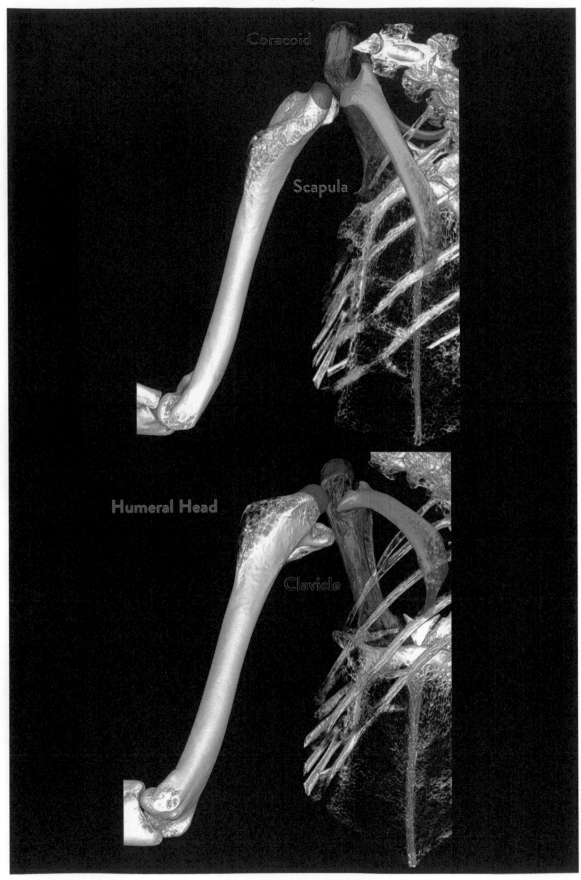

Ventral and Cranial Shoulder Girdle

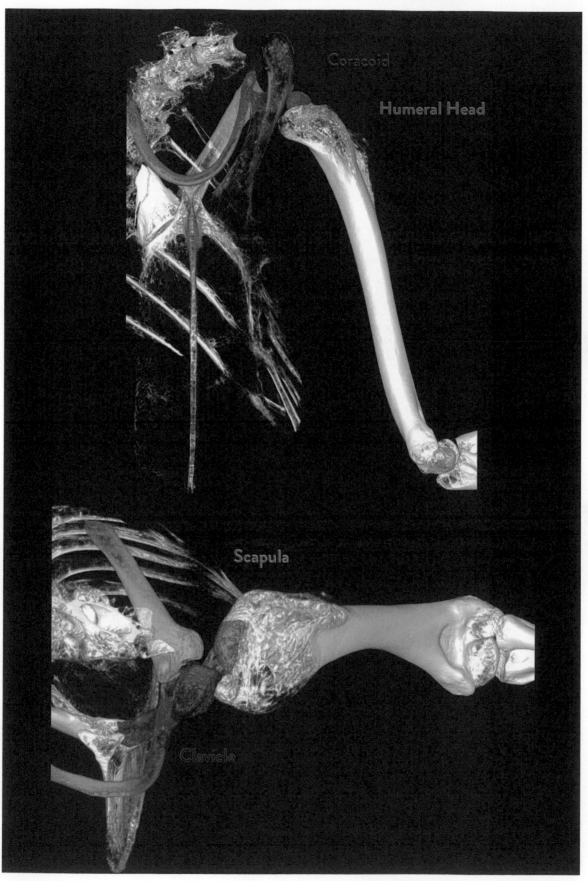

Military Macaw (*Ara militaris*)
Dorsal, Dorsal Cranial Oblique and
Dorsal Caudal Oblique Shoulder Girdle

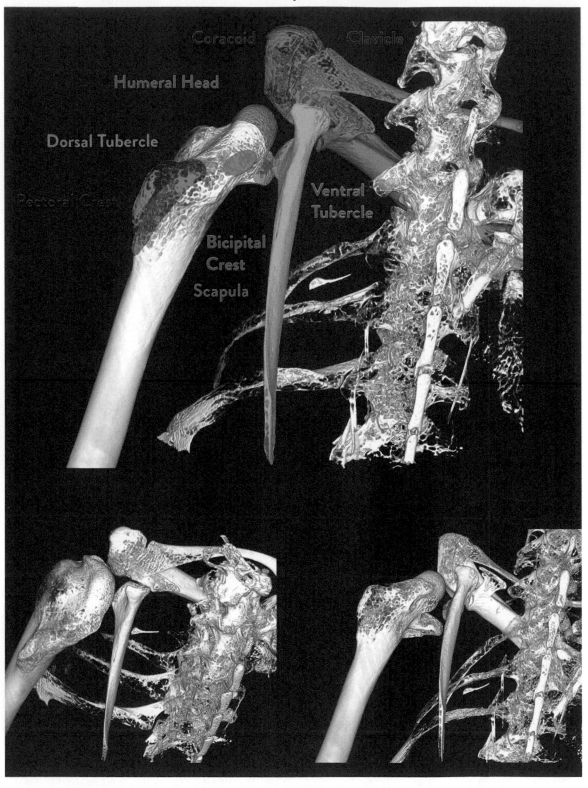

Military Macaw (*Ara militaris*)
Ventral, Ventral Cranial Oblique and Ventral Caudal Oblique Shoulder Girdle

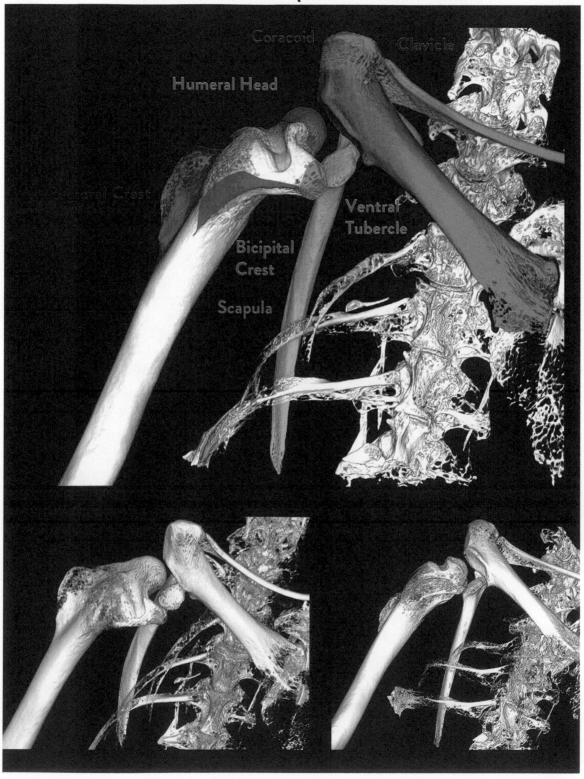

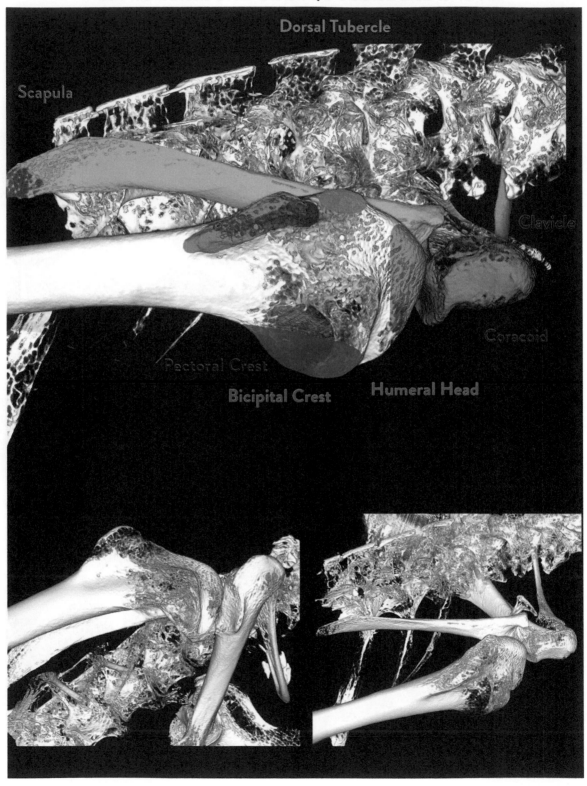

Military Macaw (*Ara militaris*)
Cranial, Cranial Dorsal Oblique and Cranial Ventral Oblique Shoulder Girdle

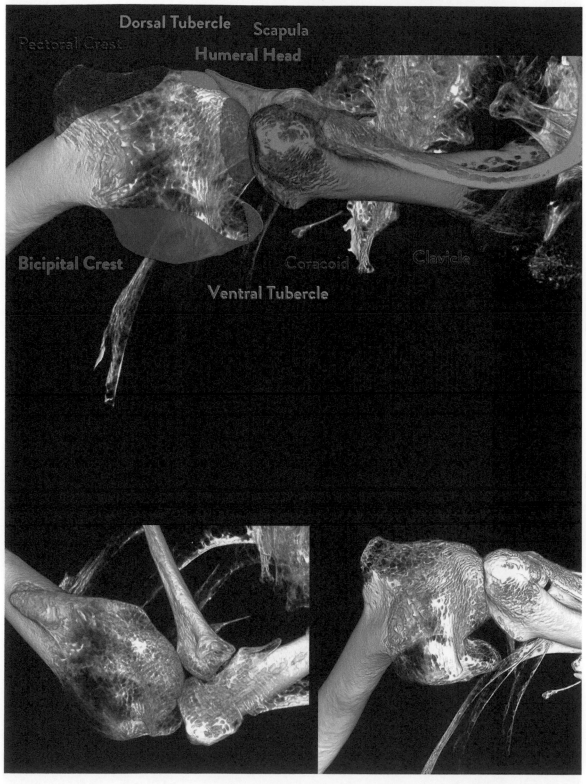

Budgerigar (*Melopsittacus undulatas*)
Dorsal and Dorsal Oblique Shoulder Girdle

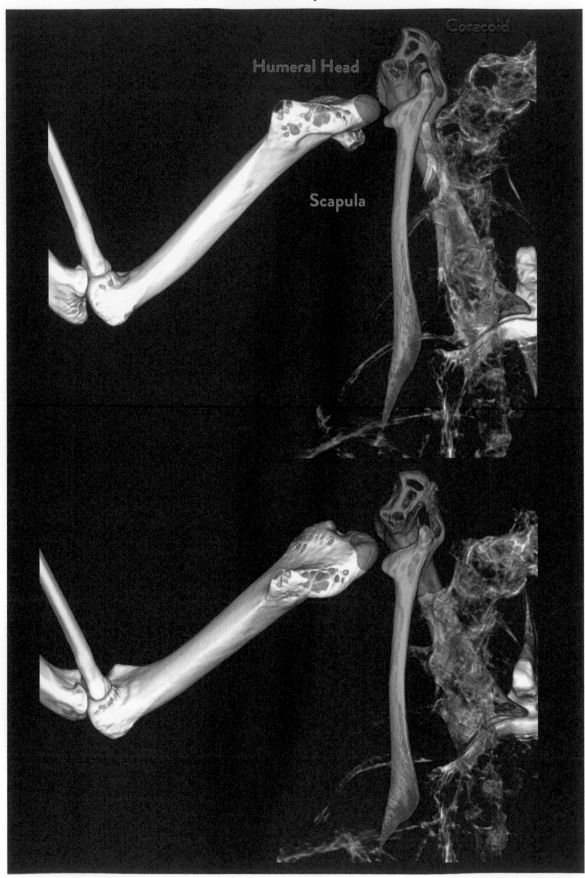

Budgerigar (*Melopsittacus undulatas*)
Ventral and Cranial Shoulder Girdle

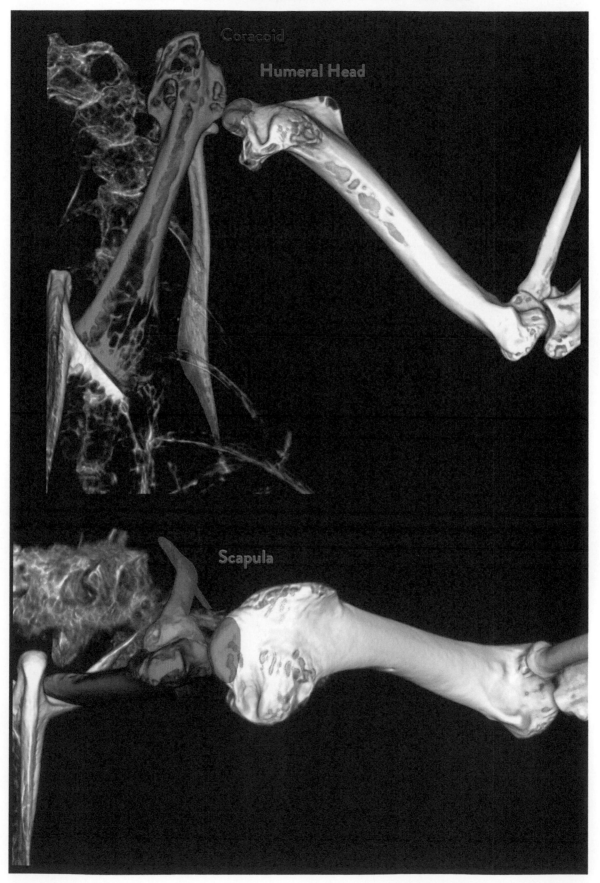

Pigeon (*Columba livia*)
Dorsal and Dorsal Oblique Shoulder Girdle

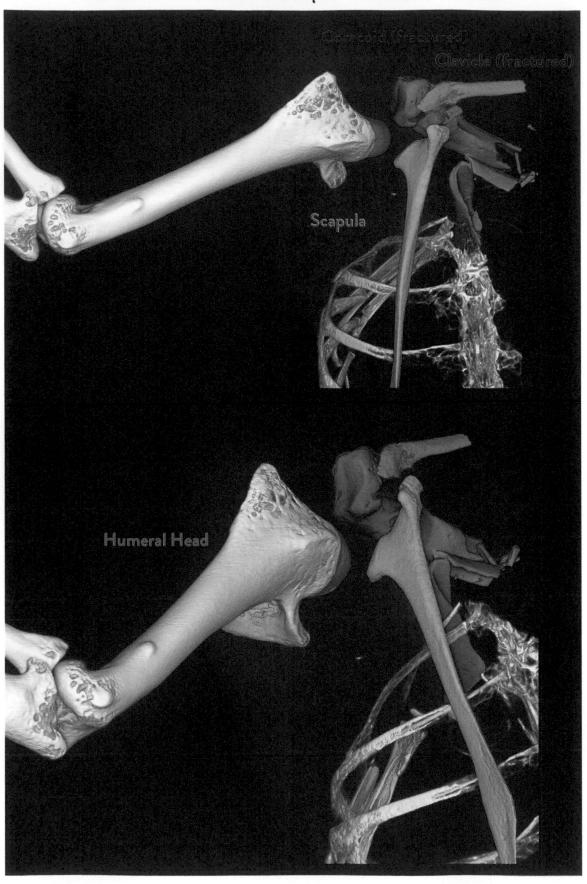

Pigeon (*Columba livia*)
Ventral and Cranial Shoulder Girdle

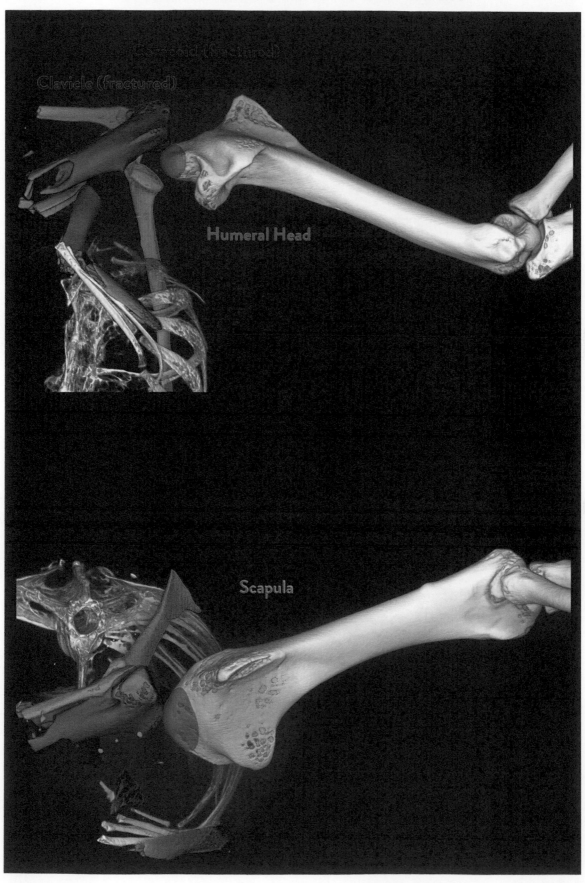

Domestic Chicken (*Gallus gallus domesticus*)
Dorsal and Dorsal Oblique Shoulder Girdle

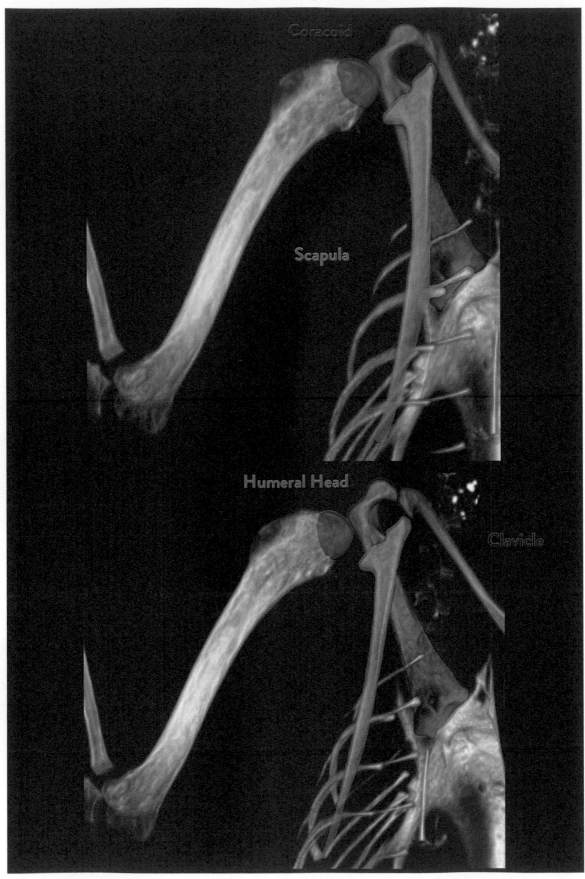

Domestic Chicken (*Gallus gallus domesticus*)
Ventral and Cranial Shoulder Girdle

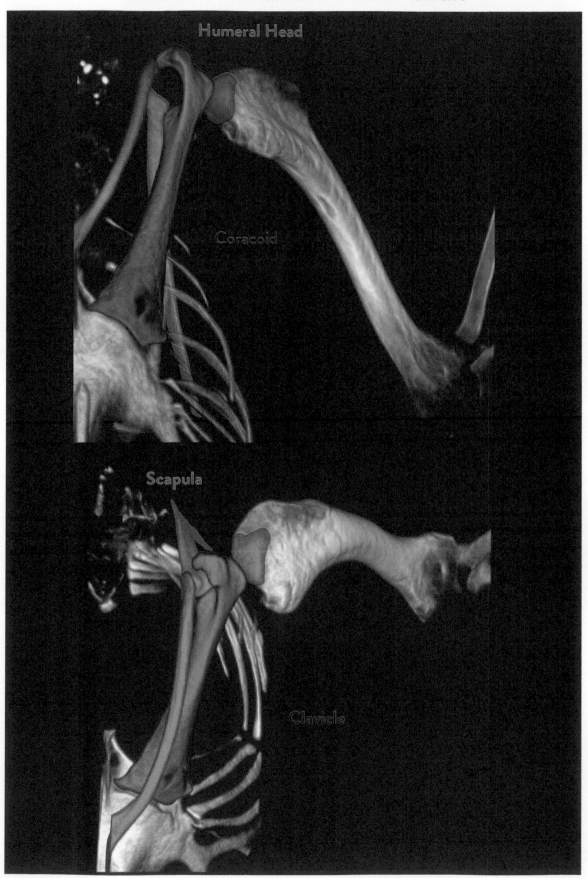

Red-tailed Hawk (*Buteo jamaicensis*)
Dorsal and Dorsal Oblique Shoulder Girdle

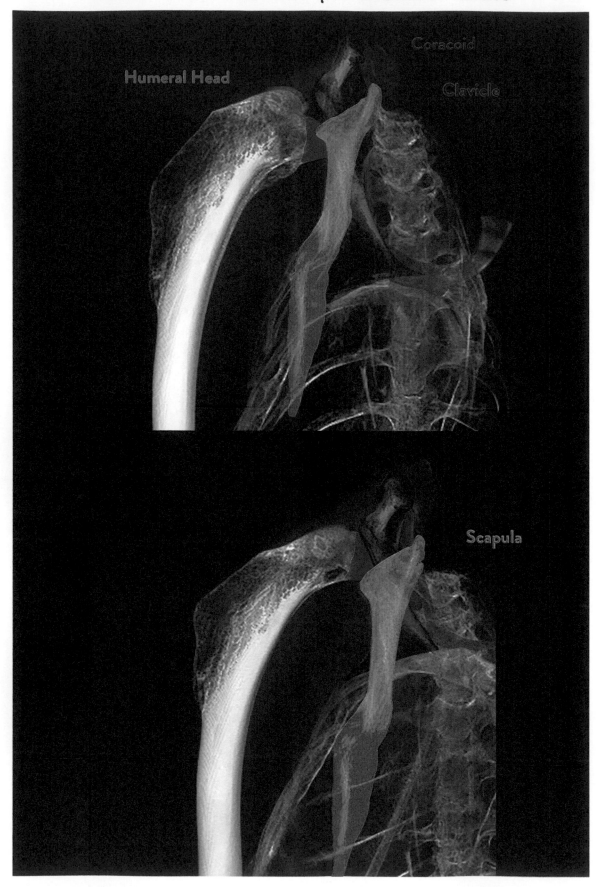

Red-tailed Hawk *(Buteo jamaicensis)*
Ventral and Cranial Shoulder Girdle

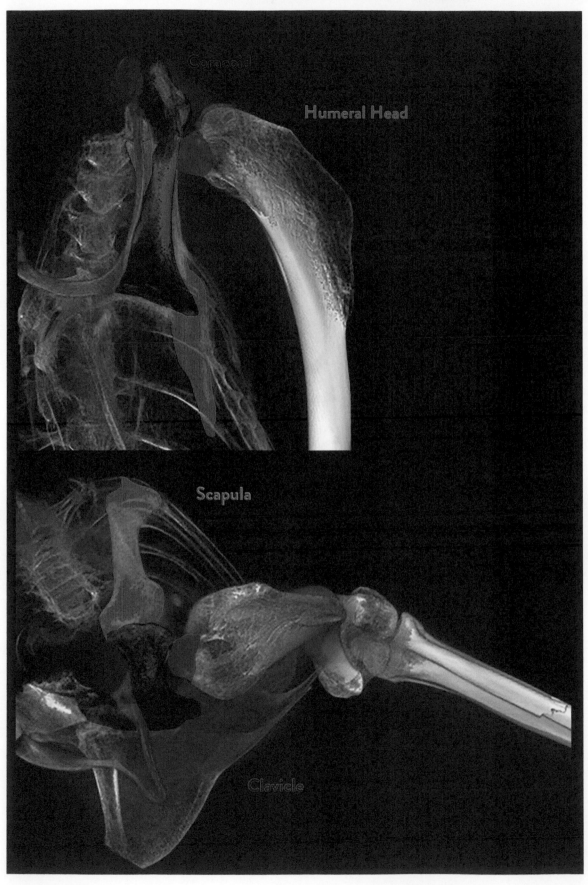

Great Horned Owl (*Bubo virginianus*)
Dorsal and Dorsal Oblique Shoulder Girdle

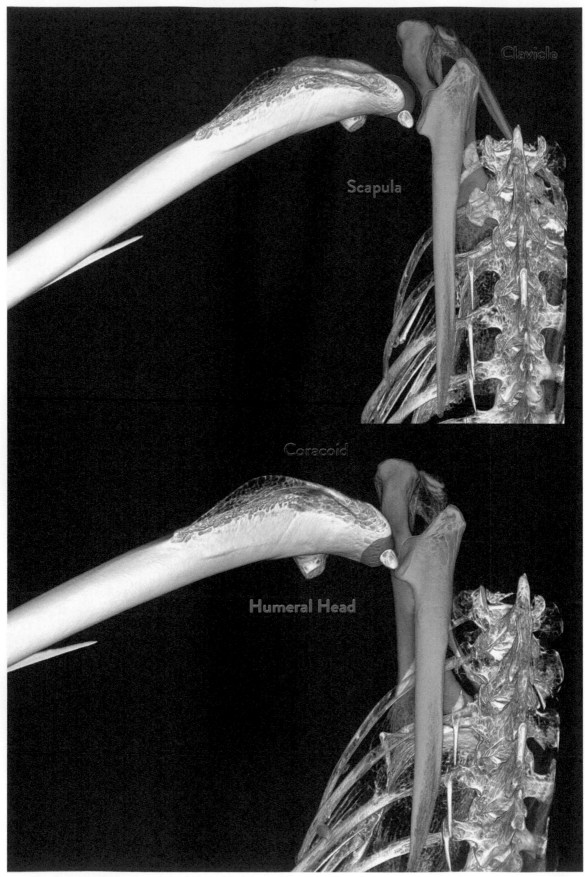

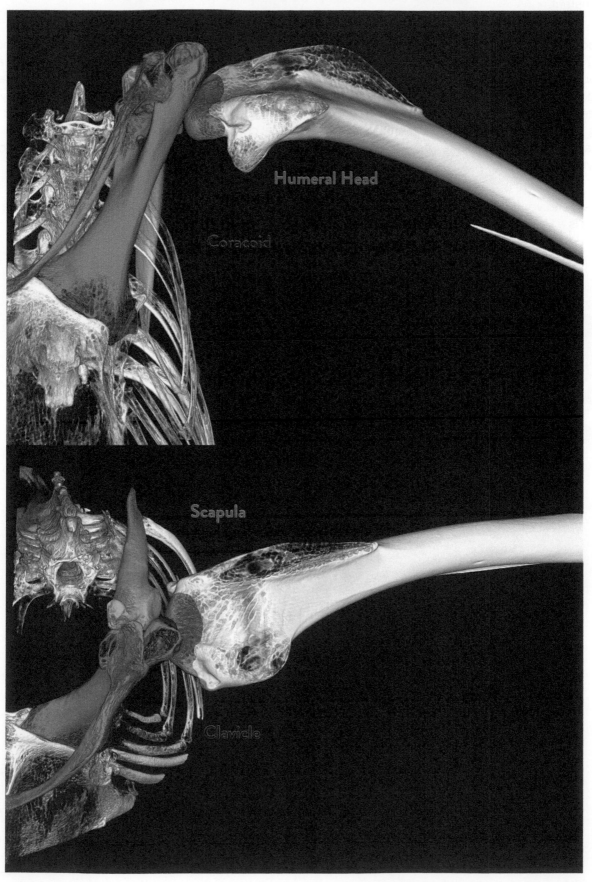

Humerus

The humerus is the bone of the pectoral limb with the largest mass. Its length, in relation to wing length, is fairly constant.

The head of the humerus articulates with the glenoid cavity of the scapula. There is a long, cranially directed pectoral crest [crista pectoralis] or deltoid crest. Between the crest and the head of the humerus is a small protuberance, the dorsal tubercle (major tubercle in dogs). The ventral or minor tubercle is bounded by a fossa on the dorsal caudal surface of the humerus and the bicipital crest. Distally, the dorsal and ventral condyles articulate with the radius and ulna. The dorsal condyle is homologous to the lateral condyle in domestic animals, and the ventral condyle is homologous to the medial condyle. The extrathoracic portion of the clavicular air sac has extensions into the medullary cavity of the humerus, as well as into the coracoid, scapula, and clavicle. Pneumaticity with the clavicular air sac varies among species.

The dorsal and ventral condyles are more evident on the ventral surface of the humerus. Proximal to the condyles is a triangular depression, the brachial fossa.

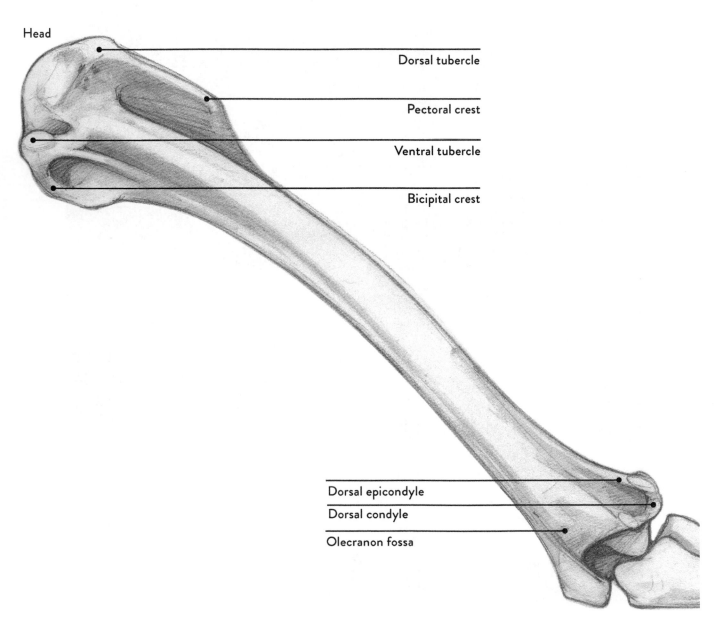

Head

Dorsal tubercle

Pectoral crest

Ventral tubercle

Bicipital crest

Dorsal epicondyle

Dorsal condyle

Olecranon fossa

Dorsal view of the humerus

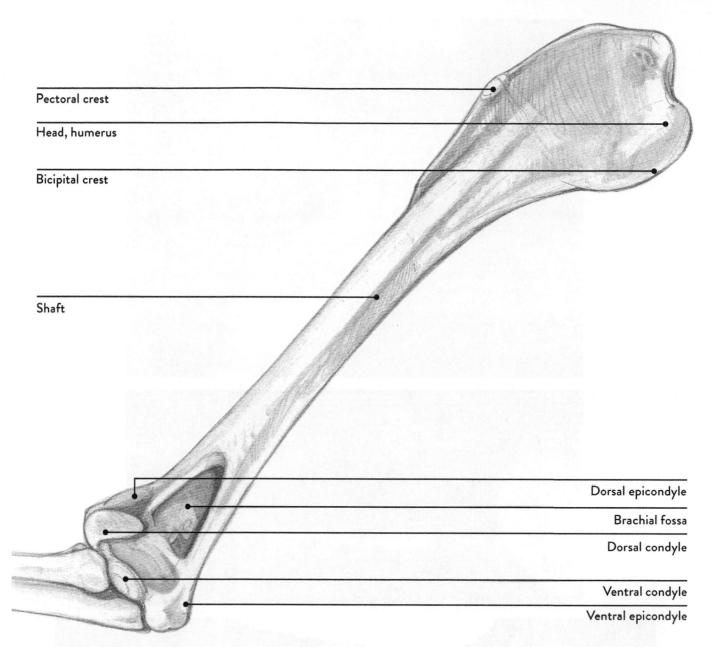

Pectoral crest

Head, humerus

Bicipital crest

Shaft

Dorsal epicondyle

Brachial fossa

Dorsal condyle

Ventral condyle

Ventral epicondyle

Ventral view of the humerus

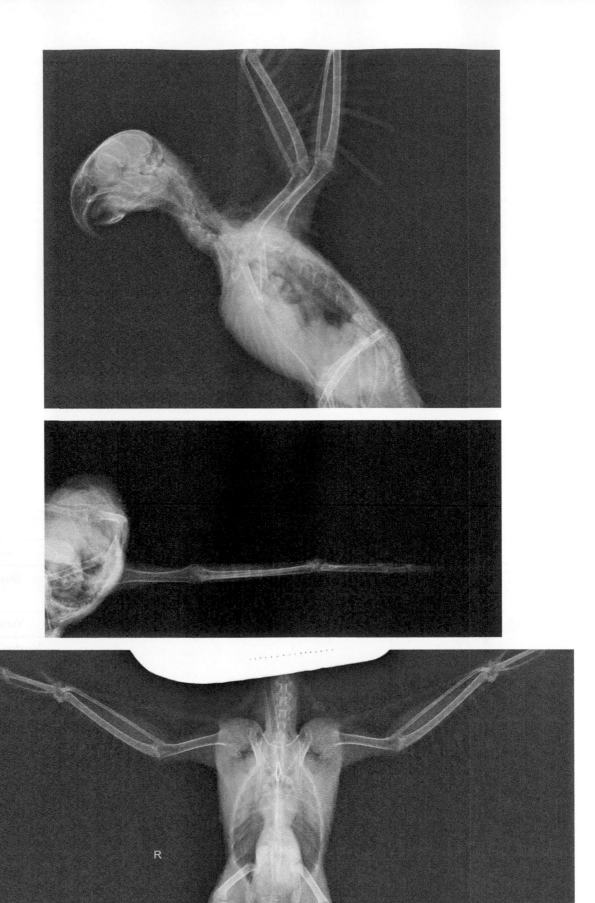

Radiographs of a 23-year old male orange-winged Amazon (*Amazona amazonica*). Lateral whole body, anterior-posterior of the wing and ventral-dorsal whole body.

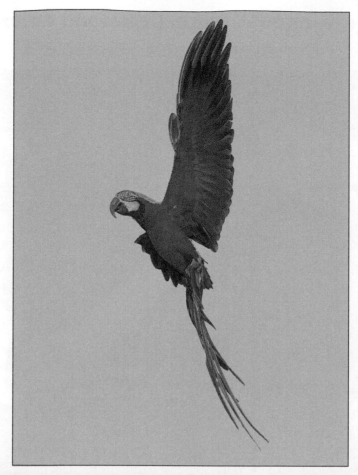

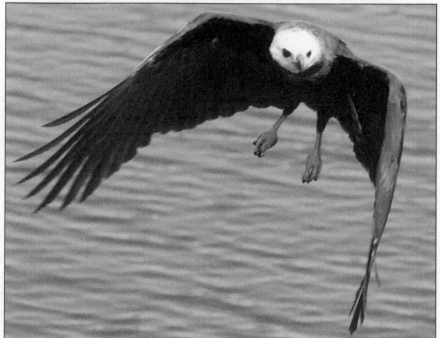

Humerus: CT Images

Computed tomography images of the humerus are presented for the orange-winged Amazon (*Amazona amazonica*), umbrella cockatoo (*Cacatua alba*), budgerigar (*Melopsittacus undulatus*), pigeon (*Columba livia*), domestic chicken (*Gallus gallus domesticus*), red-tailed hawk (*Buteo jamaicensis*), and great horned owl (*Bubo virginianus*). The military macaw and golden eagle were not imaged because they were too large for the scanner to capture in their entirety. Structures are color-coded, allowing easy recognition and ready comparison across species.

Orange-winged Amazon (*Amazona amazonica*)
Dorsal and Cranial Humerus

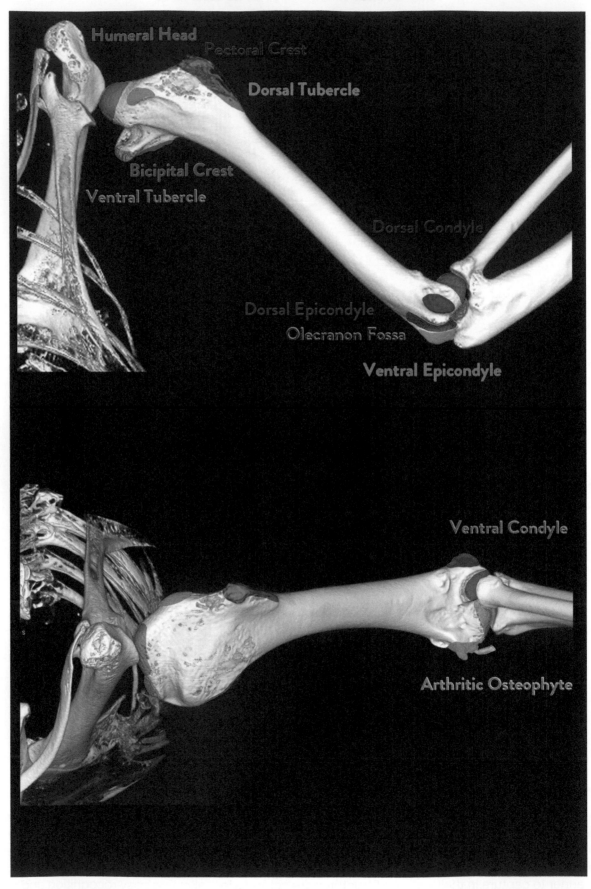

Orange-winged Amazon (*Amazona amazonica*)
Ventral and Caudal Humerus

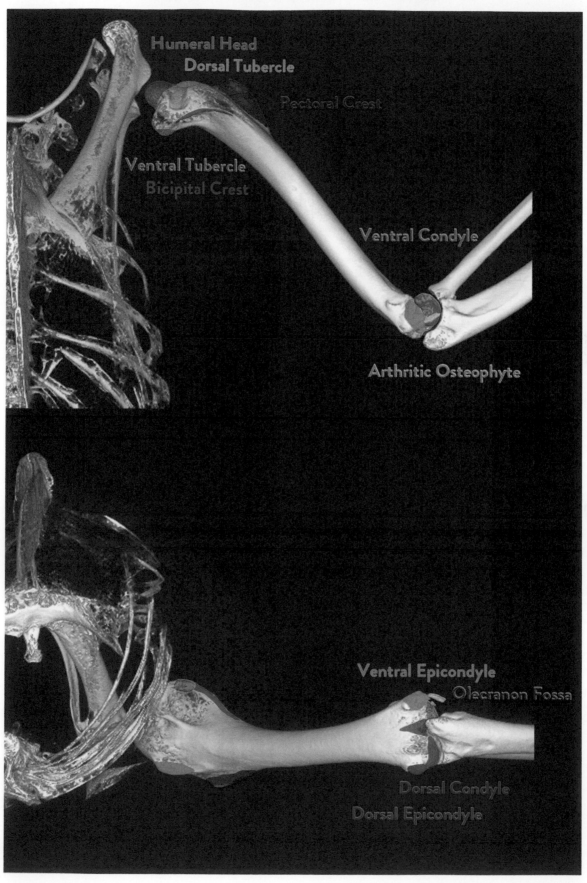

Umbrella Cockatoo (*Cacatua alba*)
Dorsal and Cranial Humerus

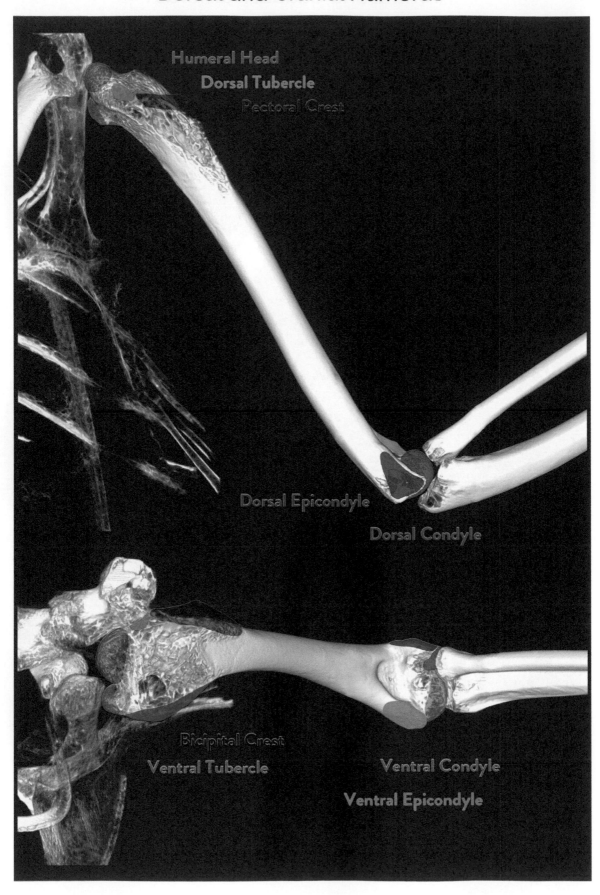

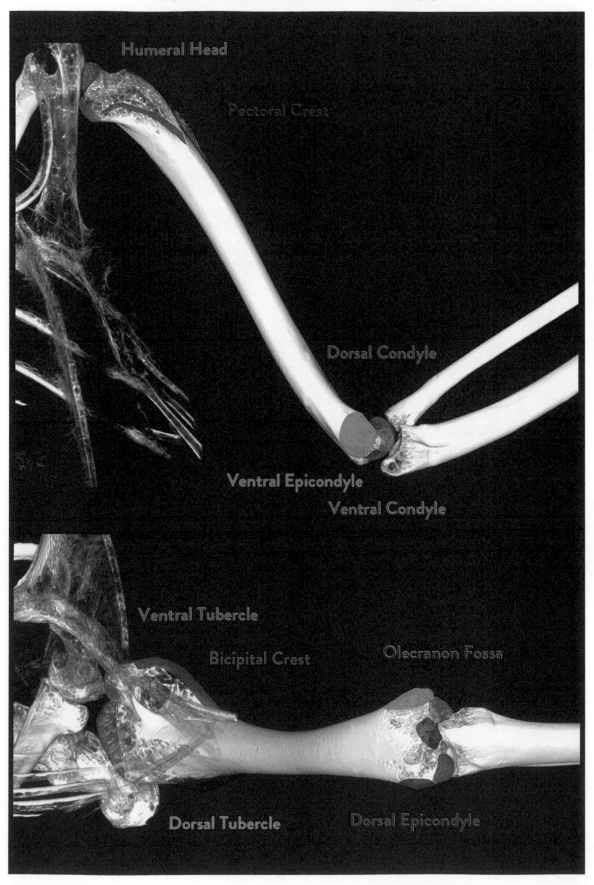

Budgerigar (*Melopsittacus undulatus*)
Dorsal and Cranial Humerus

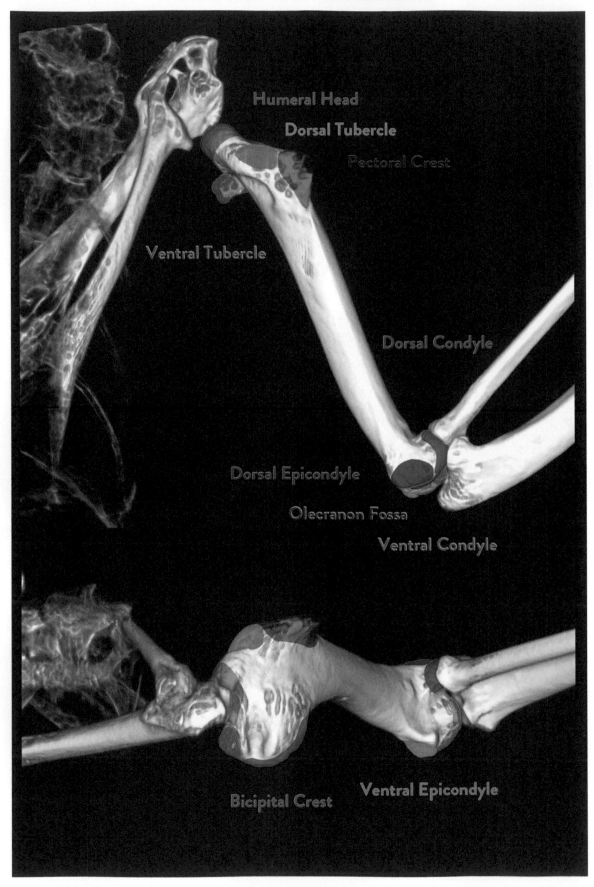

Humeral Head

Dorsal Tubercle

Pectoral Crest

Ventral Tubercle

Dorsal Condyle

Dorsal Epicondyle

Olecranon Fossa

Ventral Condyle

Bicipital Crest

Ventral Epicondyle

Budgerigar (*Melopsittacus undulatus*)
Ventral and Caudal Humerus

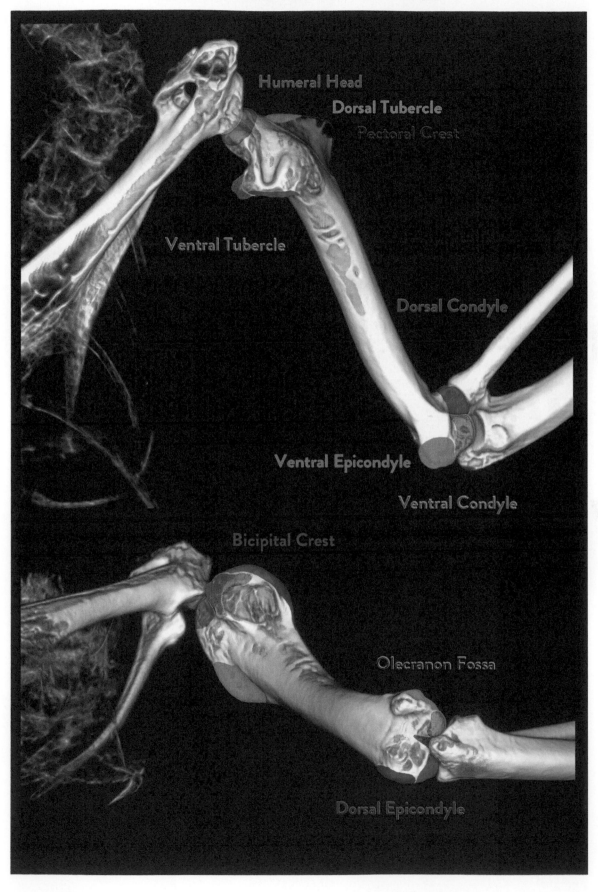

Pigeon (*Columba livia*)
Dorsal and Cranial Humerus

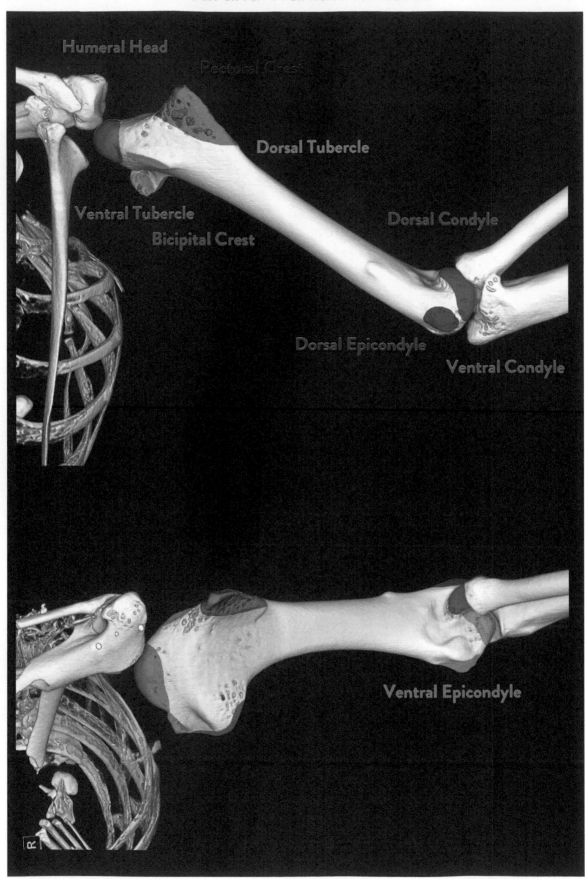

90

Pigeon (*Columba livia*)
Ventral and Caudal Humerus

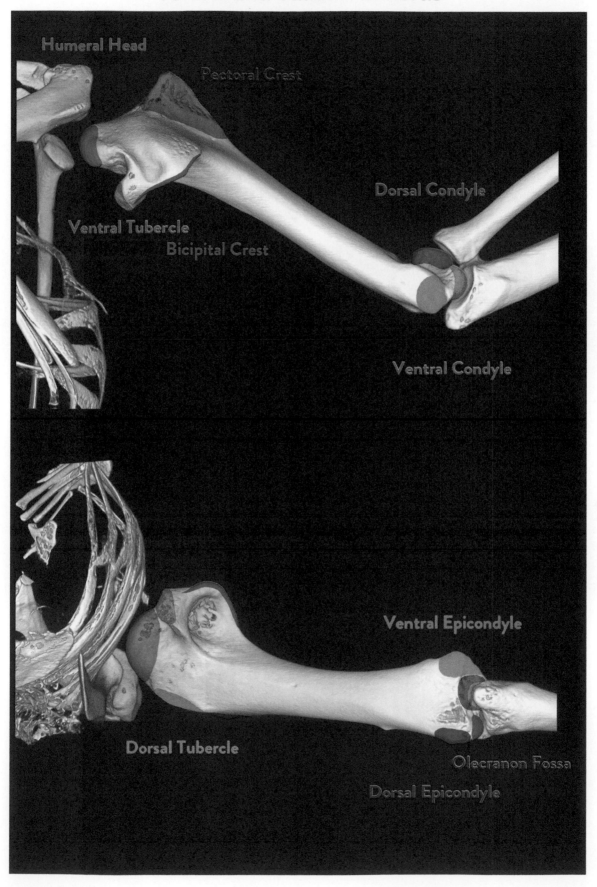

Humeral Head

Pectoral Crest

Dorsal Condyle

Ventral Tubercle

Bicipital Crest

Ventral Condyle

Ventral Epicondyle

Dorsal Tubercle

Olecranon Fossa

Dorsal Epicondyle

Domestic Chicken (*Gallus gallus domesticus*)
Dorsal and Cranial Humerus

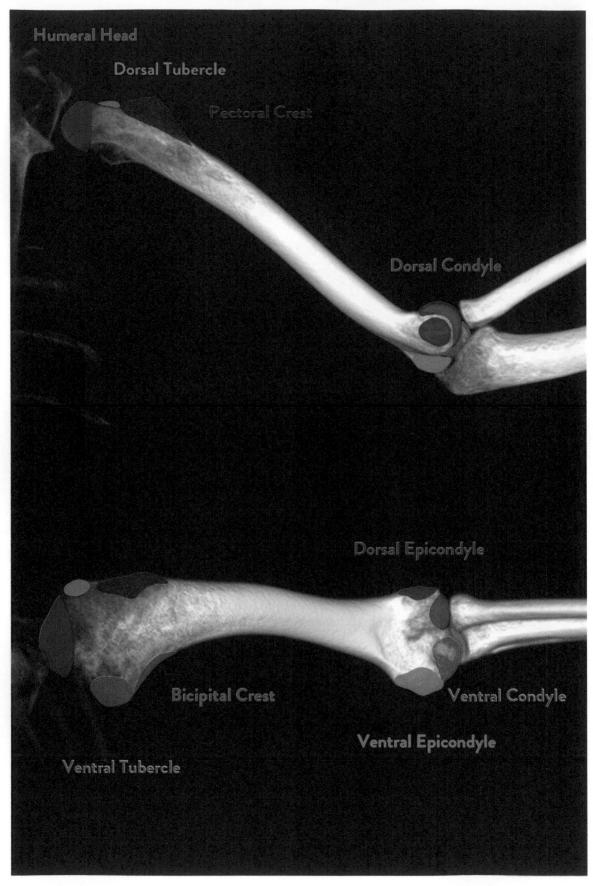

Domestic Chicken (*Gallus gallus domesticus*)
Ventral and Caudal Humerus

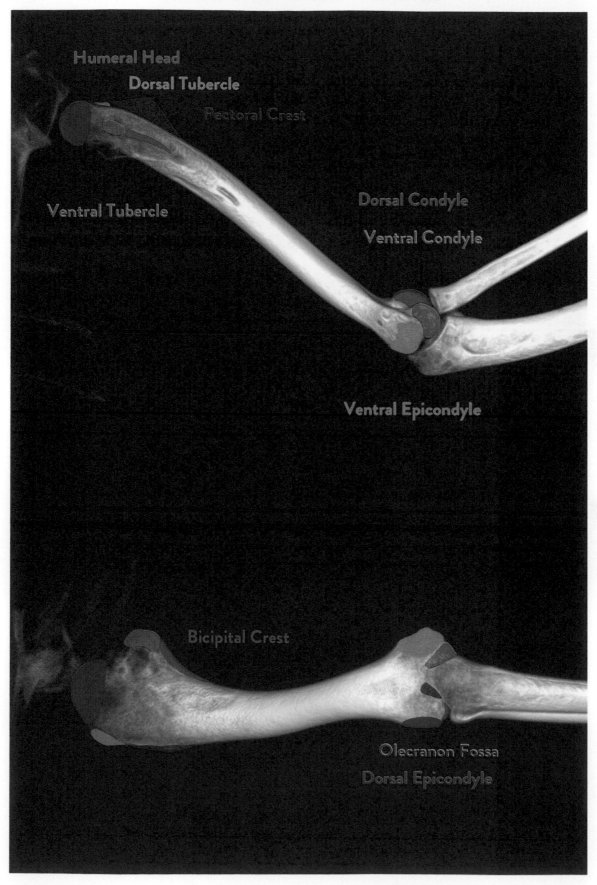

Humeral Head

Dorsal Tubercle

Pectoral Crest

Ventral Tubercle

Dorsal Condyle

Ventral Condyle

Ventral Epicondyle

Bicipital Crest

Olecranon Fossa

Dorsal Epicondyle

Red-tailed Hawk (*Buteo jamaicensis*)
Dorsal and Cranial Humerus

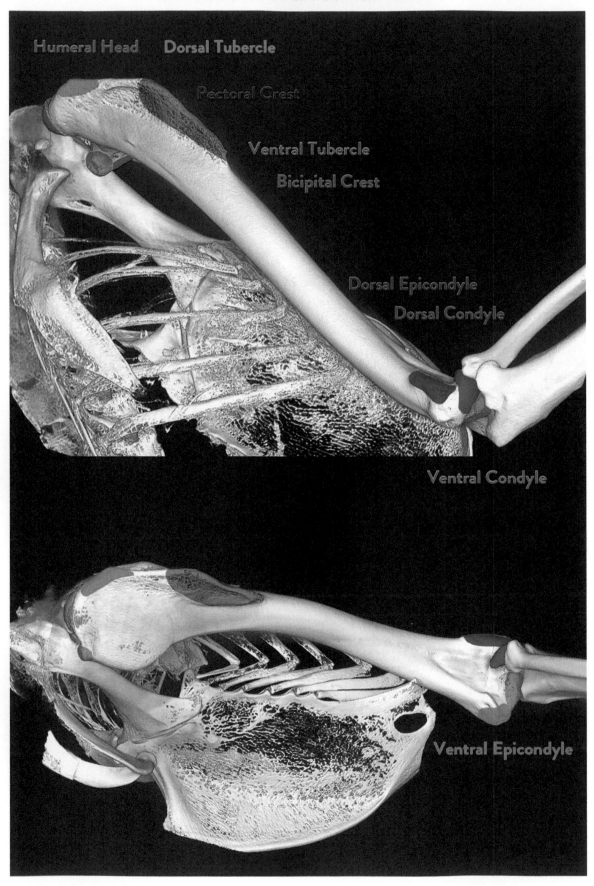

Humeral Head   Dorsal Tubercle

Pectoral Crest

Ventral Tubercle

Bicipital Crest

Dorsal Epicondyle

Dorsal Condyle

Ventral Condyle

Ventral Epicondyle

Red-tailed Hawk *(Buteo jamaicensis)*
Ventral and Caudal Humerus

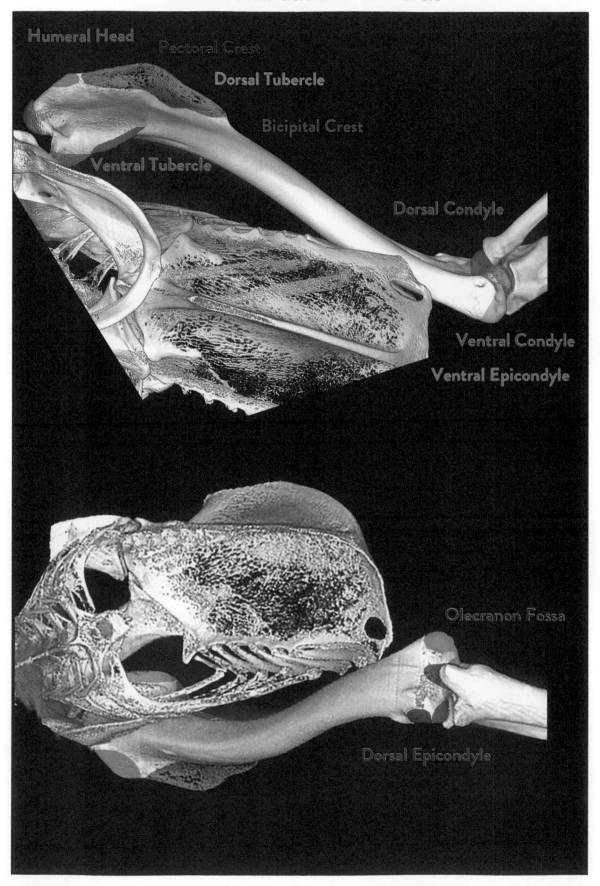

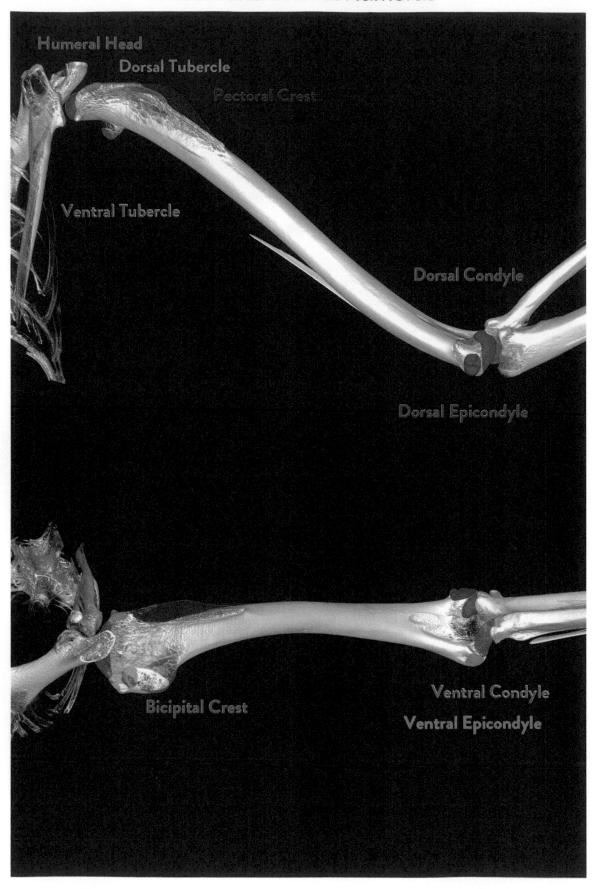

Great Horned Owl (*Bubo virginianus*)
Ventral and Caudal Humerus

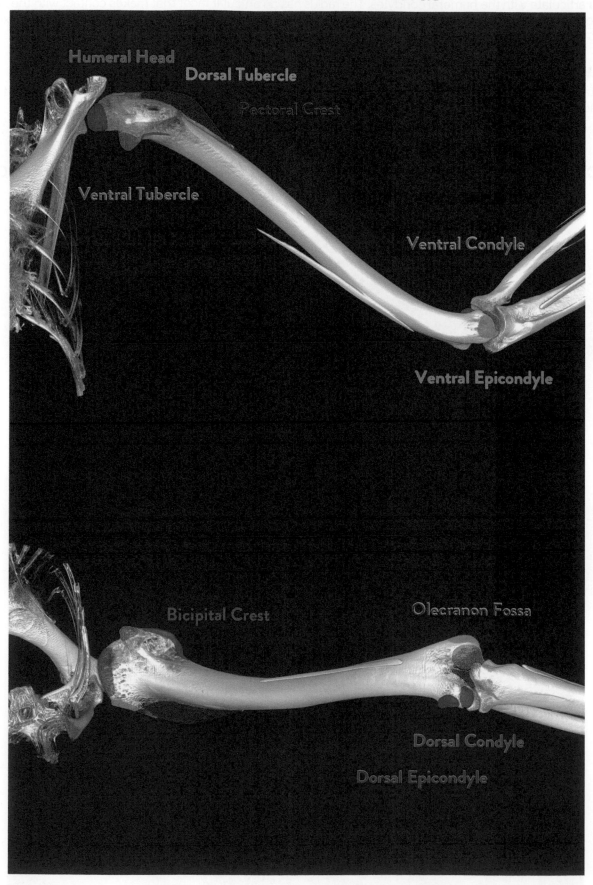

Humeral Head

Dorsal Tubercle

Pectoral Crest

Ventral Tubercle

Ventral Condyle

Ventral Epicondyle

Bicipital Crest

Olecranon Fossa

Dorsal Condyle

Dorsal Epicondyle

Elbow

The elbow consists of the articulation of the humerus with the radius cranially and the ulna caudally. The radius and ulna articulate with the humeral condyles. The radius has an articular facet that makes contact with the smaller dorsal condyle. The ulna has a concave surface for articulation with the ventral condyle with an olecranon extension.

Elbow: CT Images

Computed tomography images of the distal wing are presented for the military macaw (*Ara militaris*) and golden eagle (*Aquila chrysaetos*).

Military Macaw (*Ara militaris*)
Dorsal, Dorsal Cranial Oblique and Dorsal Caudal Oblique Elbow

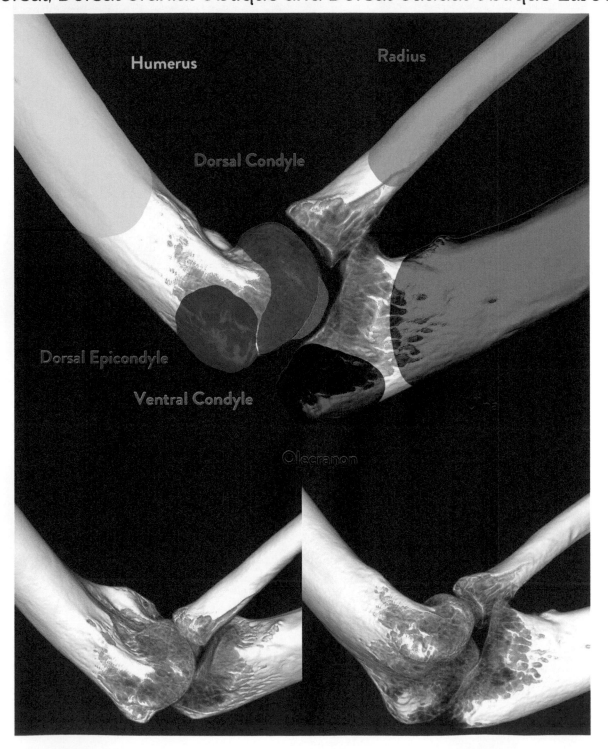

Military Macaw (*Ara militaris*)
Ventral, Ventral Cranial Oblique and Ventral Caudal Oblique Elbow

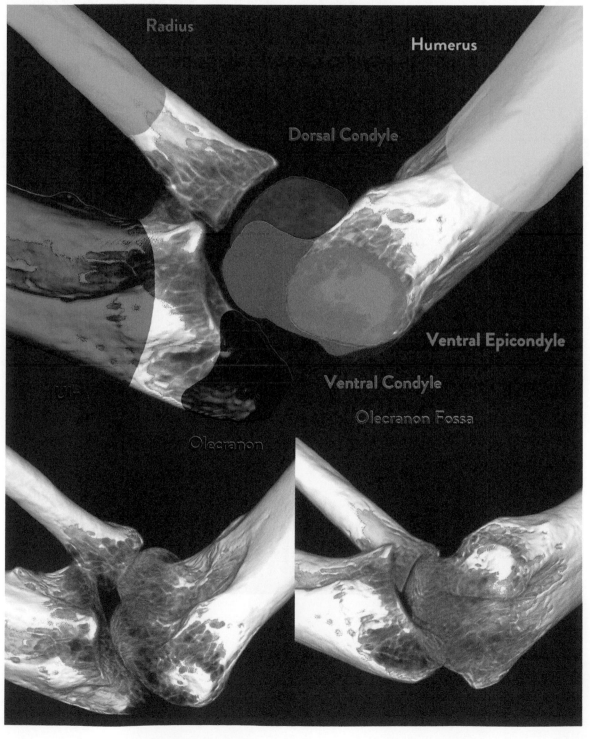

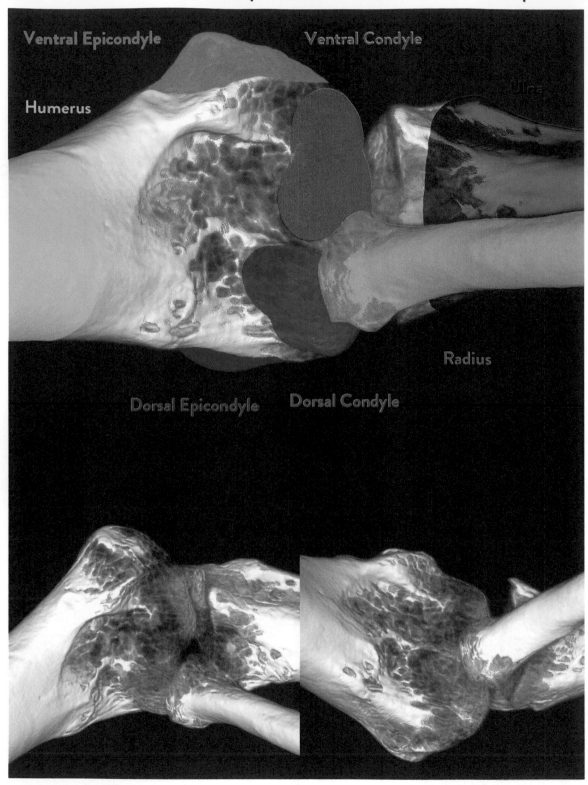

Military Macaw (*Ara militaris*)
Caudal, Caudal Ventral Oblique and Caudal Dorsal Oblique Elbow

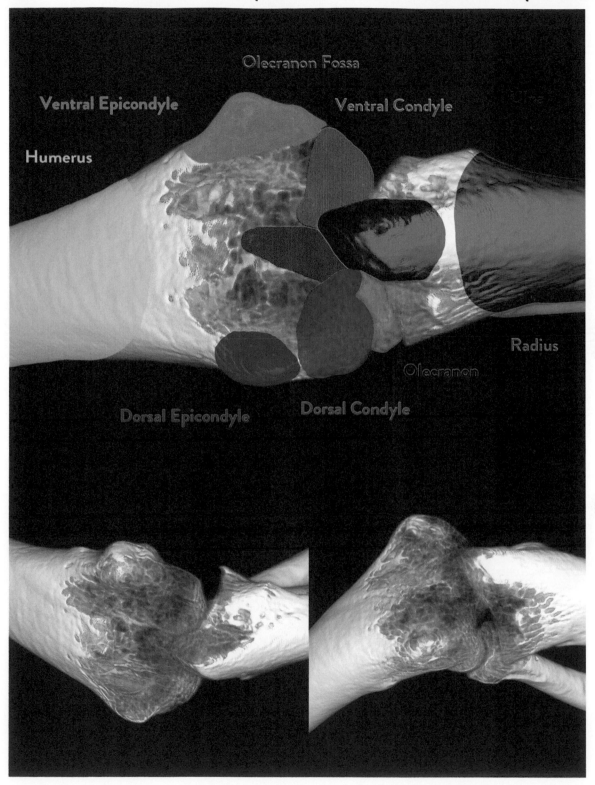

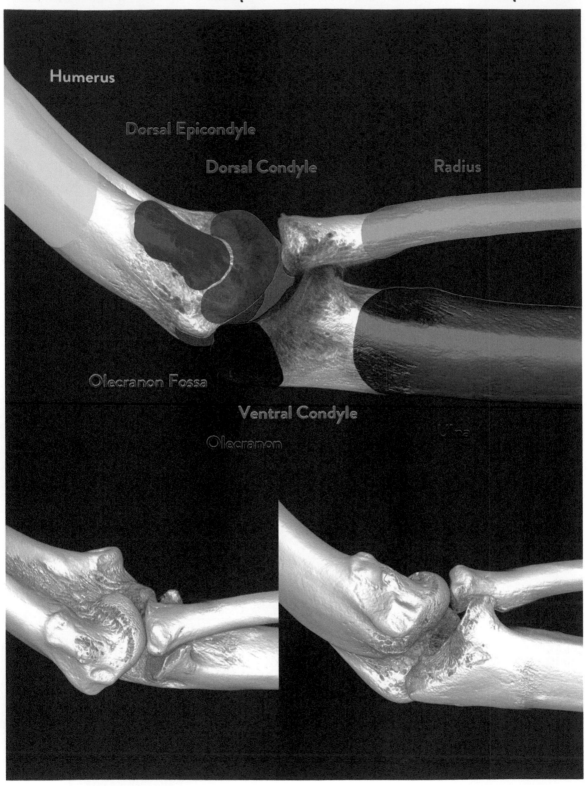

Golden Eagle (*Aquila chrysaetos*)
Ventral, Ventral Cranial Oblique and Ventral Caudal Oblique Elbow

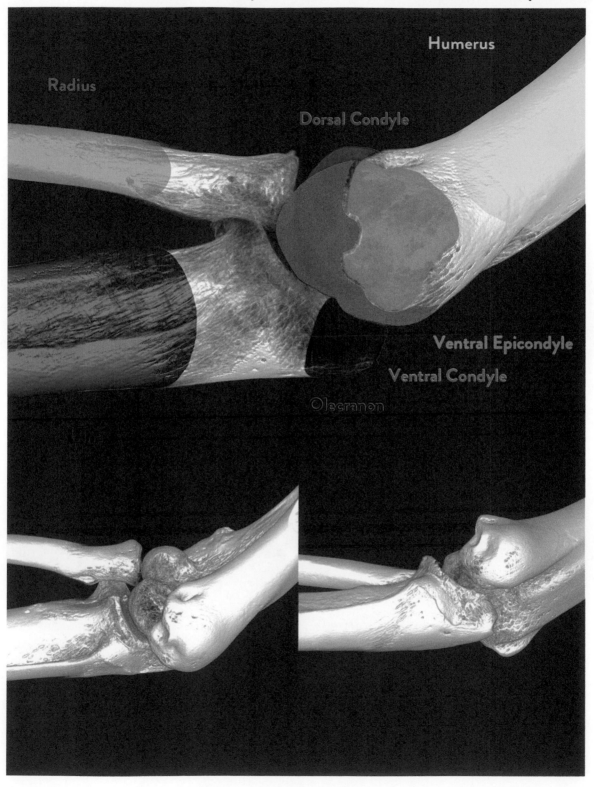

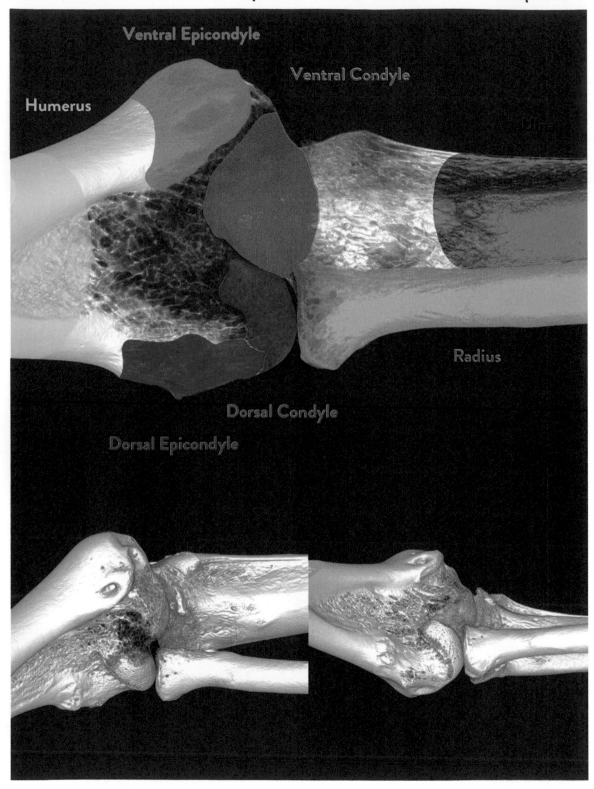

104

Golden Eagle (*Aquila chrysaetos*)
Caudal, Caudal Ventral Oblique and Caudal Dorsal Oblique Elbow

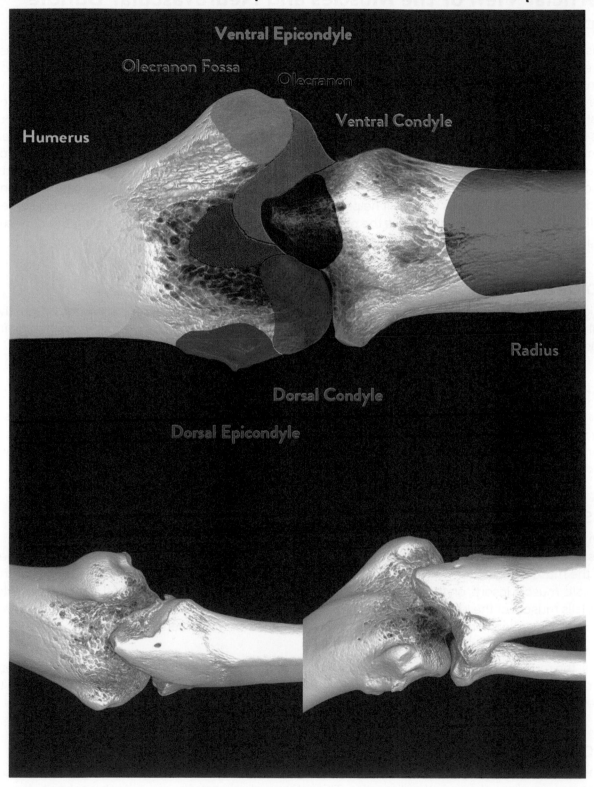

Dorsal Humerus

Superficial View of the Muscles and Neurovascular Bundle

The Propatagialis Complex (Tensor propatagialis)

The muscles that compose this mass over the cranial margin of the shoulder have various degrees of fusion; it is therefore convenient to describe them as the propatagialis complex. This muscle mass and its tendons of insertion are closely associated with the propatagial skin fold. There are two primary tendons of insertion: the pars brevis tendon, which inserts onto the tendon of origin of the extensor metacarpi radialis, as well as onto a fascial attachment running dorsally on the ulna; and the pars longus tendon, which inserts onto the extensor process of the metacarpus. The dermotensor patagii or the dermo-cleido dorsalis (Shufeldt 1890, Kaupp, 1918) is a dermo-osseous muscle that attaches to the skeleton and the skin and resembles a slip of muscle from the cucullaris of reptiles (Getty 1975). It has also been called the cucullaris cervicis and this muscle inserts in part onto the humeral feather tracts. In some vultures (Fischer 1946) and psittacines (Getty 1975), it becomes continuous with the pars longus tendon. It helps extend the metacarpus and digits while providing some flexion of the elbow. The complex can also tense the propatagium, an important factor in controlling the curvature of the wing for lift (Fischer 1946). These muscles are innervated by the axillary nerve.

Deltoideus major

The major deltoid muscle originates from the scapula and inserts along the shaft of the humerus from the pectoral crest distally. The muscle pulls the wing caudally and dorsally, and it is therefore important for flapping flight (Fischer 1946).

Triceps brachii

In cathartids, the triceps muscle is composed of three muscle bellies, one of which originates from the scapula. In many species, it has two heads: one from the scapula and another from the humerus (Getty 1975). The scapular (long) head acts to draw the humerus caudally when the wing is extended and helps to maintain the semiflexed position important for flex gliding (Fischer 1946).

Latissimus dorsi

This thin and flattened muscle is usually divided into two independent heads, the cranialis and caudalis muscles. The cranial head arises from several caudal cervical and cranial thoracic spinous processes; the caudal head of the muscle arises from caudal thoracic vertebrae down to and sometimes including the synsacrum. The cranialis muscle inserts on the head of the humerus between two of the bellies of the triceps muscle. The caudalis muscle of the latissimus dorsi may be lacking in some birds (pigeons and finches) or may have a variable site of insertion (International Committee on Avian Anatomical Nomenclature 1979).

In raptors, the muscle is closely associated with two cutaneous bands of muscle that insert onto the area of the scapular coverts, namely the cutaneus costohumeralis. These muscular slips arise from the ribs, ventral to the uncinate processes, and swing dorsally. They correlate with the cutaneous trunci of mammals.

Blood Supply and Innervation

Branches of the subscapular artery and vein appear between muscle fascicles of the rhomboideus muscles which are deep and not shown in the dissection. This artery and vein provide muscular branches to the propatagialis complex and deltoideus muscles. The axillary nerve is found between the deltoideus major and minor muscles. After supplying these muscles, it continues dorsally to innervate the propatagialis complex. Commonly, the radial nerve emerges between the distal end of the deltoideus major and the triceps brachii muscles, where it innervates the latter muscle. It serves as an important landmark for identification and preservation in mid-shaft diaphyseal humeral fractures.

Dorsal Humerus
Deep Layer of Muscles (Propatagialis Complex Removed)
Deltoideus minor

This muscle is found deep to the propatagialis complex of muscles and proximal to the deltoideus major muscle. It originates from both the scapula and clavicle and inserts on the proximal humerus, thereby lifting the humerus and pulling it cranially. This may be important in the recovery stroke of the wing in flight (Fischer 1946).

Biceps brachii

This muscle, a strong flexor of the elbow, originates on the cranial border of the proximal humerus. The tendon of the biceps muscle divides, with the proximal, larger tendon inserting on the proximal radius. The other tendon inserts on the ulna and may include a small slip of fibers that forms part of the tensor propatagialis pars brevis tendon of insertion (Getty 1975). This muscle is innervated by the bicipital nerve, a branch from the medianoulnar nerve.

Brachialis

This small muscle is found between the humerus and radius in the flexor space. It inserts on the ventral surface of the proximal ulna. Although the brachialis flexes the elbow, it is thought to maintain the forearm (or forewing) in a horizontal position in flight during gusts of wind (Fischer 1946).

Coracobrachialis cranialis *(Coracobrachialis dorsalis)*

This triangular muscle fills part of the space between the coracoid and the head of the humerus dorsally. As the name implies, it takes origin from the head of the coracoid bone, but it inserts on the ventral side of the humeral head. During the initial phase of the downstroke, it may function to pull the wing cranially (Fischer 1946).

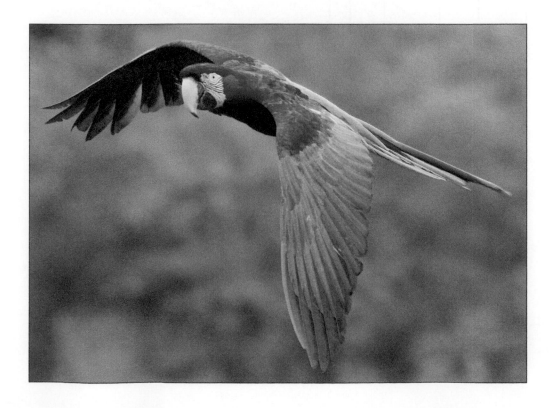

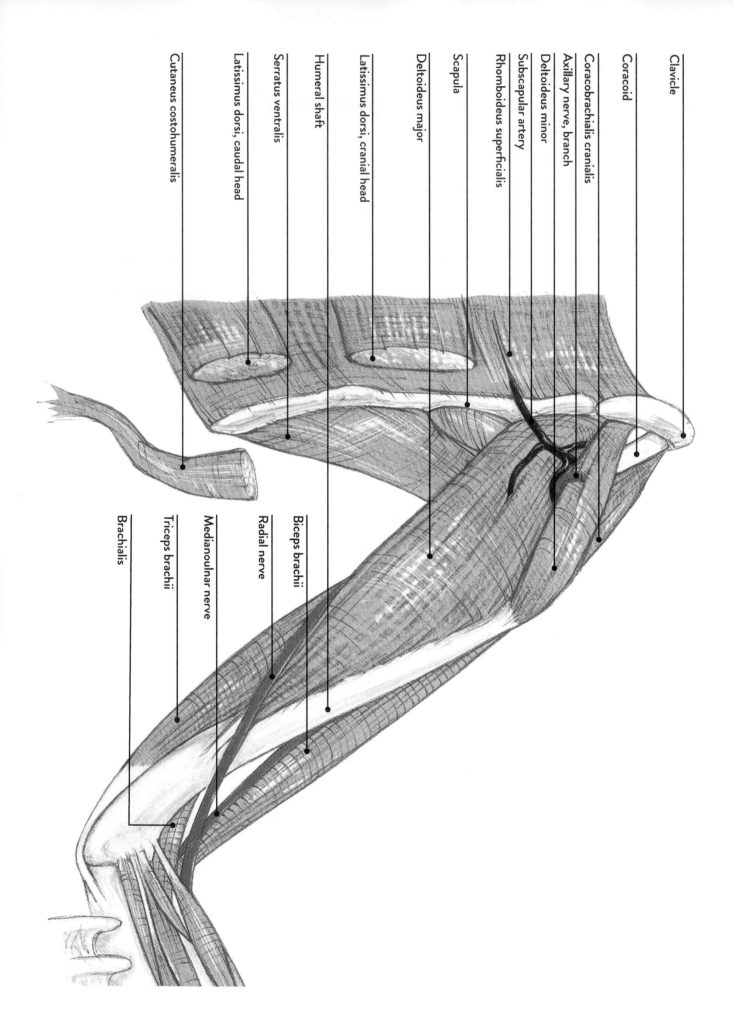

Clavicle

Coracoid

Coracobrachialis cranialis

Axillary nerve, branch

Deltoideus minor

Subscapular artery

Rhomboideus superficialis

Scapula

Deltoideus major

Latissimus dorsi, cranial head

Humeral shaft

Serratus ventralis

Latissimus dorsi, caudal head

Cutaneus costohumeralis

Brachialis

Triceps brachii

Medianoulnar nerve

Radial nerve

Biceps brachii

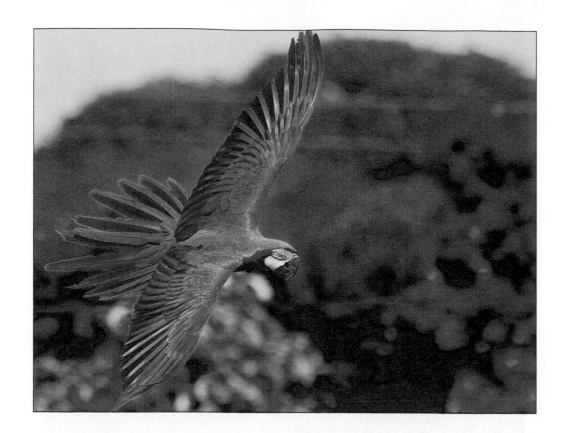

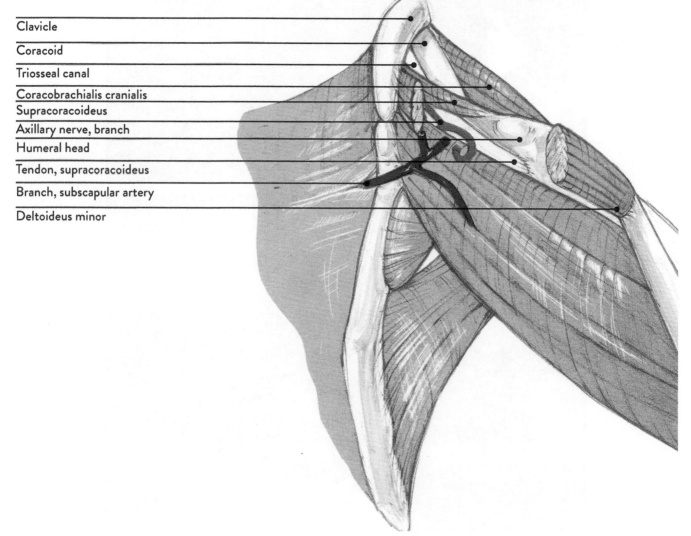

Clavicle

Coracoid

Triosseal canal

Coracobrachialis cranialis

Supracoracoideus

Axillary nerve, branch

Humeral head

Tendon, supracoracoideus

Branch, subscapular artery

Deltoideus minor

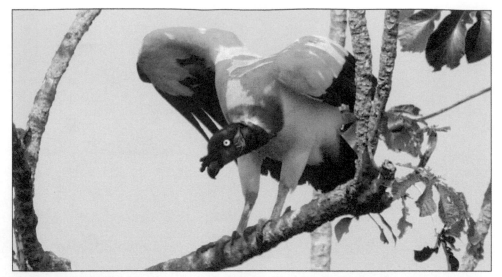

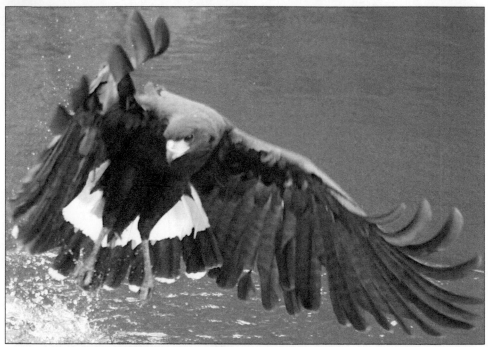

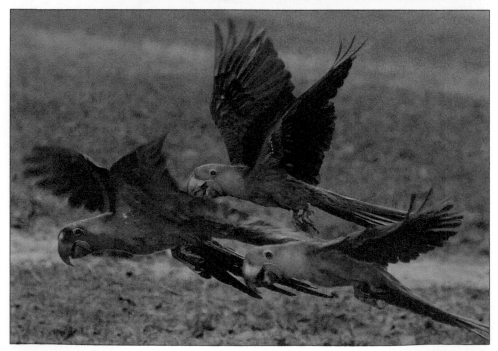

Proximal Dorsal Humerus

The orientation diagram on the right is intended to show the region depicted in the anatomical dissections below. It is not intended to represent a surgical approach.

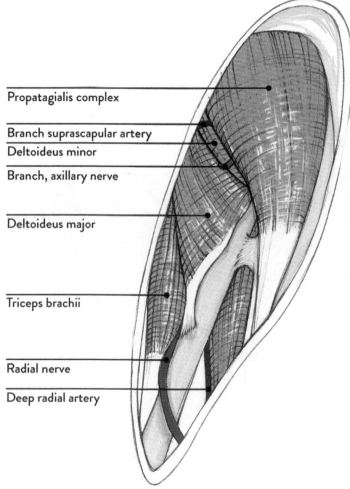

Propatagialis complex

Branch suprascapular artery

Deltoideus minor

Branch, axillary nerve

Deltoideus major

Triceps brachii

Radial nerve

Deep radial artery

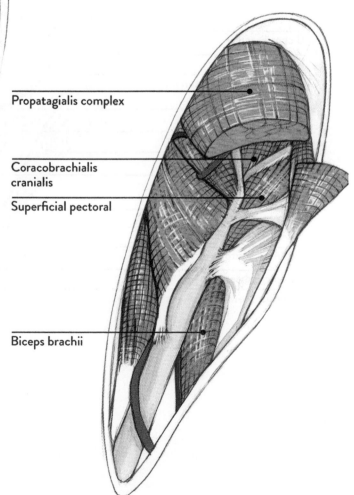

Propatagialis complex

Coracobrachialis cranialis

Superficial pectoral

Biceps brachii

Dorsal Distal Humerus, Detail

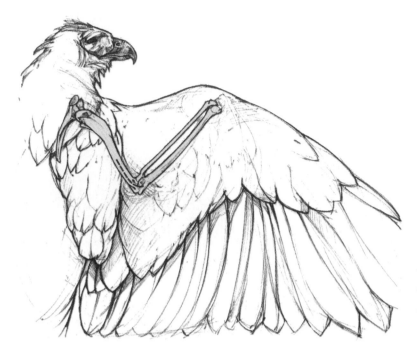

The orientation diagram on the left is intended to show the region depicted in the anatomical dissections below. It is not intended to represent a surgical approach.

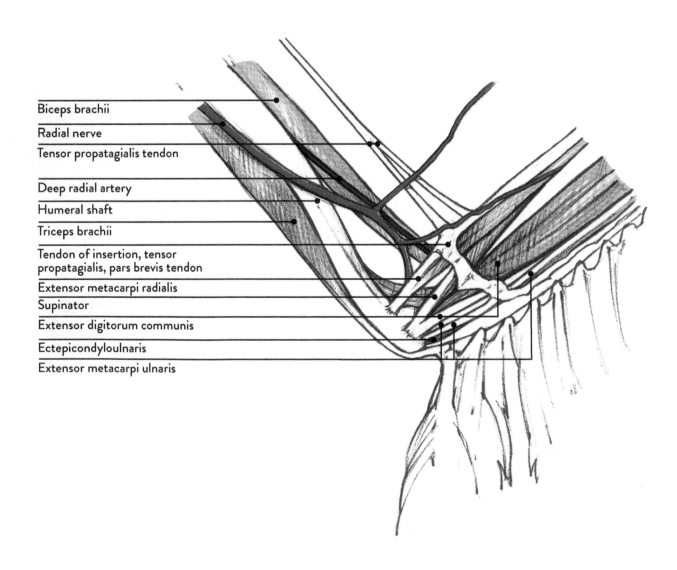

Biceps brachii

Radial nerve

Tensor propatagialis tendon

Deep radial artery

Humeral shaft

Triceps brachii

Tendon of insertion, tensor propatagialis, pars brevis tendon

Extensor metacarpi radialis

Supinator

Extensor digitorum communis

Ectepicondyloulnaris

Extensor metacarpi ulnaris

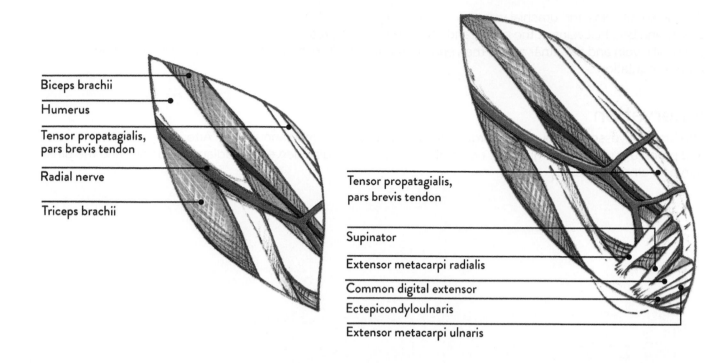

Biceps brachii
Humerus
Tensor propatagialis, pars brevis tendon
Radial nerve
Triceps brachii

Tensor propatagialis, pars brevis tendon
Supinator
Extensor metacarpi radialis
Common digital extensor
Ectepicondyloulnaris
Extensor metacarpi ulnaris

Ventral Humerus
Superficial View of the Muscles and the Neurovascular Supply
Superficial Pectoral Muscle *(Pectoralis)*

There is considerable variation in the pectoral muscle mass among species of birds. Descriptions of these muscles also vary. For veterinary purposes, it is easier to describe two muscles, one superficial and the other deep. The superficial muscle is closely associated with the propatagial complex of muscles. Vanden Berge, in Sisson and Grossman's Anatomy of the Domestic Animals (Getty 1975) refers to a portion of the superficial pectoral muscle that inserts into the propatagium as the pars propatagialis.

The superficial pectoral muscle covers the ventral surface of the sternum and represents most of the muscle mass that is palpated in a physical examination. Most of the muscle originates from the keel and inserts along the pectoral crest and the proximal humerus. Psittacines and many of the raptors appear to have a single, large muscle mass without the superficial and deep divisions. However, in vultures that glide, the muscle can be divided into a superficial and deep pectoral muscle. The large, powerful superficial pectoral muscle is important in flapping flight. It is responsible for the downstroke, as well as for depressing the leading edge of the wing to reduce turbulence across the wing (Fischer 1946).

Biceps brachii

This muscle originates on the cranial border of the proximal humerus. The tendon of the biceps muscle divides, with the proximal, larger tendon inserting on the proximal cranial radius. The other tendon inserts on the ventral ulna. It is a strong flexor of the elbow.

Blood Supply

The major vessels and nerves to the thoracic limb are located proximally between the biceps and triceps brachii muscles. The most superficial vessel is a cutaneous vein often used for venipunctures: the basilic vein [v. basilica]. It provides the major drainage of venous blood from the wing to the axillary vein. The brachial artery divides into the ulnar and radial arteries in the proximal arm. These arteries course along the caudal margin of the biceps brachii, with the ulnar artery superficial and cranial to the radial. The radial artery runs with the medianoulnar nerve.

Several small veins, the brachial veins, run with these arteries. Venous anastomoses are found between the basilic and brachial veins at the elbow and the proximal humerus. In addition, there are anastomoses between the basilic vein and the ulnar artery, the venae commitantes. These structures may play a role in counter-current thermoregulation.

Innervation
The brachial vessels surround the large medianoulnar nerve (n. medianoulnaris). After supplying the muscles and propatagium in that region, the nerve divides into the median nerve (n. medianus) cranially and the ulnar nerve (n. ulnaris) caudally.

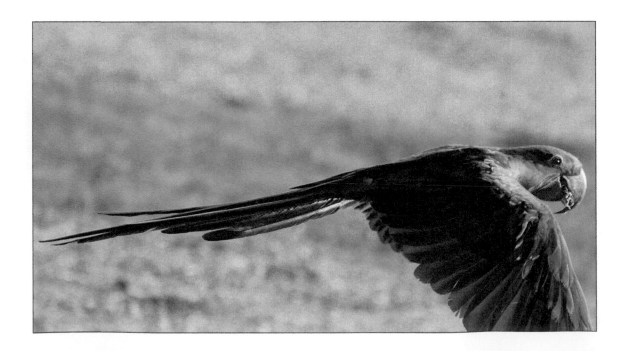

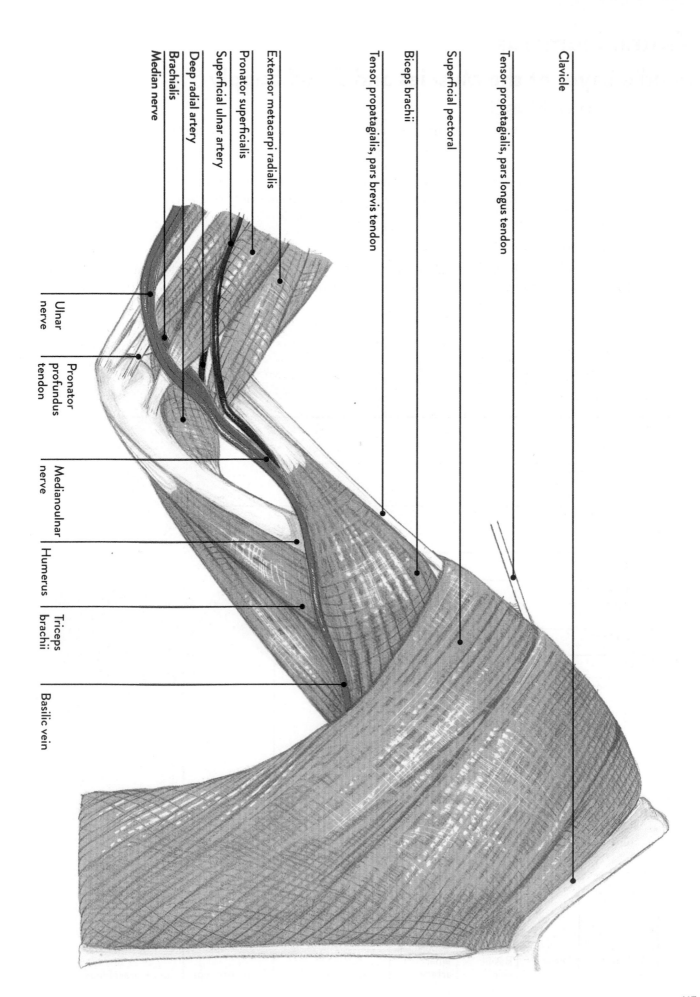

Clavicle

Tensor propatagialis, pars longus tendon

Superficial pectoral

Biceps brachii

Tensor propatagialis, pars brevis tendon

Extensor metacarpi radialis

Pronator superficialis

Superficial ulnar artery

Deep radial artery

Brachialis

Median nerve

Ulnar nerve

Pronator profundus tendon

Medianoulnar nerve

Humerus

Triceps brachii

Basilic vein

Ventral Humerus
Middle Layer of the Muscles and Blood Supply
Deep Pectoral Muscle
The deep pectoral muscle is found in vultures and may occur in other longer winged bird species. The muscle originates from the keel and the clavicle, deep to the origin of the superficial pectoral muscle. Its insertion is along the ventral side of the pectoral crest. The deep pectoral muscle's tendon continues ventrally to the proximal humerus. It is thought that this muscle is responsible for the forward motion of the wing immediately prior to the downstroke. Psittacines, hawks, and owls do not have a well-defined deep pectoral muscle.

Blood Supply
The brachial artery gives off the deep brachial artery before dividing into the ulnar and radial arteries. The deep brachial artery runs along the caudal surface of the scapular (long) head of the triceps with the radial nerve.

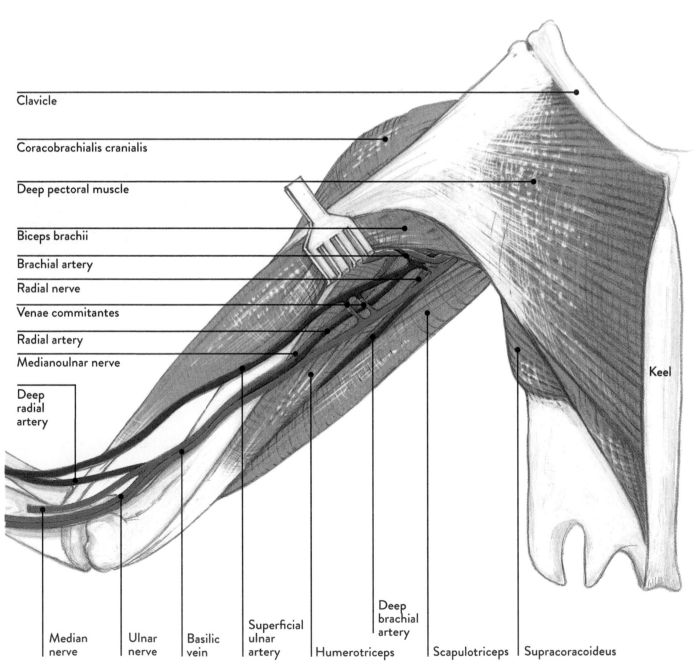

Clavicle

Coracobrachialis cranialis

Deep pectoral muscle

Biceps brachii

Brachial artery

Radial nerve

Venae commitantes

Radial artery

Medianoulnar nerve

Deep radial artery

Keel

Median nerve

Ulnar nerve

Basilic vein

Superficial ulnar artery

Humerotriceps

Deep brachial artery

Scapulotriceps

Supracoracoideus

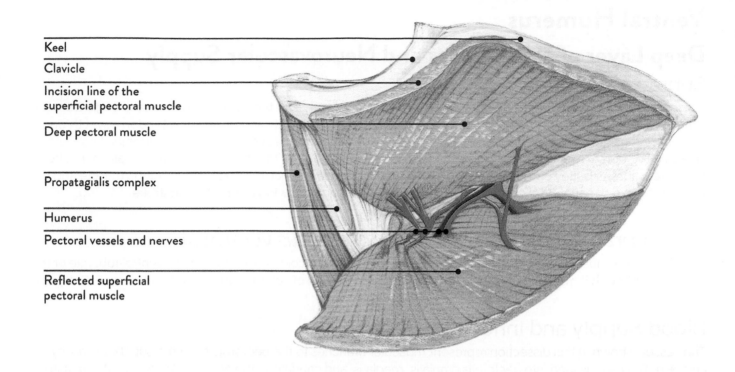

Keel

Clavicle

Incision line of the
superficial pectoral muscle

Deep pectoral muscle

Propatagialis complex

Humerus

Pectoral vessels and nerves

Reflected superficial
pectoral muscle

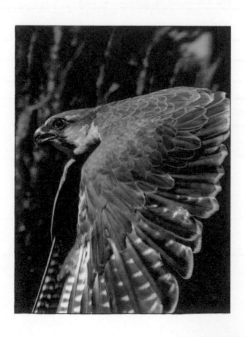

Ventral Humerus
Deep Layer of the Muscles and Neurovascular Supply
Supracoracoideus

This muscle is extensive in many species as it can cover a large area of the keel. It can also take origin from the surfaces of the clavicle and coracoid (Getty,1975). A muscular slip and its accompanying tendon travel through the triosseal canal in a synovial sheath where they abruptly change direction over the shoulder joint capsule to insert on the dorsal tubercle of the humerus. Often there is a ligament that holds the tendon in place and helps to create a fibrous pulley of the tendon. By traversing the triosseal canal, the supracoracoideus muscle and its tendon change direction to elevate the humerus, thereby raising the wing during the upstroke.

Coracobrachialis caudalis *(Coracobrachialis ventralis)*

This short, thick muscle covers the ventrolateral surface of the coracoid and inserts on the ventral tubercle of the humerus. Although it may help to depress the wing, its mechanism of action is uncertain (Fischer 1946, Getty 1975).

Blood Supply and Innervation

The vessels shown in this dissection represent muscular branches to the pectorals from the subclavian artery and vein. They are divided into pectoralis cranialis, medialis, and caudalis in the *Nomina Anatomica Avium* (International Committee on Avian Anatomical Nomenclature 1993). The muscular branches of the pectoral nerves *[n. pectoralis cranialis and caudalis]* arise from the brachial plexus and supply the superficial and deep pectoral muscles. The supracoracoideus muscle is supplied by its own nerve from the brachial plexus. The coracobrachialis caudalis muscle is innervated by a ventral branch of the brachial plexus.

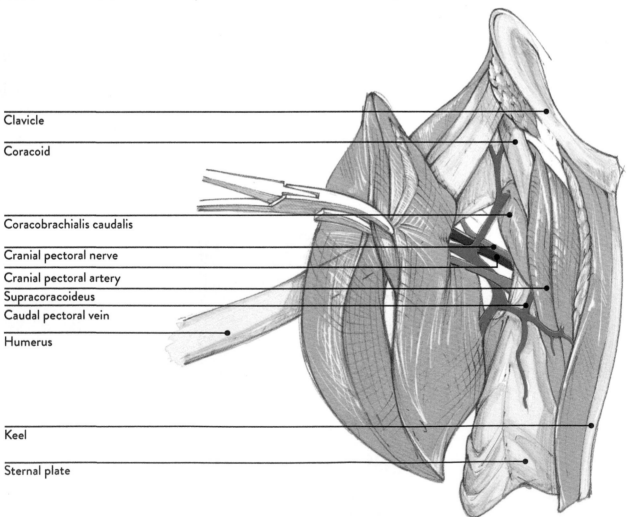

Clavicle

Coracoid

Coracobrachialis caudalis

Cranial pectoral nerve

Cranial pectoral artery

Supracoracoideus

Caudal pectoral vein

Humerus

Keel

Sternal plate

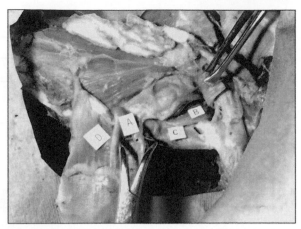

Dissection of a turkey vulture *(Cathartes aura)* showing the dorsal, cranial shoulder, and the triosseal canal. *"A"* is the deltoideus minor muscle that has been cut exposing the head of the humerus that is white. *"B"* is the supracoracoideus muscle, visualized in the triosseal canal before its insertion on the dorsal tubercle of the humerus. *"C"* is the coracobrachialis cranialis muscle. *"D"* is the cut muscle of the tensor propatagialis muscle.

Ventral Shoulder and Humerus: Anatomical Detail

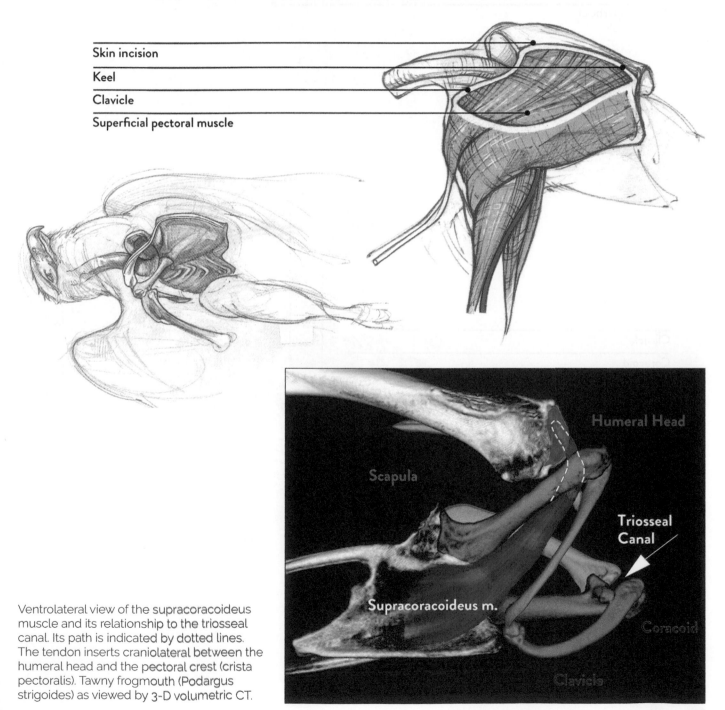

Skin incision

Keel

Clavicle

Superficial pectoral muscle

Humeral Head

Scapula

Triosseal Canal

Supracoracoideus m.

Coracoid

Clavicle

Ventrolateral view of the supracoracoideus muscle and its relationship to the triosseal canal. Its path is indicated by dotted lines. The tendon inserts craniolateral between the humeral head and the pectoral crest (crista pectoralis). Tawny frogmouth (Podargus strigoides) as viewed by 3-D volumetric CT.

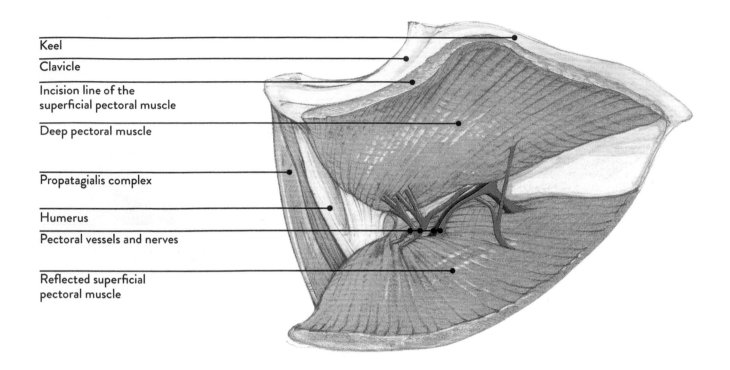

Keel

Clavicle

Incision line of the
superficial pectoral muscle

Deep pectoral muscle

Propatagialis complex

Humerus

Pectoral vessels and nerves

Reflected superficial
pectoral muscle

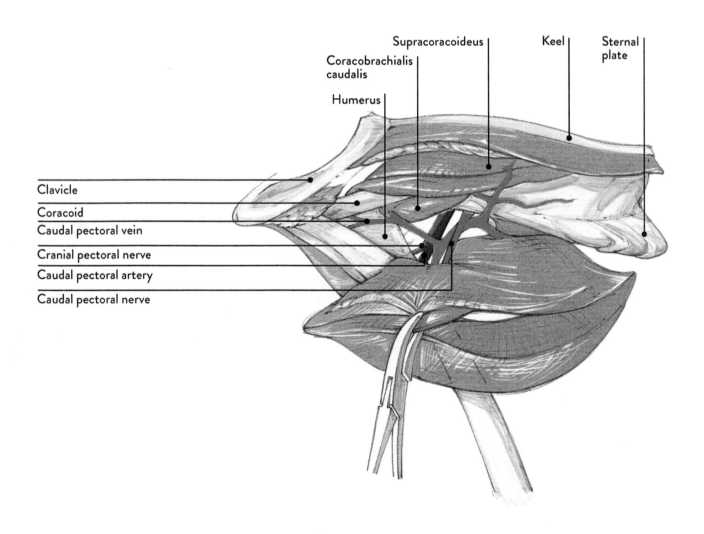

Coracobrachialis
caudalis

Supracoracoideus

Humerus

Keel

Sternal
plate

Clavicle

Coracoid

Caudal pectoral vein

Cranial pectoral nerve

Caudal pectoral artery

Caudal pectoral nerve

Ventral Distal Humerus

The orientation diagram to the right is intended to show the region depicted in the anatomical dissections below. It is not intended to represent a surgical approach.

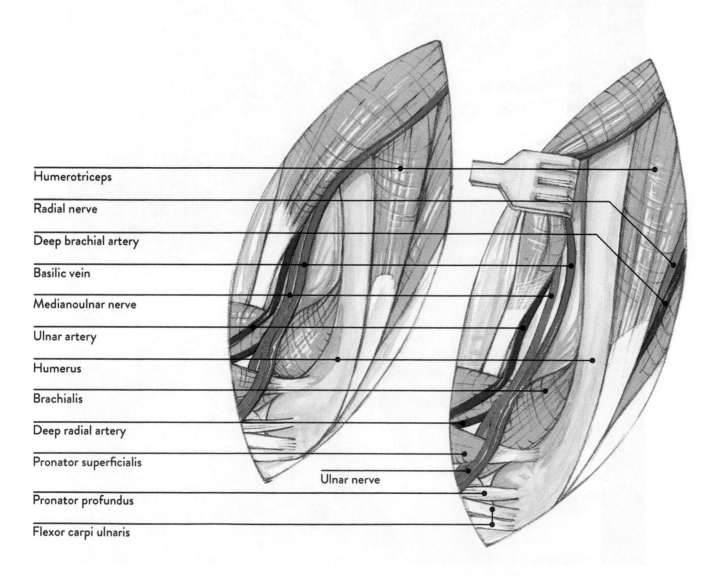

Humerotriceps

Radial nerve

Deep brachial artery

Basilic vein

Medianoulnar nerve

Ulnar artery

Humerus

Brachialis

Deep radial artery

Pronator superficialis

Ulnar nerve

Pronator profundus

Flexor carpi ulnaris

Vasculature Contrast Images of the Shoulder Girdle and Humerus

Vasculature contrast images of the proximal wing (shoulder, humerus, and elbow) are presented for four species: the pigeon *(Columba livia)*, barn owl *(Tyto alba)*, painted stork *(Mycteria leucoephala)*, and the African goose *(Anser anser domesticus)*.

Pigeon (*Columba livia*)
Dorsal and Dorsal Oblique Shoulder Girdle

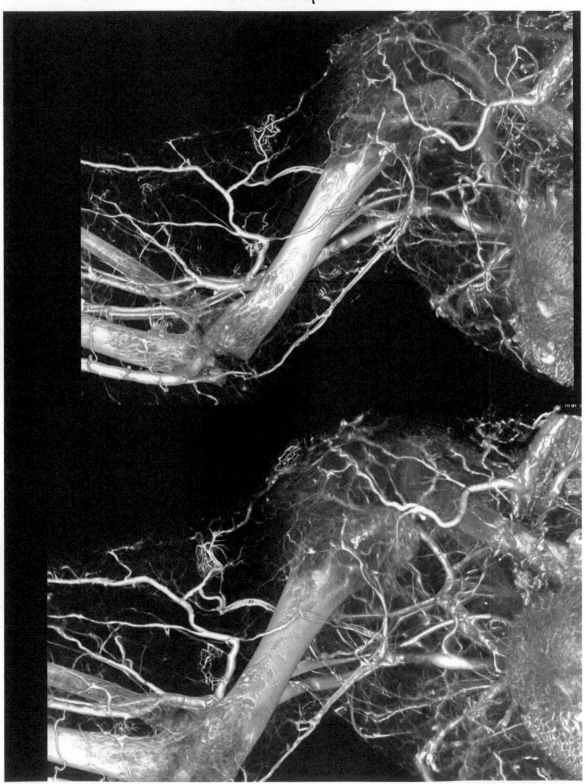

Pigeon (*Columba livia*)
Ventral and Cranial Shoulder Girdle

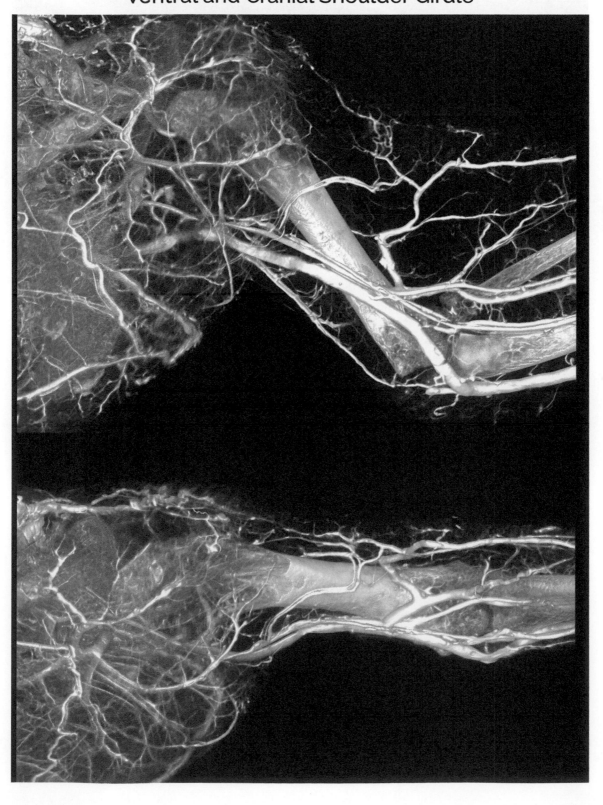

Pigeon (*Columba livia*)
Dorsal and Cranial Elbow

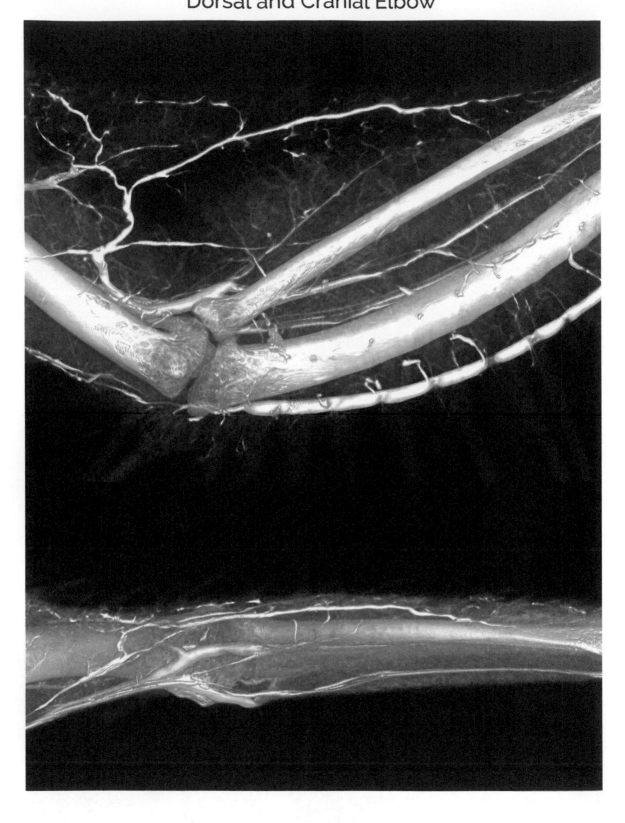

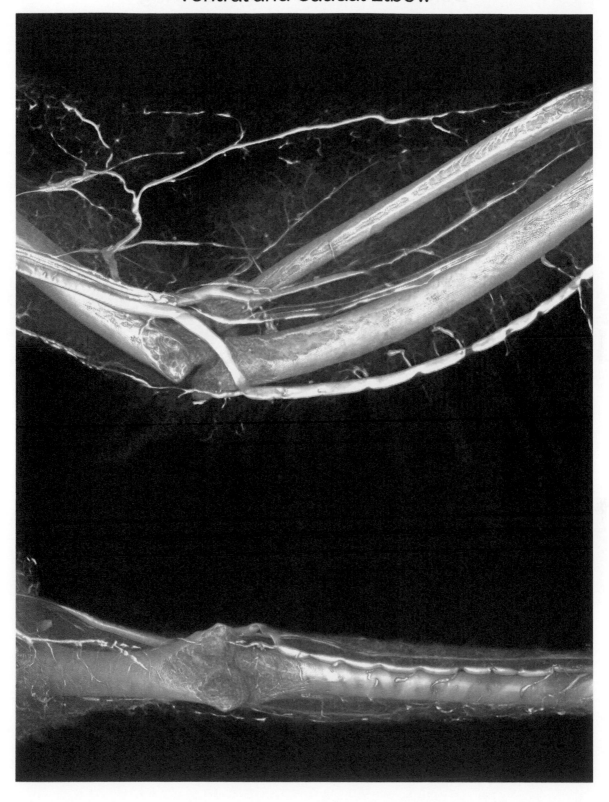

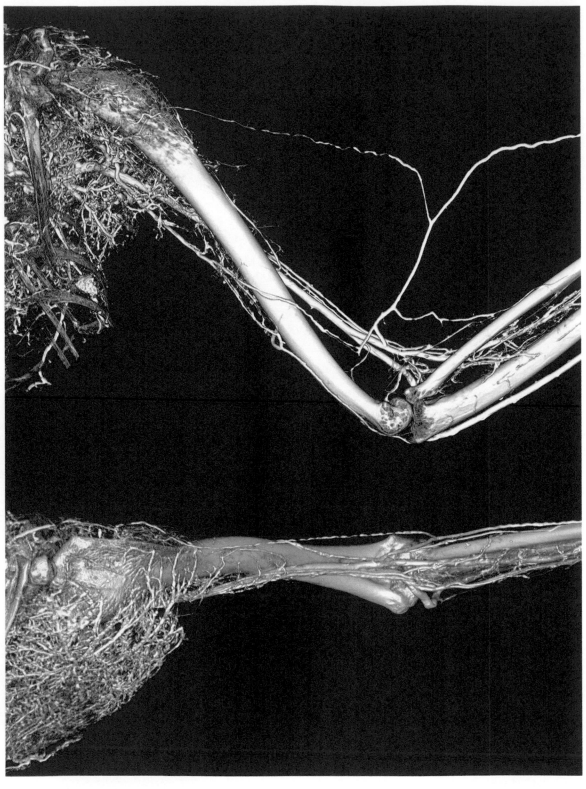

Barn Owl (*Tyto alba*)
Ventral and Caudal Proximal Wing

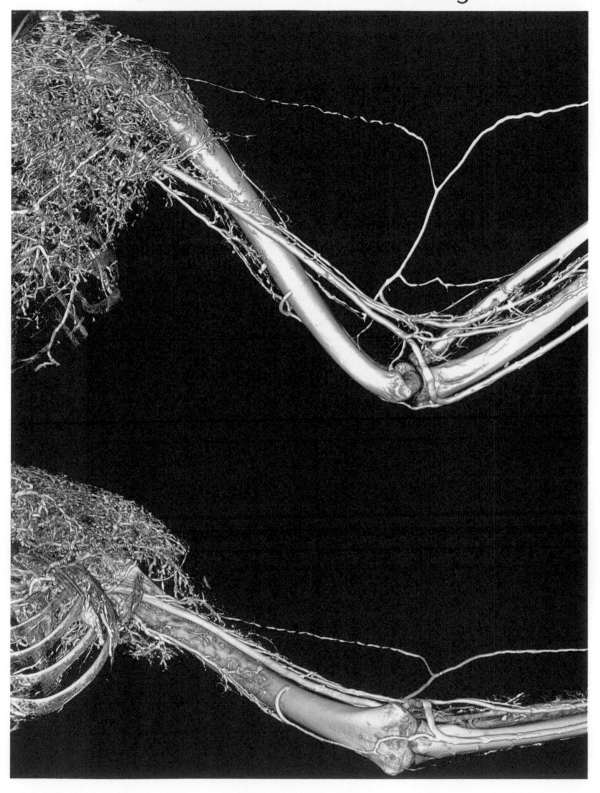

Painted Stork (*Mycteria leucocephala*)
Dorsal and Cranial Proximal Wing

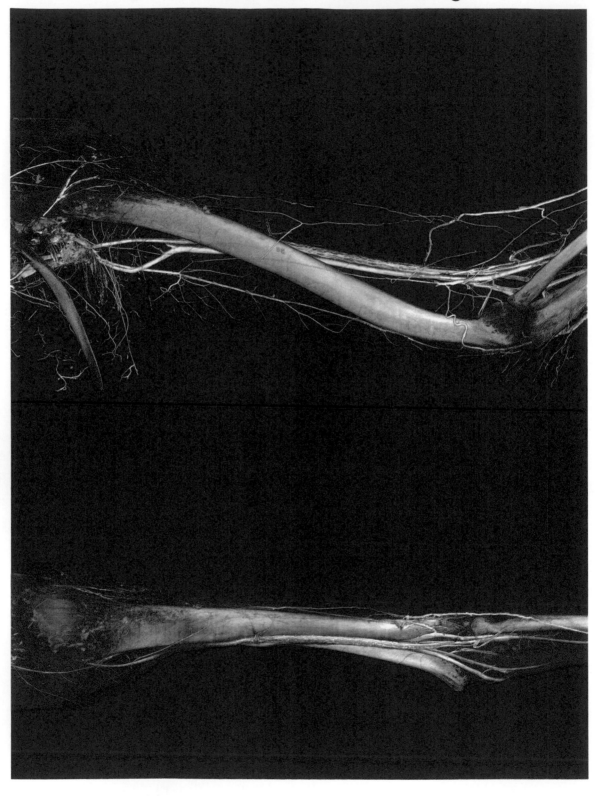

Painted Stork (*Mycteria leucocephala*)
Ventral and Caudal Proximal Wing

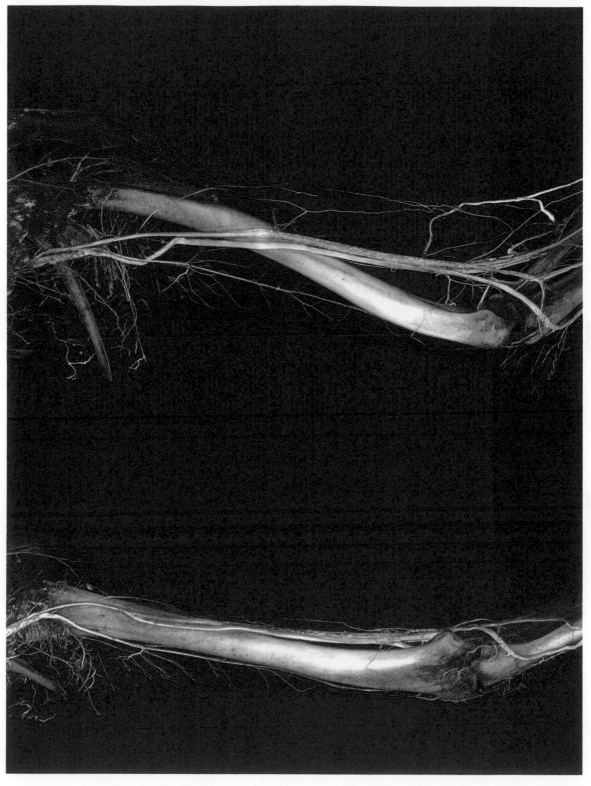

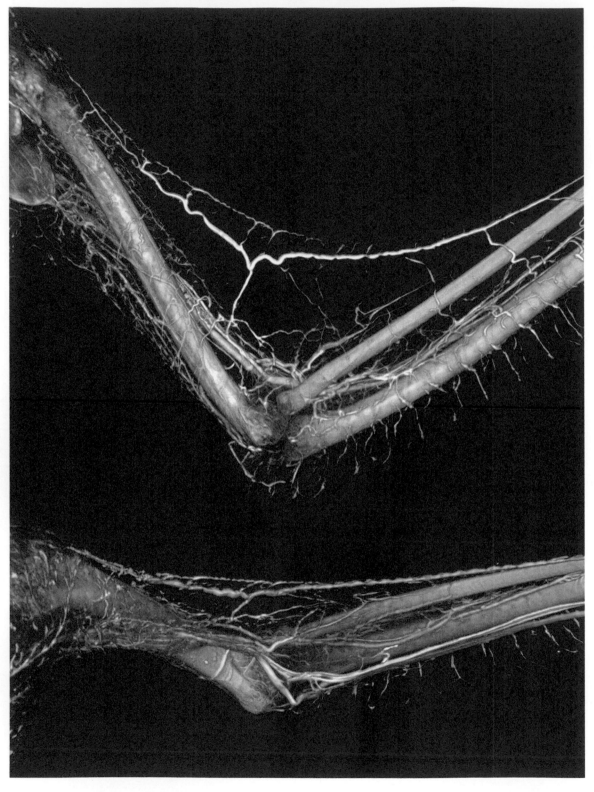

African Goose (*Anser anser domesticus*)
Ventral and Caudal Proximal Wing

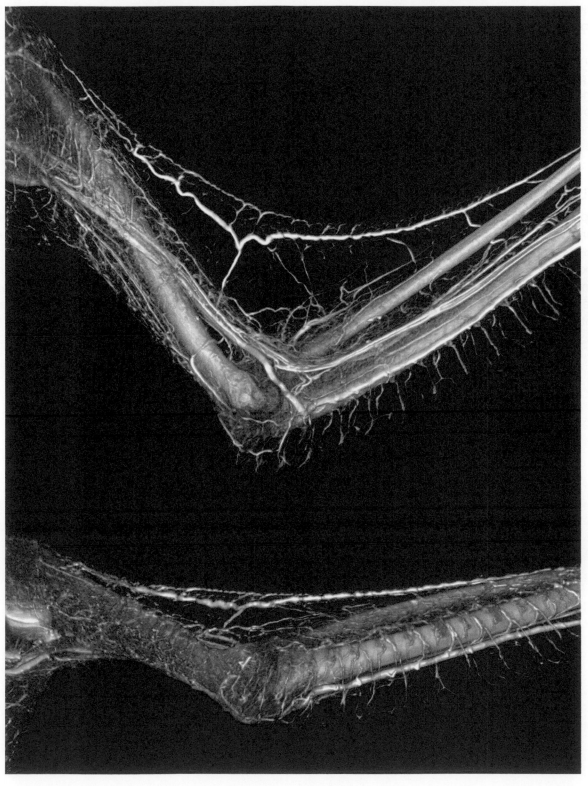

Dorsal Distal Skeleton of the Wing

Radius and Ulna

The bones of the forearm or antebrachium are the radius and ulna. They are of comparable length, and the bones may have a convex curve depending on the species in their midshaft. The degree of curvature varies with species. Those that soar, tend to be relatively straight in comparison to those that have a more powerful flapping flight. Unlike mammals, the ulna in birds has a small olecranon for articulation with the humeral condyle, which is more pronounced in accipiters (Fischer 1946). In contrast to mammals, the ulna is larger than the radius in birds. The radius and ulna act in concert to extend or flex the manus or hand in relation to the forearm. Flexion of the elbow joint results in flexion of the carpal joint. This reciprocal mechanism is dependent on the ligamentous attachments from the carpus to the radius and ulna (Baumel 1983). As the elbow is extended, the radius slides with the ligamentous attachments to pull the metacarpus into extension.

Carpus, Carpometacarpus

The carpus consists of two bones: the radial and ulnar carpal bones. The radial carpal bone is cranial, and the ulnar carpal bone is caudal. The carpometacarpus is composed of metacarpal bones partially fused to a distal row of carpal bones. These bones have important flight related functions. During the downstroke, the ulnar carpal bone prevents hyperpronation of the manus by transmitting forces to the ulna to stabilize it. When taking off or landing, there can be a flick of the manus. The upward component of the flick results from the interplay of the ventral portion of the ulnar carpal bone with the ventral ridge of the carpometacarpal bone and its ligamentous attachments (Vazquez 1992).

Metacarpal I

This is a small, cranially directed protuberance—the extensor process *[processus extensorius]*. The major metacarpal *[osmetacarpale majus]* and minor metacarpal *[osmetacarpale minus]* bones are fused both proximally and distally, forming an intermetacarpal space *[spatium intermetacarpale]* or interosseous space. These bones are flattened so that the primary remiges or primary flight feathers can take origin dorsally from this flattened carpometacarpus.

The alular digit *[phalanx digiti alulae]* is important to redirect airflow, thereby preventing separation of the flow of air during high angles of attack to prevent stalling. It usually has one phalanx, phalanx digiti alulae. The major digit normally has two phalanges, *phalanx proximalis digiti majoris* and *phalanx distalis digiti majoris*. The minor digit normally has one phalanx, *phalanx digiti minoris*.

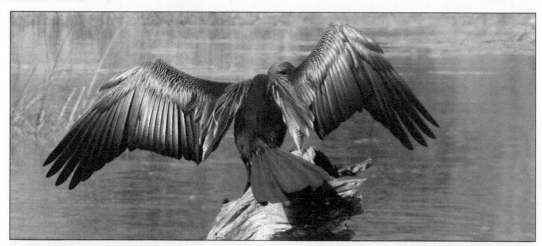

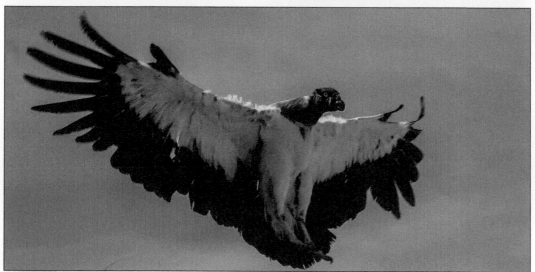

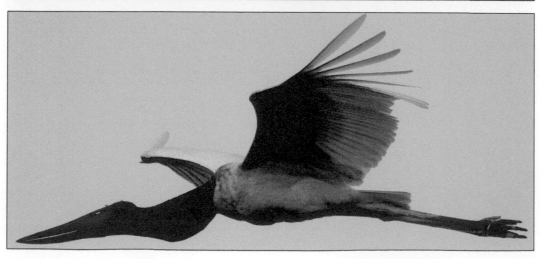

Dorsal Distal Skeleton

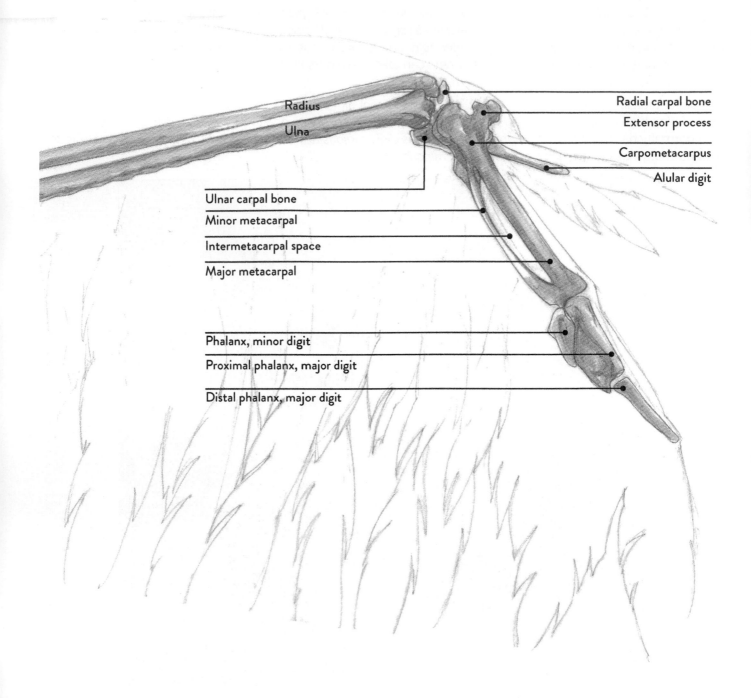

Radius

Ulna

Radial carpal bone

Extensor process

Carpometacarpus

Alular digit

Ulnar carpal bone

Minor metacarpal

Intermetacarpal space

Major metacarpal

Phalanx, minor digit

Proximal phalanx, major digit

Distal phalanx, major digit

Dorsal Distal Wing
Carpometacarpus and Digits

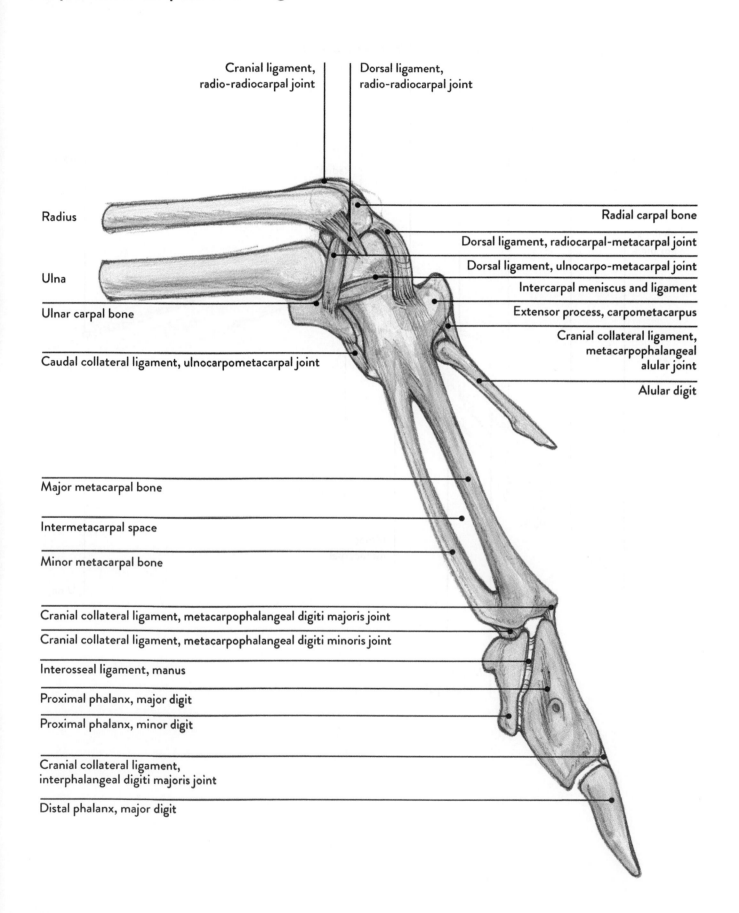

Cranial ligament, radio-radiocarpal joint

Dorsal ligament, radio-radiocarpal joint

Radius

Ulna

Ulnar carpal bone

Caudal collateral ligament, ulnocarpometacarpal joint

Radial carpal bone

Dorsal ligament, radiocarpal-metacarpal joint

Dorsal ligament, ulnocarpo-metacarpal joint

Intercarpal meniscus and ligament

Extensor process, carpometacarpus

Cranial collateral ligament, metacarpophalangeal alular joint

Alular digit

Major metacarpal bone

Intermetacarpal space

Minor metacarpal bone

Cranial collateral ligament, metacarpophalangeal digiti majoris joint

Cranial collateral ligament, metacarpophalangeal digiti minoris joint

Interosseal ligament, manus

Proximal phalanx, major digit

Proximal phalanx, minor digit

Cranial collateral ligament, interphalangeal digiti majoris joint

Distal phalanx, major digit

Ventral Distal Skeleton of the Wing

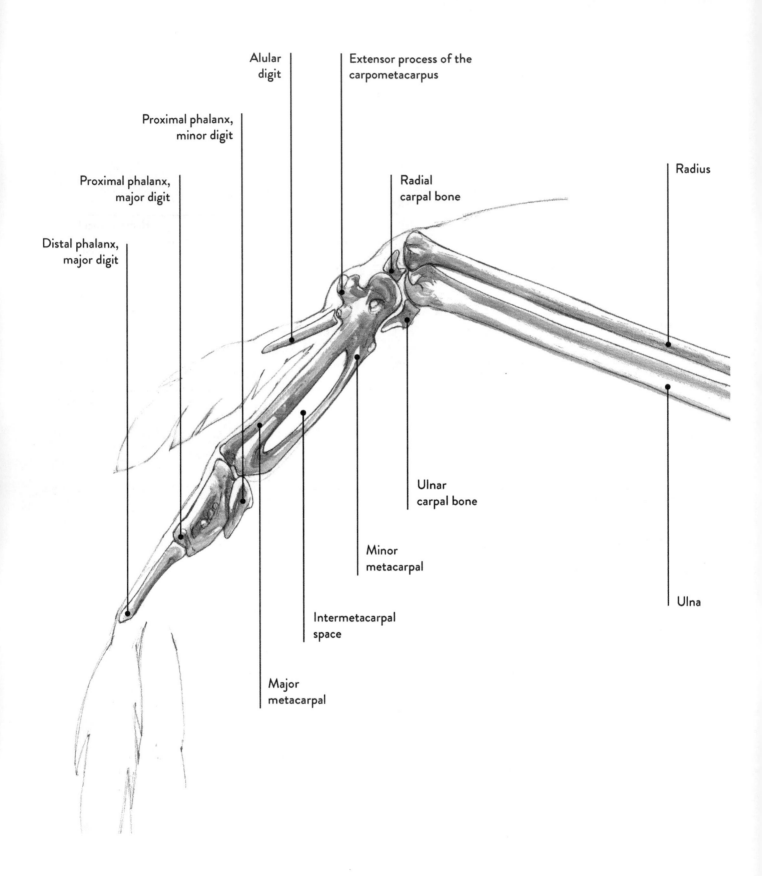

Alular digit

Proximal phalanx, minor digit

Proximal phalanx, major digit

Distal phalanx, major digit

Extensor process of the carpometacarpus

Radial carpal bone

Radius

Ulnar carpal bone

Minor metacarpal

Intermetacarpal space

Ulna

Major metacarpal

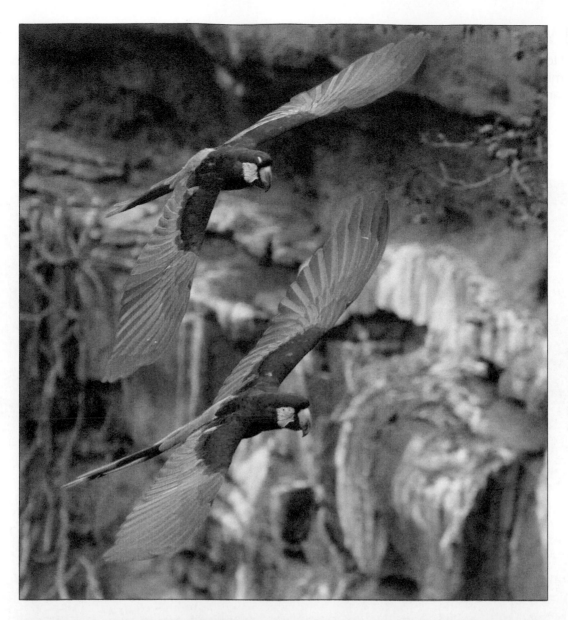

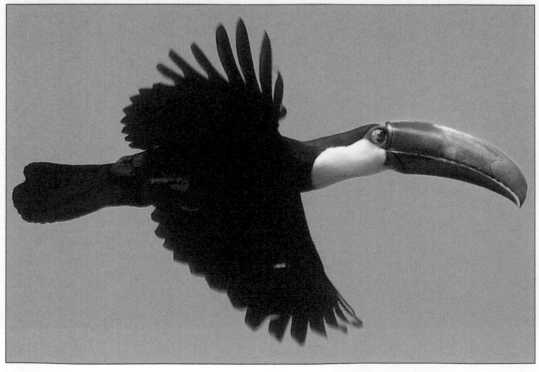

Distal Wing

Computed tomography images of the distal wing are presented for the orange-winged Amazon, umbrella cockatoo, military macaw, budgerigar, pigeon, chicken, red-tailed hawk, great horned owl, and golden eagle. Structures are color-coded, allowing easy recognition and ready comparison across species.

Orange-winged Amazon (*Amazona amazonica*)
Dorsal and Cranial Distal Wing

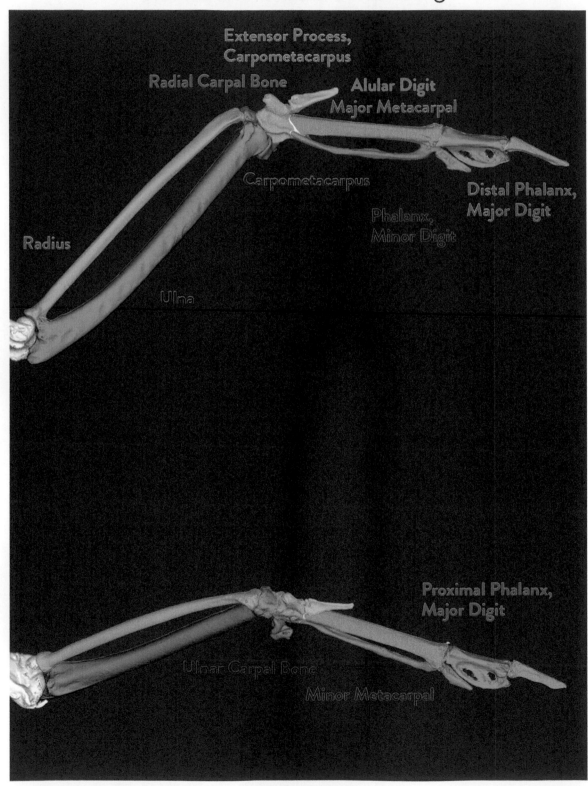

Orange-winged Amazon (*Amazona amazonica*)
Ventral and Caudal Distal Wing

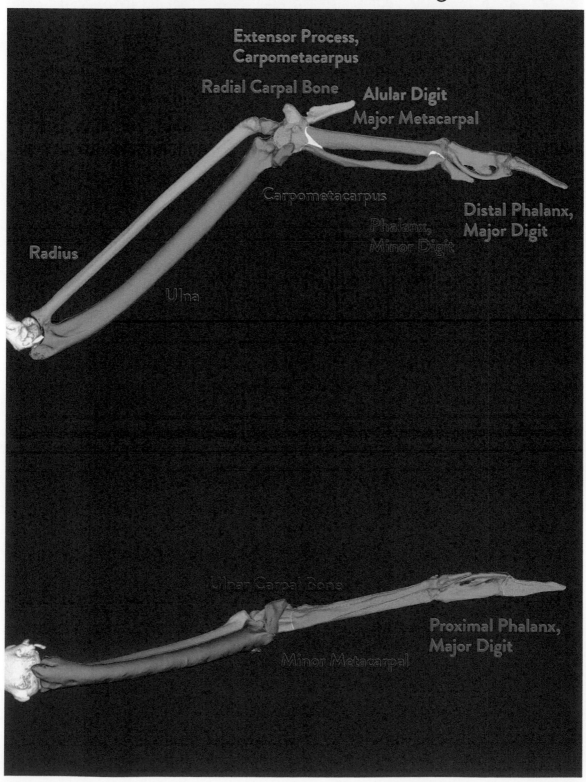

Umbrella Cockatoo (*Cacatua alba*)
Dorsal and Cranial Distal Wing

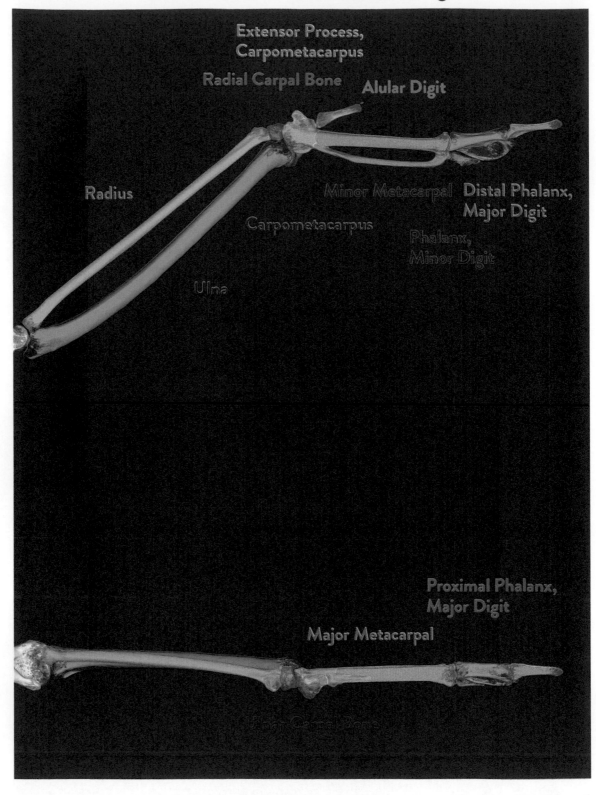

Umbrella Cockatoo *(Cacatua alba)*
Ventral and Caudal Distal Wing

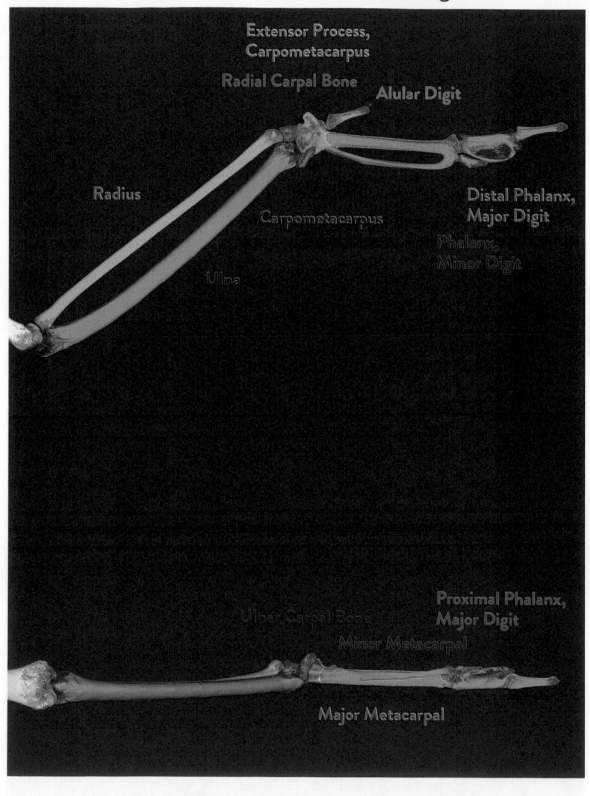

Military Macaw (*Ara militaris*)
Multiple Views of Distal Wing

Dorsal Cranial Oblique, Dorsal and Dorsal Caudal Oblique Distal Wing

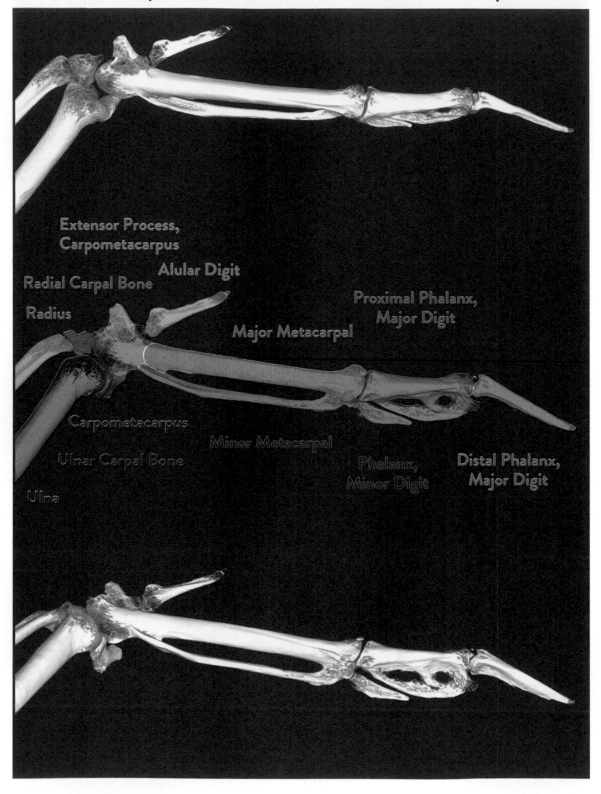

Military Macaw (*Ara militaris*)
Ventral Cranial Oblique, Ventral and Ventral Caudal Oblique Distal Wing

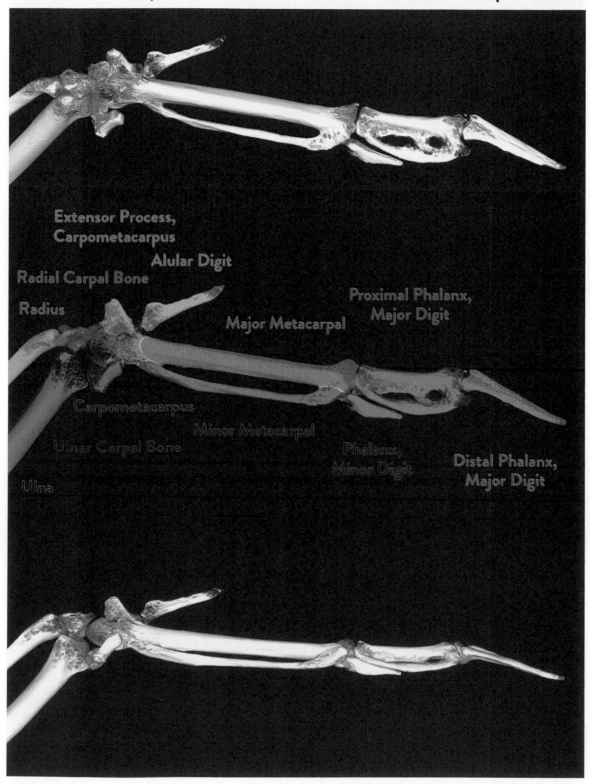

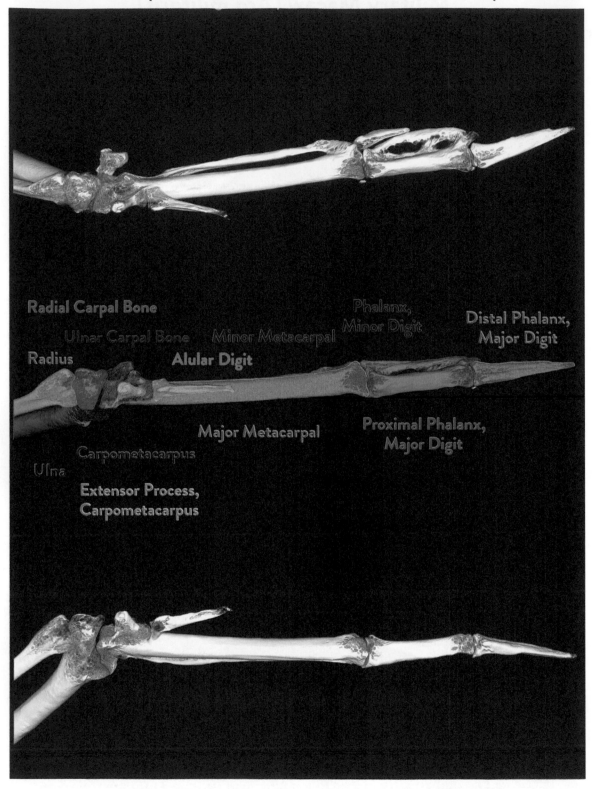

Military Macaw (*Ara militaris*)
Caudal Ventral Oblique, Caudal and Caudal Dorsal Oblique Distal Wing

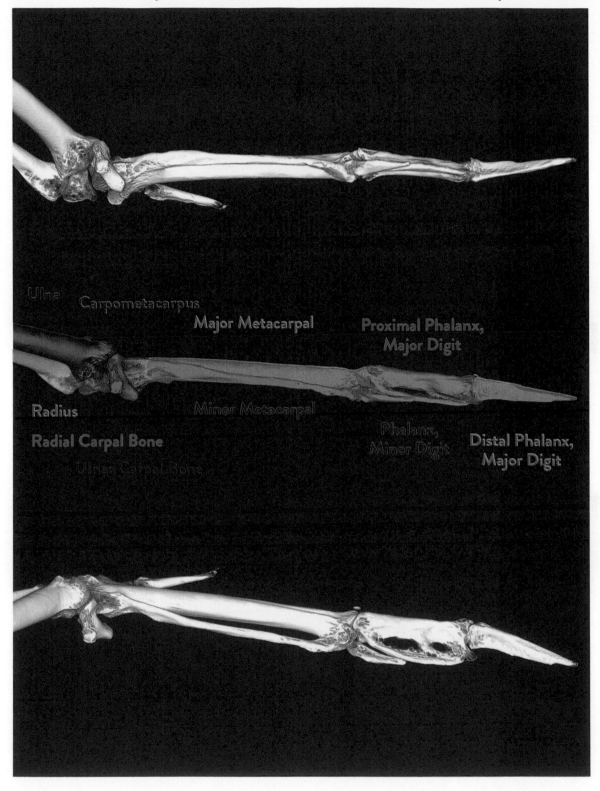

Ulna

Carpometacarpus

Major Metacarpal

Proximal Phalanx,
Major Digit

Radius

Minor Metacarpal

Radial Carpal Bone

Phalanx,
Minor Digit

Distal Phalanx,
Major Digit

Ulnar Carpal Bone

Budgerigar (*Melopsitticus undulatus*)
Dorsal and Cranial Distal Wing

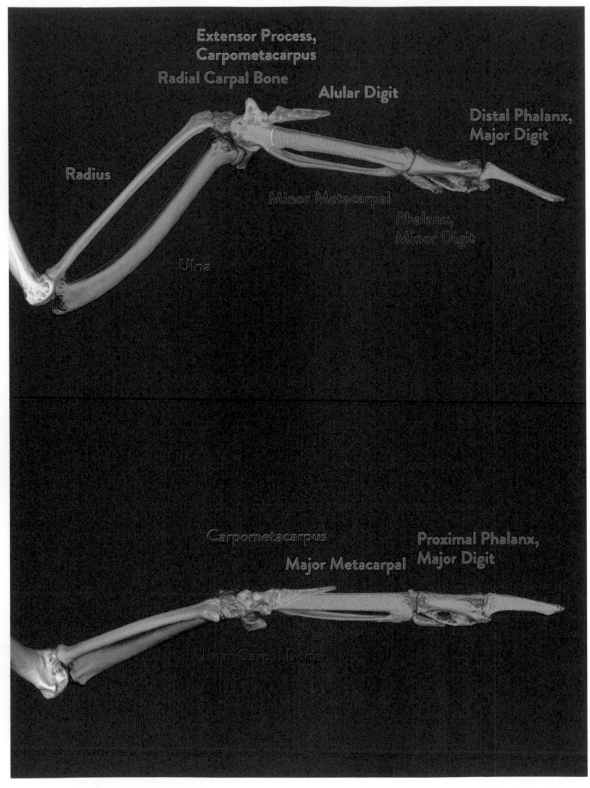

Budgerigar (*Melopsitticus undulatus*)
Ventral and Caudal Distal Wing

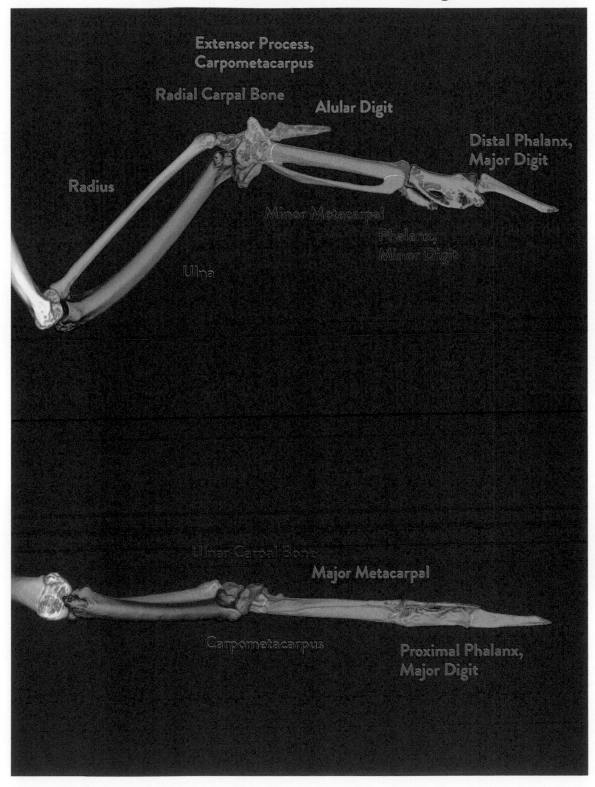

Pigeon (*Columba livia*)
Dorsal and Cranial Distal Wing

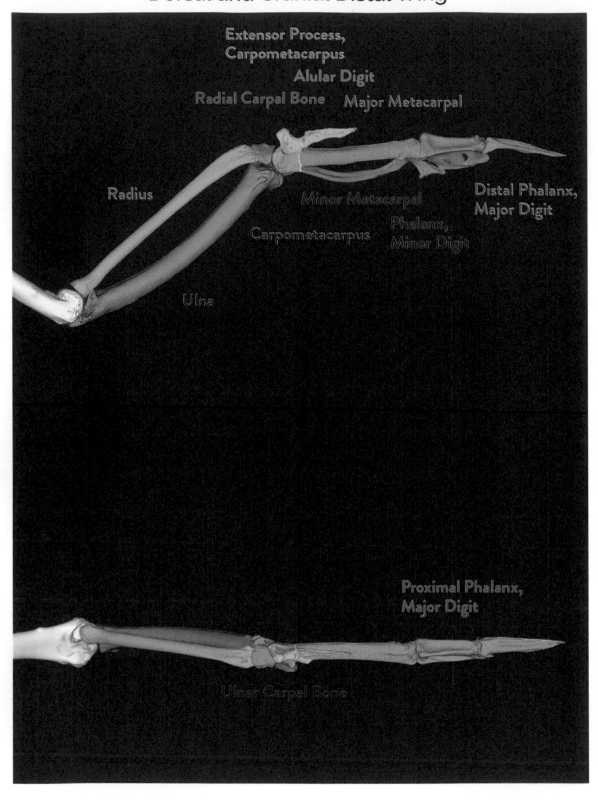

Extensor Process, Carpometacarpus

Alular Digit

Radial Carpal Bone

Major Metacarpal

Radius

Minor Metacarpal

Distal Phalanx, Major Digit

Carpometacarpus

Phalanx, Minor Digit

Ulna

Proximal Phalanx, Major Digit

Ulnar Carpal Bone

Pigeon (*Columba livia*)
Ventral and Caudal Distal Wing

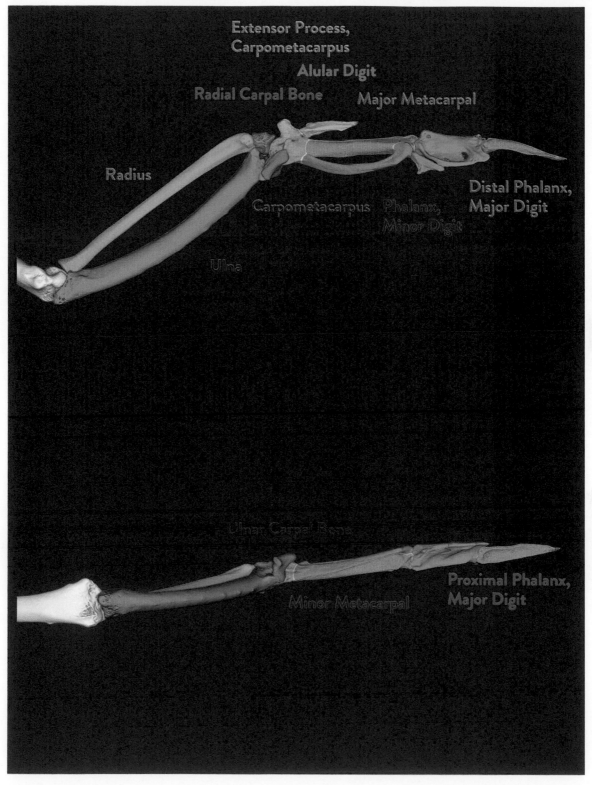

Extensor Process, Carpometacarpus

Alular Digit

Radial Carpal Bone

Major Metacarpal

Radius

Carpometacarpus

Phalanx, Minor Digit

Distal Phalanx, Major Digit

Ulna

Ulnar Carpal Bone

Minor Metacarpal

Proximal Phalanx, Major Digit

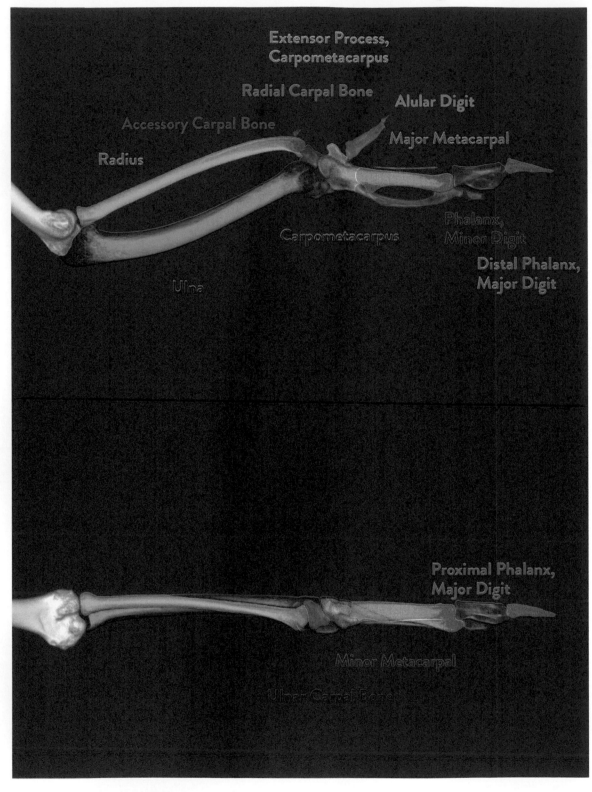

Domestic Chicken (*Gallus gallus domesticus*)
Ventral and Caudal Distal Wing

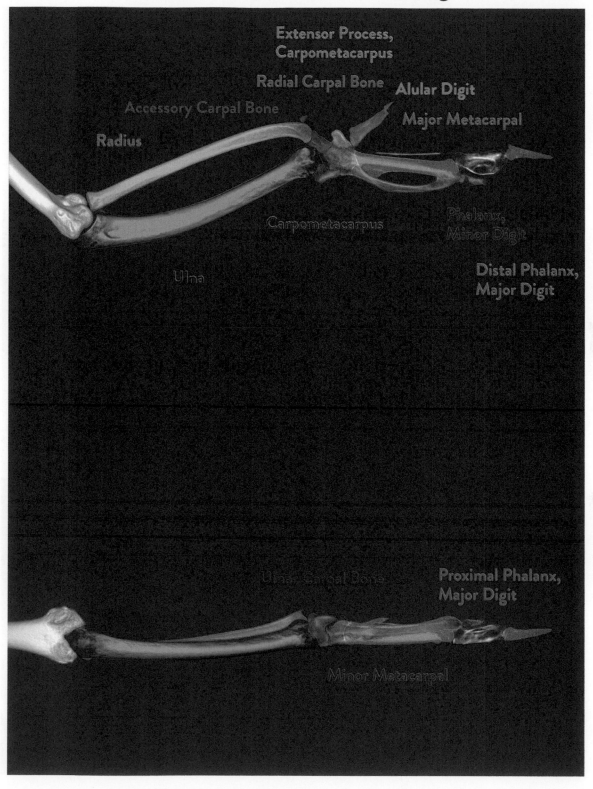

Red-tailed Hawk (*Buteo jamaicensis*)
Dorsal and Cranial Distal Wing

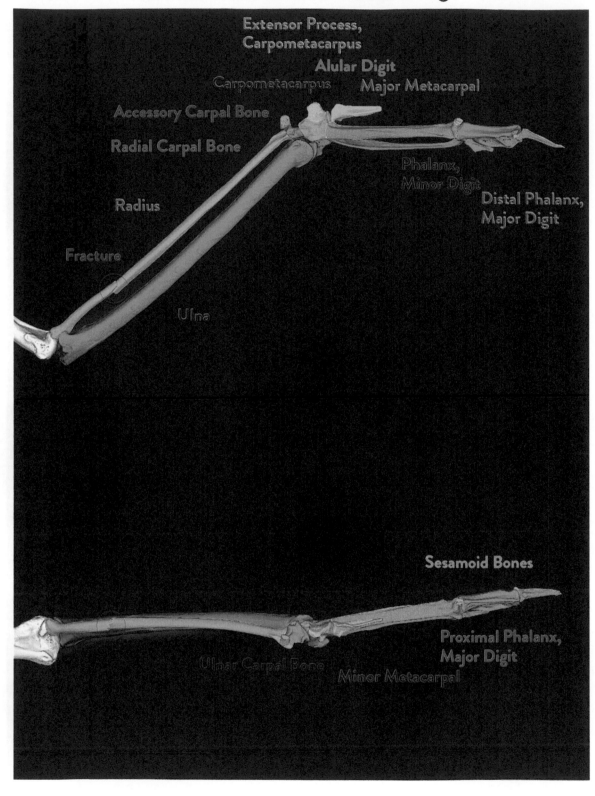

Extensor Process, Carpometacarpus

Alular Digit

Carpometacarpus

Major Metacarpal

Accessory Carpal Bone

Radial Carpal Bone

Phalanx, Minor Digit

Distal Phalanx, Major Digit

Radius

Fracture

Ulna

Sesamoid Bones

Proximal Phalanx, Major Digit

Ulnar Carpal Bone

Minor Metacarpal

Red-tailed Hawk *(Buteo jamaicensis)*
Ventral and Caudal Distal Wing

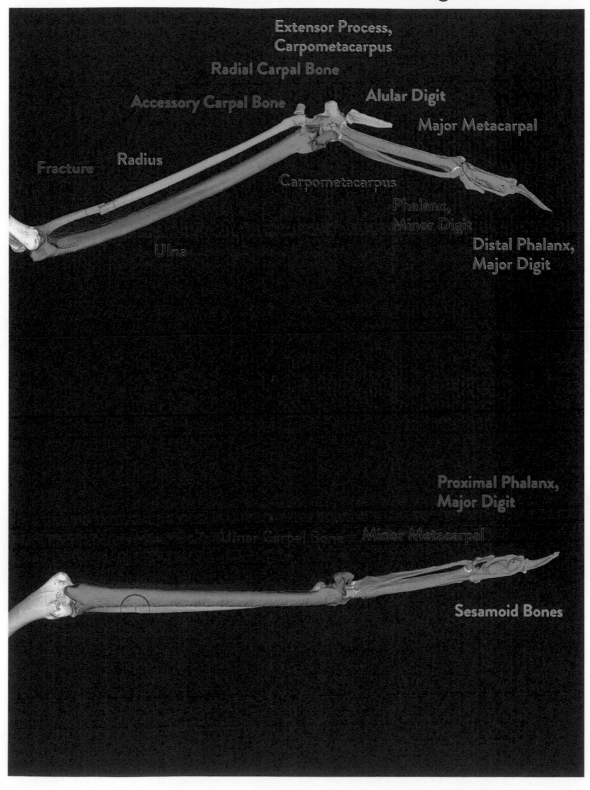

Great Horned Owl (*Bubo virginianus*)
Dorsal and Cranial Distal Wing

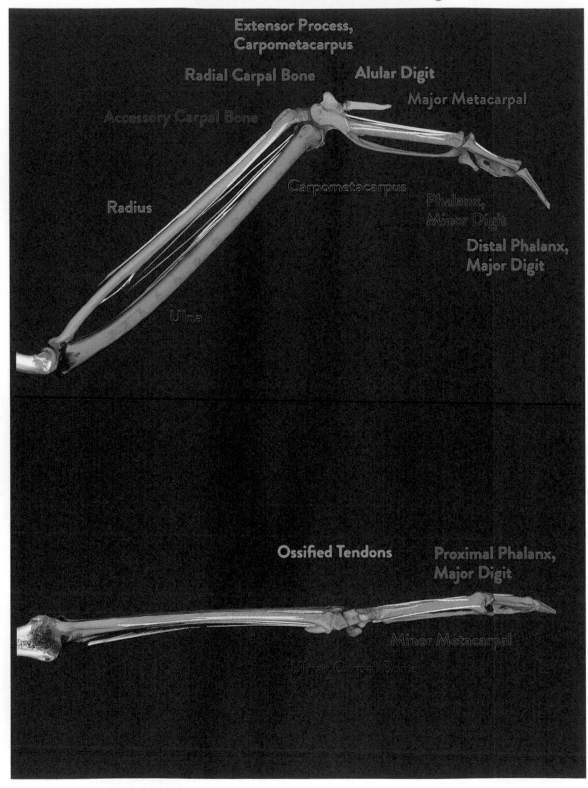

Extensor Process, Carpometacarpus

Radial Carpal Bone

Alular Digit

Major Metacarpal

Accessory Carpal Bone

Radius

Carpometacarpus

Phalanx, Minor Digit

Distal Phalanx, Major Digit

Ulna

Ossified Tendons

Proximal Phalanx, Major Digit

Minor Metacarpal

Ulnar Carpal Bone

Great Horned Owl (*Bubo virginianus*)
Ventral and Caudal Distal Wing

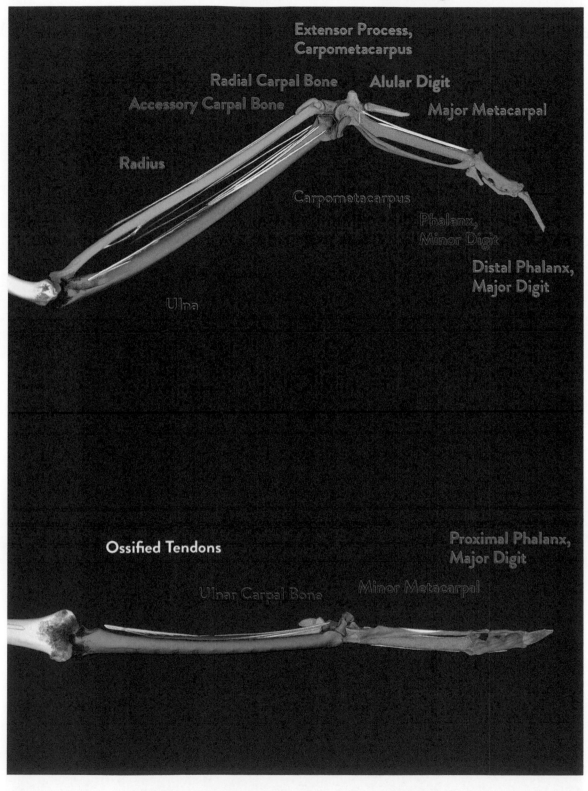

Extensor Process, Carpometacarpus

Radial Carpal Bone

Accessory Carpal Bone

Alular Digit

Major Metacarpal

Radius

Carpometacarpus

Phalanx, Minor Digit

Distal Phalanx, Major Digit

Ulna

Ossified Tendons

Proximal Phalanx, Major Digit

Ulnar Carpal Bone

Minor Metacarpal

Golden Eagle (*Aquila chrysaetos*)
Multiple Views of Distal Wing

Dorsal Cranial Oblique, Dorsal and Dorsal Caudal Oblique Distal Wing

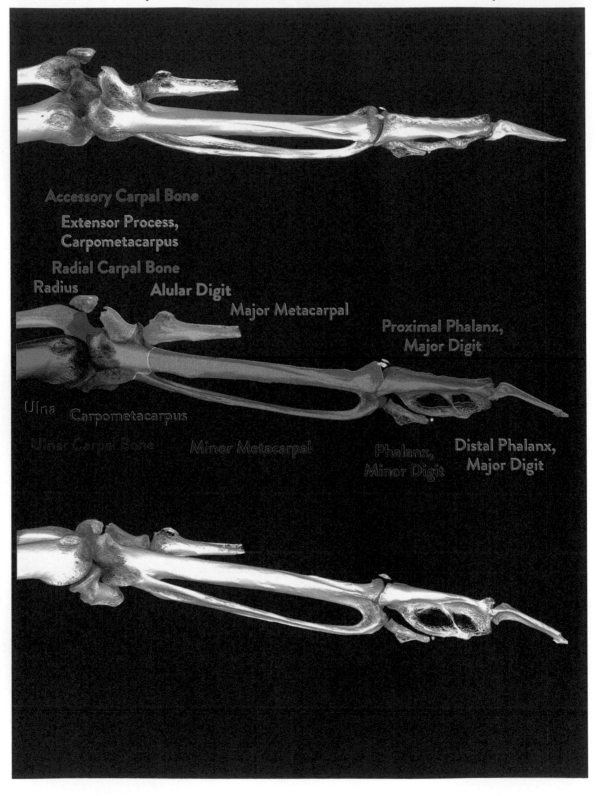

Golden Eagle *(Aquila chrysaetos)*
Ventral Cranial Oblique, Ventral and Ventral Caudal Oblique Distal Wing

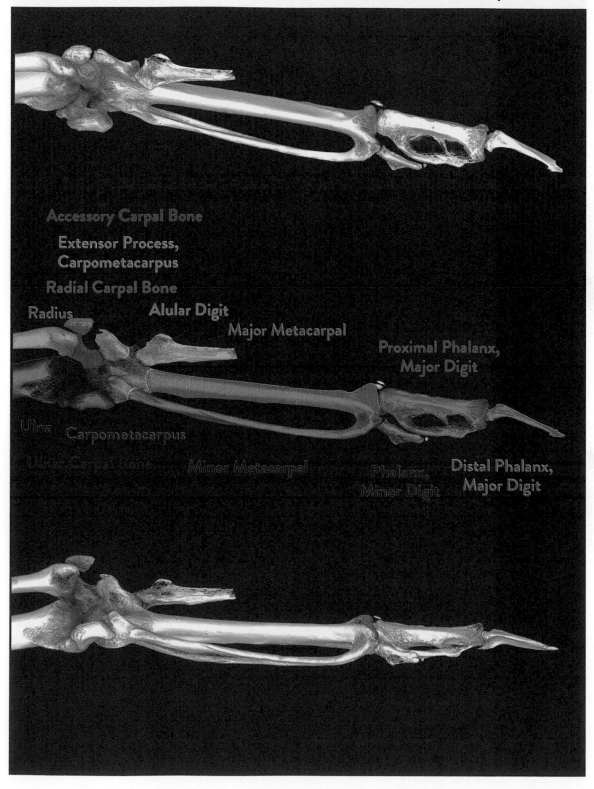

Accessory Carpal Bone

Extensor Process, Carpometacarpus

Radial Carpal Bone

Radius

Alular Digit

Major Metacarpal

Proximal Phalanx, Major Digit

Ulna

Carpometacarpus

Ulnar Carpal Bone

Minor Metacarpal

Phalanx, Minor Digit

Distal Phalanx, Major Digit

Golden Eagle (*Aquila chrysaetos*)
Cranial Ventral Oblique, Cranial and Cranial Dorsal Oblique Distal Wing

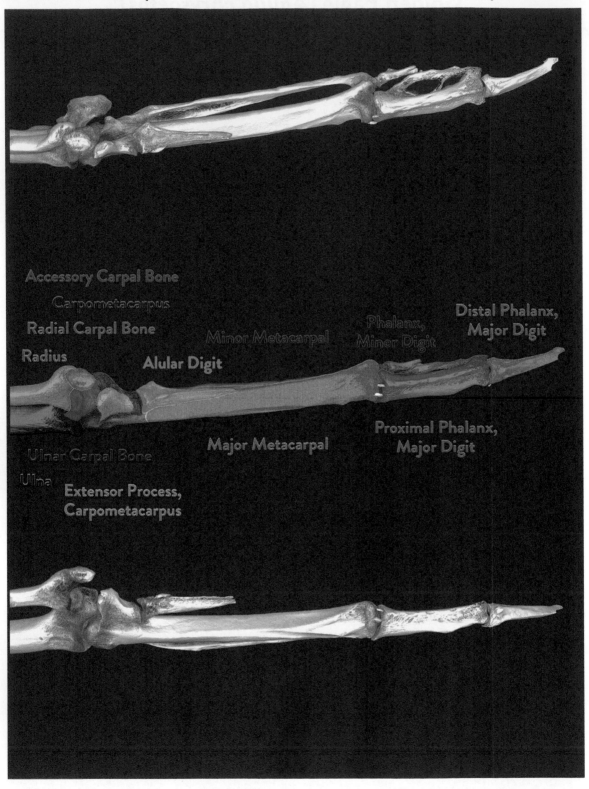

Accessory Carpal Bone

Carpometacarpus

Radial Carpal Bone

Radius

Alular Digit

Minor Metacarpal

Phalanx, Minor Digit

Distal Phalanx, Major Digit

Ulnar Carpal Bone

Ulna

Extensor Process, Carpometacarpus

Major Metacarpal

Proximal Phalanx, Major Digit

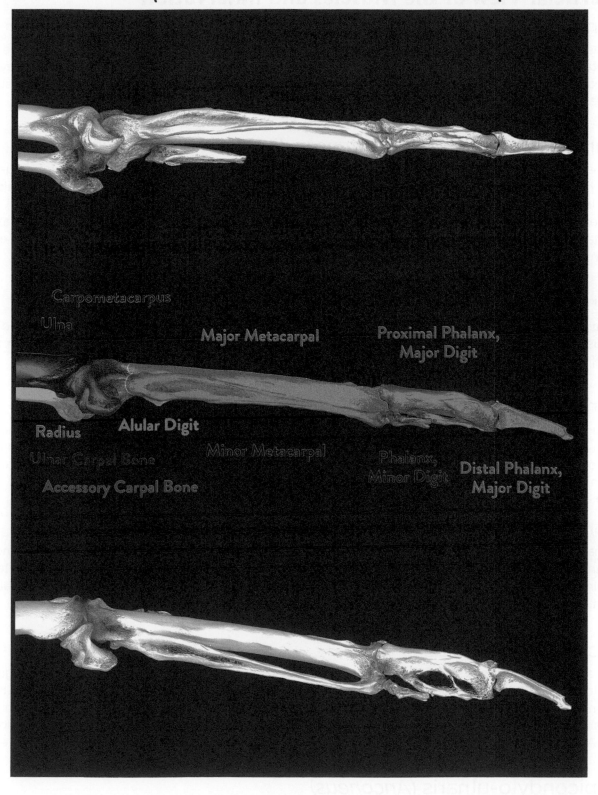

Carpometacarpus

Ulna

Major Metacarpal

Proximal Phalanx, Major Digit

Radius

Alular Digit

Minor Metacarpal

Ulnar Carpal Bone

Phalanx, Minor Digit

Distal Phalanx, Major Digit

Accessory Carpal Bone

Dorsal Distal Wing
Superficial View of the Muscles and Innervation
Extensor metacarpi radialis

This muscle is composed of two heads that insert as a common tendon onto the extensor process of the first metacarpal bone. Because it acts to extend the carpus and metacarpus, a portion of this tendon may be removed to deflight some species of birds. However, this may not work in others. In addition to its extension of the distal wing, it flexes the elbow.

Common digital extensor *(Extensor digitorum communis)*

This muscle takes origin at the same point as the supinator muscle on the dorsal condyle of the humerus. The muscle has a short tendon that inserts on the base of the alular digit [phalanx digiti alulae], while the major tendon inserts onto the base of the proximal phalanx of the major digit [phalanx proximalis digiti majoris]. It acts to extend the manus or the distal end of the wing, especially when the forearm is extended. It may assist in maintaining the position of the alula against the metacarpus during flight or stabilize the position of the alula (Fischer 1946, Getty 1975).

Supinator

The supinator usually takes origin with the extensor digitorum communis on the dorsal epicondyle of the humerus. It facilitates supination of the manus because it also elevates the cranial border of the forearm. It may help to flex the elbow (Fischer 1946, Getty 1975).

Extensor metacarpi ulnaris *(Ulnaris lateralis)*

This muscle is the caudal-most muscle of the 3 superficial muscles on the dorsal proximal aspect of the forearm or distal forewing. The tendinous origin of the extensor metacarpi ulnaris muscle is in common with the ectepicondylo-ulnaris or anconeus on the dorsal condyle of the humerus. While its name suggests an extensor function, this muscle flexes both the elbow and the manus when the wing is extended.

Ulnometacarpalis dorsalis *(Flexor metacarpi caudalis)*

This small muscle fills in the flexor space between the ulna and carpometacarpus. It inserts onto the minor metacarpal bone and onto the base of the primaries by tendinous slips. Just distal to this muscle is the flexor digiti minoris, which inserts onto the minor digit. The ulnometacarpalis dorsalis pulls the primaries medially or proximally to decrease the gap with the secondary flight feathers (Fischer 1946).

Muscles of the Manus

Soaring and gliding flight is associated with several small muscles of the carpus, carpometacarpus, and digits for fine motor control. The extensor brevis alulae extends the alular digit. The extensor longus alulae is a small muscle found on the caudal border of the distal radius, and it inserts on the extensor process of the carpometacarpus. It extends the manus, not the alula. The tendon of the extensor longus digiti majoris is found in a dorsal location at the carpus. Associated with its tendon of insertion is a small muscle, the extensor brevis digiti majoris (see figure below).

Ectepicondylo-ulnaris *(Anconeus)*

The origin of this muscle may be in common with the extensor metacarpi ulnaris. It inserts along the proximal cranial surface of the ulna to flex the elbow, as well as elevate it slightly (Fischer 1946).

Innervation

The muscles that originate from the humeral epicondyle and condyle are innervated by the radial nerve.

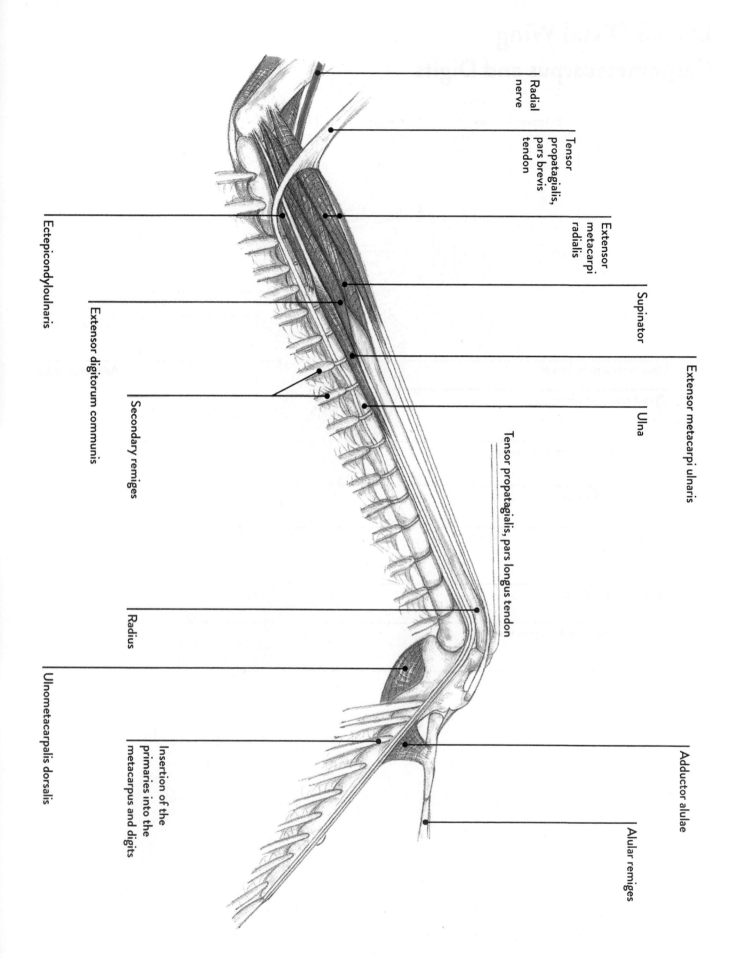

Radial nerve

Tensor propatagialis, pars brevis tendon

Extensor metacarpi radialis

Supinator

Extensor metacarpi ulnaris

Ulna

Ectepicondyloulnaris

Extensor digitorum communis

Secondary remiges

Tensor propatagialis, pars longus tendon

Radius

Ulnometacarpalis dorsalis

Insertion of the primaries into the metacarpus and digits

Adductor alulae

Alular remiges

161

Dorsal Distal Wing
Carpometacarpus and Digits

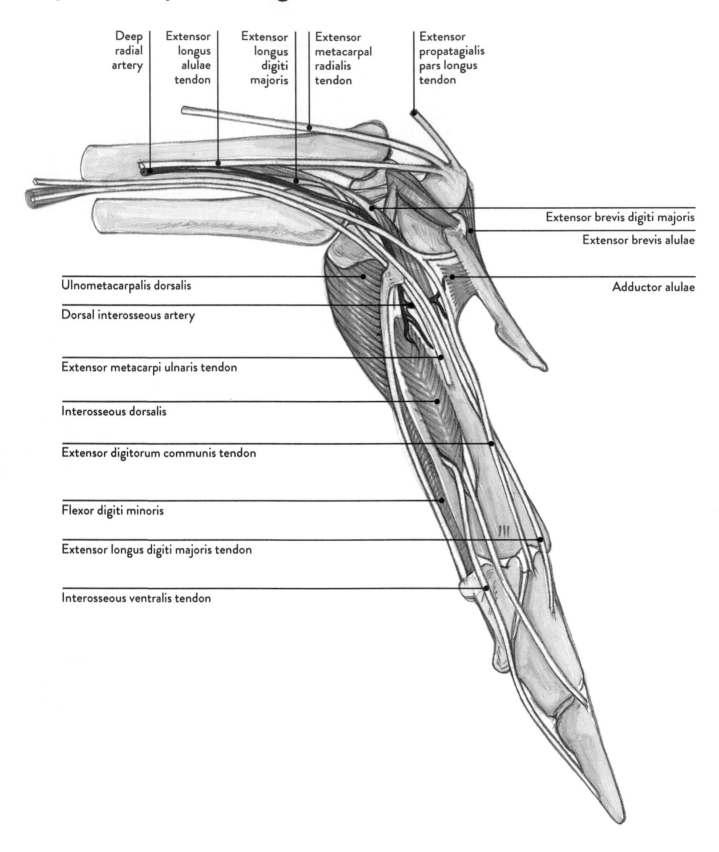

Deep radial artery

Extensor longus alulae tendon

Extensor longus digiti majoris

Extensor metacarpal radialis tendon

Extensor propatagialis pars longus tendon

Extensor brevis digiti majoris

Extensor brevis alulae

Adductor alulae

Ulnometacarpalis dorsalis

Dorsal interosseous artery

Extensor metacarpi ulnaris tendon

Interosseous dorsalis

Extensor digitorum communis tendon

Flexor digiti minoris

Extensor longus digiti majoris tendon

Interosseous ventralis tendon

Dorsal Proximal Radius and Ulna

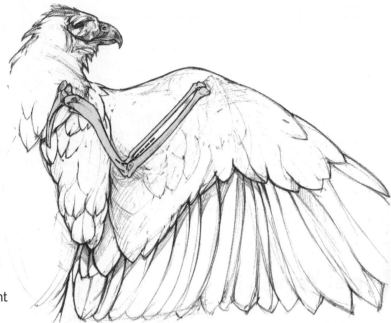

The orientation diagram to the right is intended to show the region depicted in the anatomical dissections below. It is not intended to represent a surgical approach.

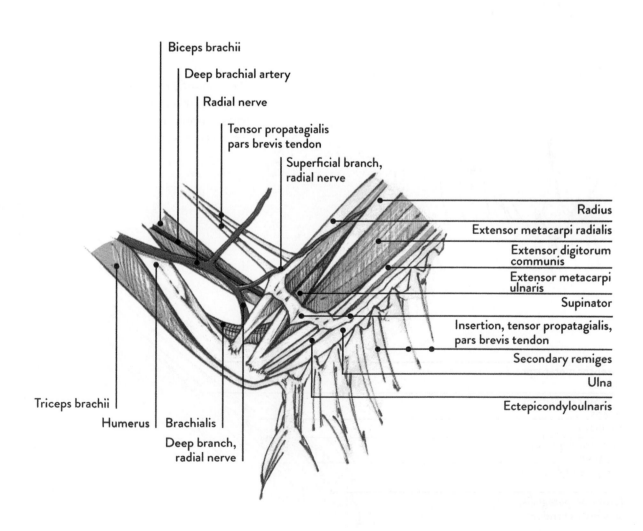

Biceps brachii

Deep brachial artery

Radial nerve

Tensor propatagialis pars brevis tendon

Superficial branch, radial nerve

Radius

Extensor metacarpi radialis

Extensor digitorum communis

Extensor metacarpi ulnaris

Supinator

Insertion, tensor propatagialis, pars brevis tendon

Secondary remiges

Ulna

Ectepicondyloulnaris

Triceps brachii

Humerus

Brachialis

Deep branch, radial nerve

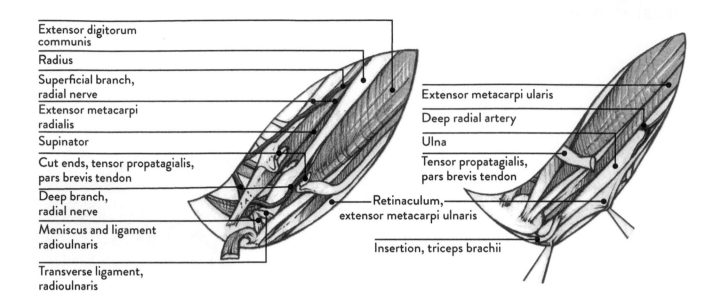

Extensor digitorum
communis

Radius

Superficial branch,
radial nerve

Extensor metacarpi
radialis

Supinator

Cut ends, tensor propatagialis,
pars brevis tendon

Deep branch,
radial nerve

Meniscus and ligament
radioulnaris

Transverse ligament,
radioulnaris

Extensor metacarpi ularis

Deep radial artery

Ulna

Tensor propatagialis,
pars brevis tendon

Retinaculum,
extensor metacarpi ulnaris

Insertion, triceps brachii

Dorsal Wing

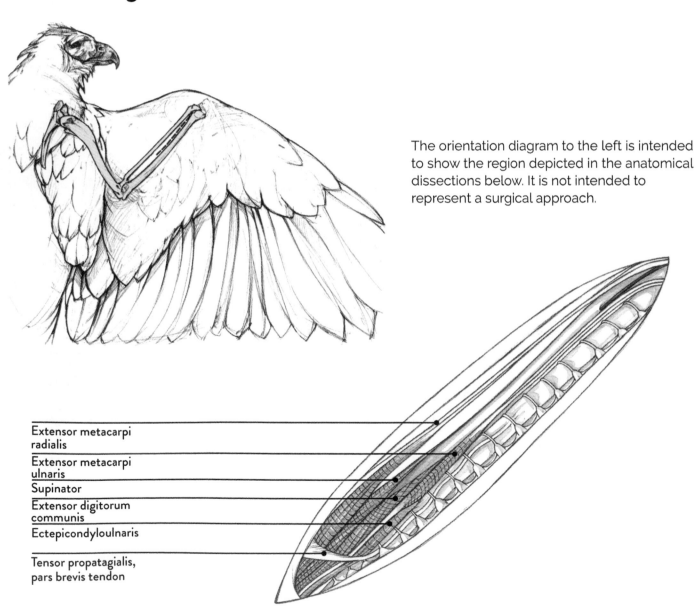

The orientation diagram to the left is intended
to show the region depicted in the anatomical
dissections below. It is not intended to
represent a surgical approach.

Extensor metacarpi
radialis

Extensor metacarpi
ulnaris

Supinator

Extensor digitorum
communis

Ectepicondyloulnaris

Tensor propatagialis,
pars brevis tendon

Ventral Distal Wing
Pronator superficialis and Pronator profundus *(Pronator brevis and longus)*

These muscles originate on the ventral epicondyle *(epicondylus ventralis)* of the humerus and insert onto the radius. These muscles are innervated by the median nerve. By pronating the wing, they depress the cranial edge (Fischer 1946).

Flexor carpi ulnaris

The flexor carpi ulnaris has been described as having three (Fischer 1946) or two (Getty 1975, International Committee on Avian Anatomical Nomenclature 1979) muscle bellies. It is probably more convenient to describe this muscle as having two muscle bellies that insert onto the ulnar carpal bone. The muscle is innervated by the ulnar nerve and functions to flex the elbow and carpal joints (Fischer 1946).

Flexor digitorum superficialis

The muscle and tendon cranial to the flexor carpi ulnaris collectively form the flexor digitorum superficialis. It crosses the carpus to insert onto the base of the distal phalanx of the major digit. It is innervated by the median nerve. When the wing is in full extension, the muscle may flex the distal end of the wing ventrally (Getty 1975). However, it may act to extend the wing (Fischer 1946).

Flexor digitorum profundus

This flexor originates from the palmar surface of the ulna and inserts onto the distal phalanx of the major digit. It is innervated by the median nerve. The muscle flexes the metacarpus and may also depress and extend the major digit. These actions are important for flex gliding (Fischer 1946).

Extensor longus digiti majoris

This muscle originates on the ventral side of the radius but crosses the carpus to insert dorsally on the distal phalanx of the major digit. It is innervated by the radial nerve. Associated with the tendon of insertion is a small muscle, the extensor brevis digiti majoris, on the dorsum of the metacarpus. The combined muscle and tendon extend the major digit and the carpus (Fischer 1946).

Abductor digiti majoris

This muscle lies between the tendons of the flexor digitorum profundus and the superficialis. It is a small muscle on the palmar side of the metacarpus that inserts on the base of the major digit. The abductor depresses the major digit ventrally and extends it (Fischer 1946).

Abductor alulae

This tiny muscle is the most cranial muscle on the palmar side of the carpus. It originates from the inserting tendon of the extensor metacarpi radialis and extends the alula (Getty 1975). It is innervated by the median nerve and pulls the alula toward the flat plane of the carpometacarpus.

Flexor alulae

The muscle lies next to the abductor. It is innervated by the deep ramus of the median nerve. It is important in keeping the alula against the carpometacarpus, as well as in flexing the digit (Fischer 1946).

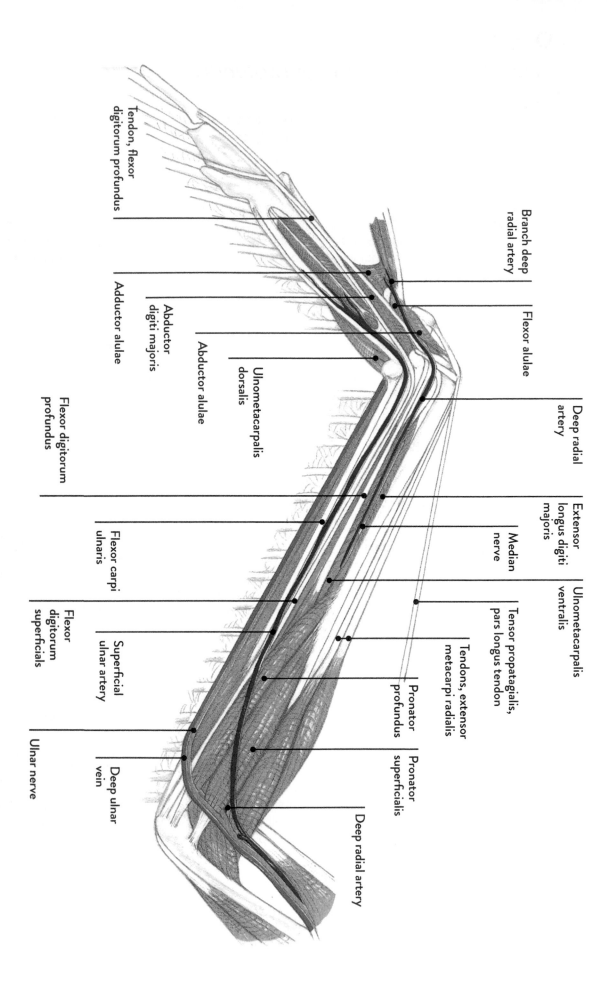

Tendon, flexor digitorum profundus

Branch deep radial artery

Flexor alulae

Adductor alulae

Abductor digiti majoris

Abductor alulae

Ulnometacarpalis dorsalis

Deep radial artery

Flexor digitorum profundus

Extensor longus digiti majoris

Median nerve

Ulnometacarpalis ventralis

Flexor carpi ulnaris

Tensor propatagialis, pars longus tendon

Tendons, extensor metacarpi radialis

Flexor digitorum superficialis

Superficial ulnar artery

Pronator profundus

Pronator superficialis

Ulnar nerve

Deep ulnar vein

Deep radial artery

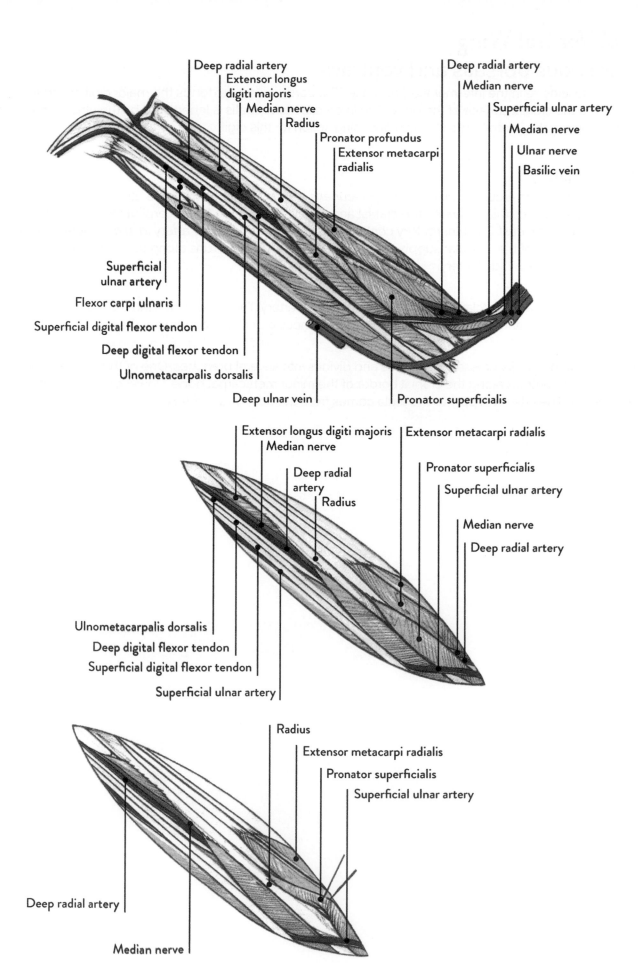

Deep radial artery
Extensor longus
digiti majoris
Median nerve
Radius
Pronator profundus
Extensor metacarpi
radialis

Deep radial artery
Median nerve
Superficial ulnar artery
Median nerve
Ulnar nerve
Basilic vein

Superficial
ulnar artery
Flexor carpi ulnaris
Superficial digital flexor tendon
Deep digital flexor tendon
Ulnometacarpalis dorsalis
Deep ulnar vein
Pronator superficialis

Extensor longus digiti majoris
Median nerve
Deep radial
artery
Radius

Extensor metacarpi radialis
Pronator superficialis
Superficial ulnar artery
Median nerve
Deep radial artery

Ulnometacarpalis dorsalis
Deep digital flexor tendon
Superficial digital flexor tendon
Superficial ulnar artery

Radius
Extensor metacarpi radialis
Pronator superficialis
Superficial ulnar artery

Deep radial artery

Median nerve

Distal Ventral Wing
Interosseous dorsalis and ventralis
These two muscles lie in the intermetacarpal space. The dorsal muscle extends the major digit owing to its insertion onto the cranial surface of the bone. The interosseous ventralis is innervated by the ulnar nerve. The caudal insertion of the ventralis results in an opposing action for this digit.

Blood Supply
In the elbow region, the recurrent ulnar artery [a. recurrens ulnaris] branches from the ulnar artery. The recurrent ulnar artery continues distally between the cranial and caudal parts of the flexor carpi ulnaris as the deep ulnar artery [a. ulnaris profundus]. The ulnar artery continues as the superficial ulnar artery [a. ulnaris superficialis], which provides most of the vascular supply to the manus. The artery that runs along the caudal, palmar surface of the radius is the deep radial artery.

Usually several veins are associated with a small, deep ulnar artery. These veins provide most of the venous drainage to the manus and antebrachium. Several small venous branches accompany the superficial ulnar artery.

The superficial ulnar artery crosses the carpus and divides into several branches. One of these dives deep to the interosseous ventralis along the cranial border of the minor metacarpal bone. However, its location may vary among species. The arterial supply to the alula comes from the deep radial artery.

Ventral Distal Wing

The red dotted lines in the drawing below illustrate the area depicted in the following section. The orientation drawing is not intended to represent a surgical approach.

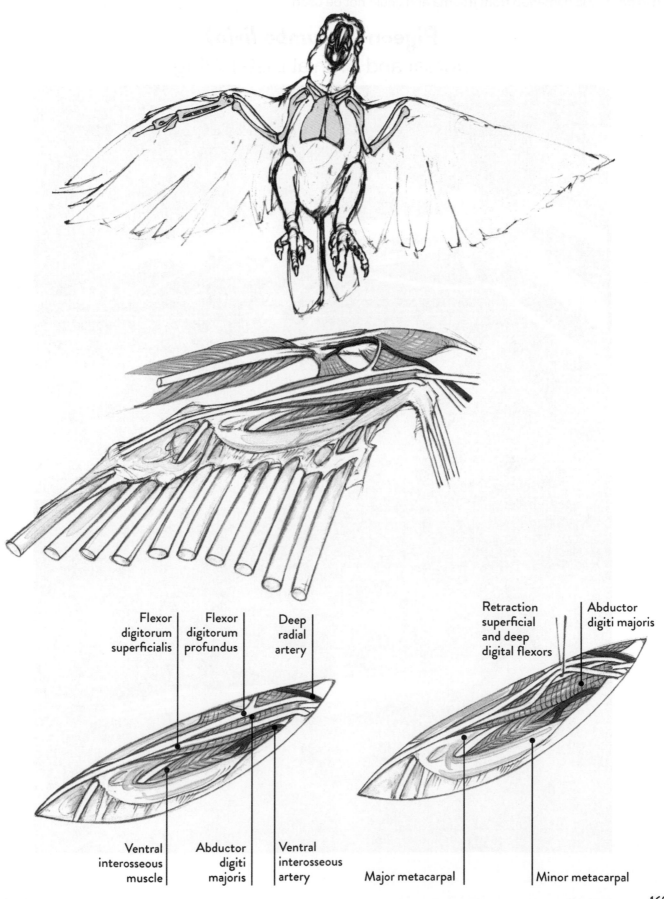

Flexor digitorum superficialis

Flexor digitorum profundus

Deep radial artery

Retraction superficial and deep digital flexors

Abductor digiti majoris

Ventral interosseous muscle

Abductor digiti majoris

Ventral interosseous artery

Major metacarpal

Minor metacarpal

Vasculature Contrast Images of the Distal Wing

Vasculature contrast images of the distal wing are presented for three species: the pigeon *(Columba livia)*, painted stork *(Mycteria leucoephala)*, and African goose *(Anser anser domesticus)*. The distal wing of a barn owl *(Tyto alba)* was damaged from trauma and could not be used.

Pigeon *(Columba livia)*
Dorsal and Cranial Distal Wing

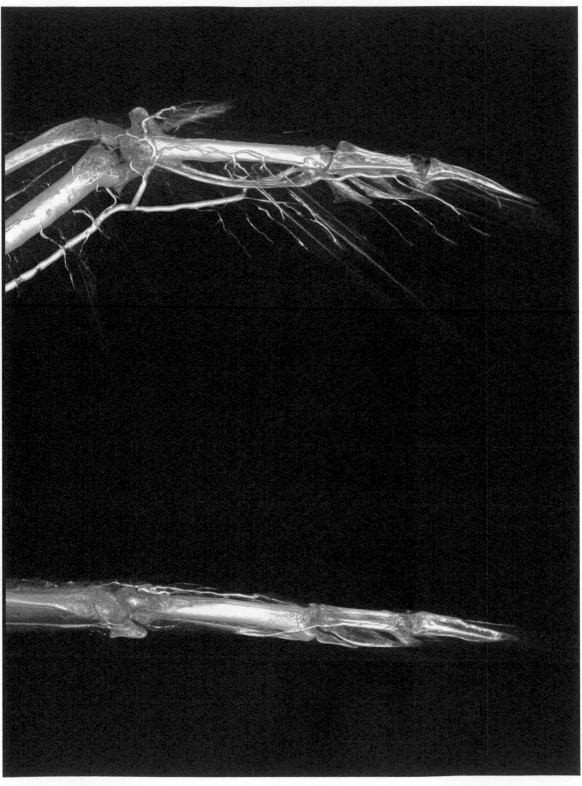

Pigeon (*Columba livia*)
Ventral and Caudal Distal Wing

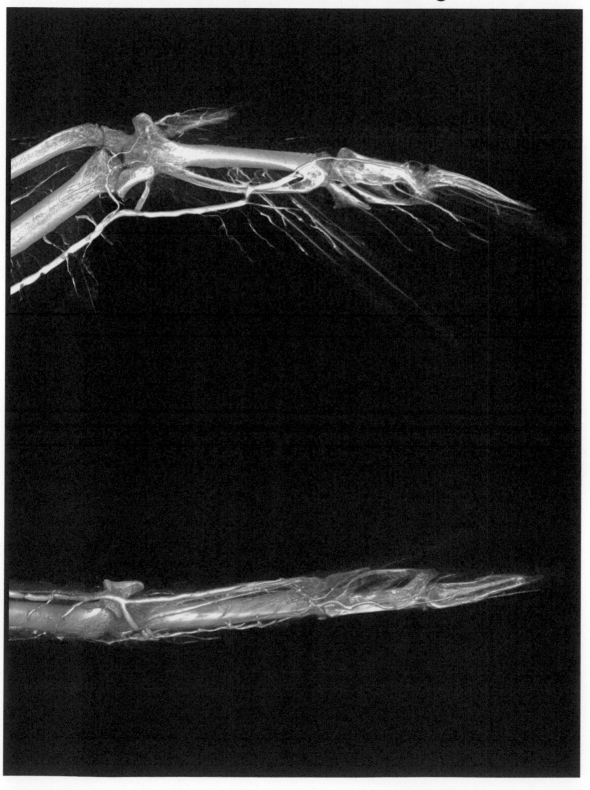

Painted Stork (*Mycteria leucocephala*)
Dorsal and Cranial Distal Wing

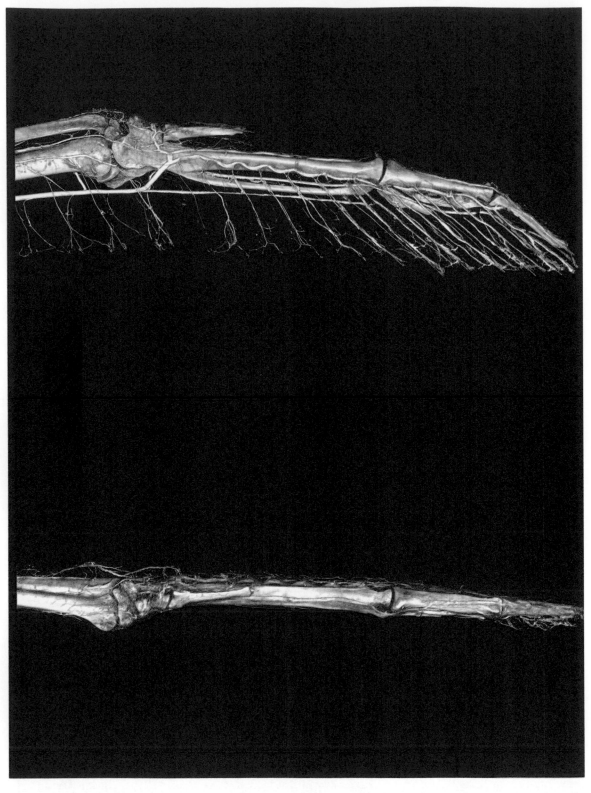

Painted Stork (*Mycteria leucocephala*)
Ventral and Caudal Distal Wing

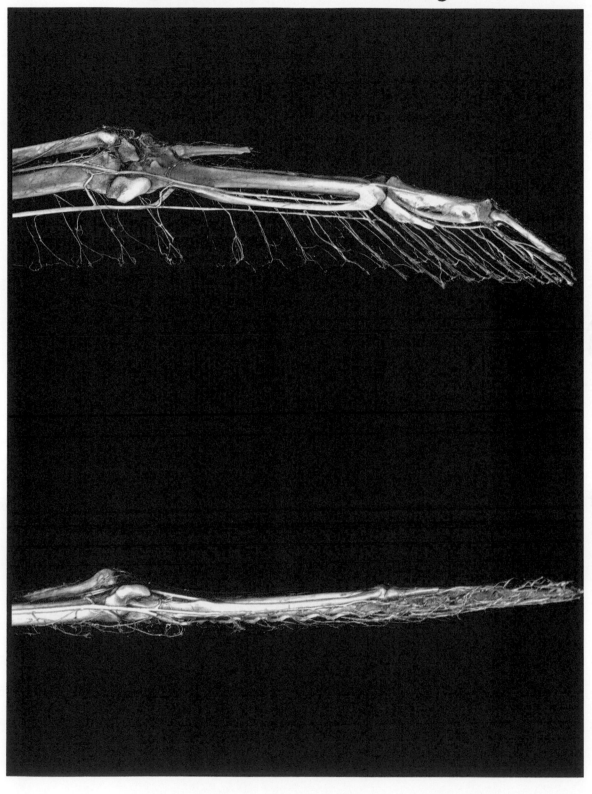

African Goose (*Anser anser domesticus*)
Dorsal and Cranial Distal Wing

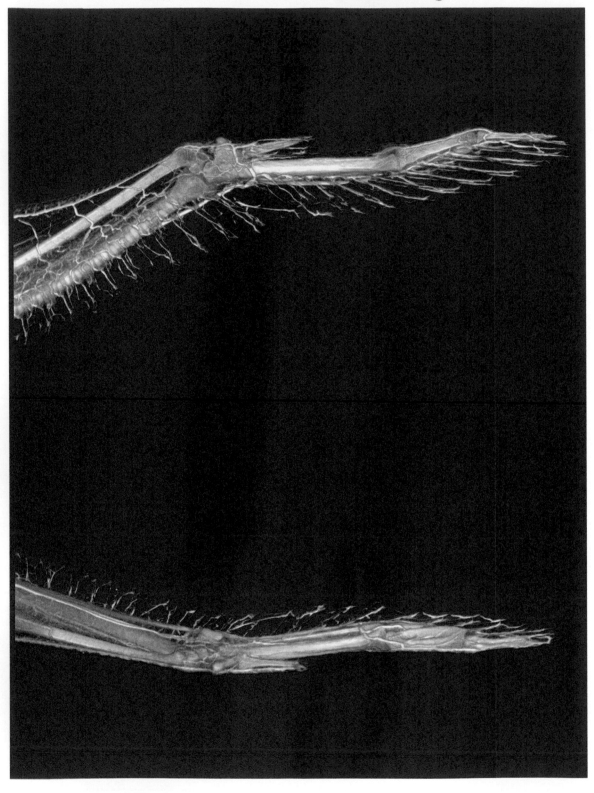

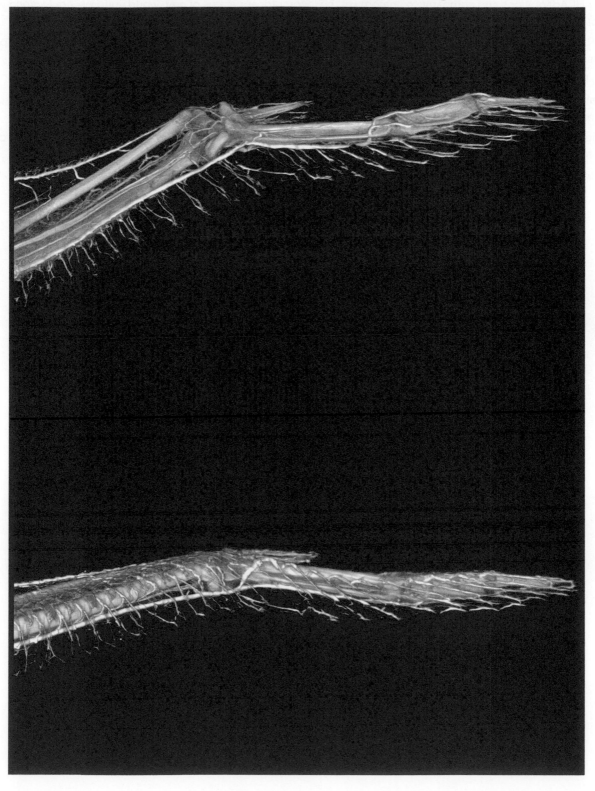

Recommended Reading

1. Baumel J. Functional anatomy of the avian thoracic limb: selected topics. *Proc Annu Conf Assoc Avian Vet.* 1983;67-70.

2. Fischer HI. Adaptations and comparative anatomy of the locomotor apparatus of new world vultures. *Am Midland Naturalist.* 1946; 35:545-727.

3. Getty R. *Sisson and Grossman's Anatomy of the Domestic Animals.* 5th ed. Vol. 2. Porcine, Carnivores, Aves. Philadelphia: WB Saunders; 1975.

4. Kaupp BF. *The Anatomy of the Domestic Fowl.* Philadelphia: WB Saunders; 1918.

5. International Committee on Avian Anatomical Nomenclature. *Nomina Anatomica Avium.* 1st ed. London: World Association of Veterinary Anatomists; 1979.

6. Shufeldt RW. The myology of the raven (*Corvus corax sinuatus*). A guide to the study of the muscular system in birds. London: MacMillan and Co; 1890. 343 pp.

7. Vazquez RJ. Functional osteology of the avian wrist and the evolution of flapping flight. *J Morphol.* 1992;211(3):259-268.

CHAPTER 6

Management of Wing Fractures

Methods of Fixation for the Humerus
General Considerations

The humerus can be divided into three zones for selection of fixation methods. The **proximal zone** extends from the head of the humerus and the dorsal tubercle to the distal extension of the pectoral crest. This proximal region has a pronounced curvature in its midsection. The **diaphyseal zone** is straight and extends from the distal end of the pectoral crest to the apex of the distal diaphyseal curvature. The **distal zone** involves the curved portion of the distal humerus proximal to the elbow joint. Fractures in the proximal and distal zones tend to be transverse while those in the diaphyseal region are often oblique, comminuted, and open. These factors affect the choice of the tie-in fixator to be used, the approach to inserting the intramedullary pin, and the choice of ancillary procedures needed to stabilize the fracture.

Application of the Tie-In Fixator to Midshaft Diaphyseal Fractures of the Humerus: The Archetypical Planform

Diaphyseal fractures of the humerus are repaired readily unless there is excessive comminution or extensive exteriorization of bone fragments. The pertinent anatomy for surgical management is presented in Chapter 5. Most diaphyseal fractures are oblique, with the proximal fragment tending to project through the dorsal surface of the wing due to the pull from the pectoral muscles. The distal fragment either projects through the skin on the ventral surface or is pulled up against the radius and ulna, owing to the contraction and/or the pull of the biceps and triceps muscles **(Figure 6-1)**.

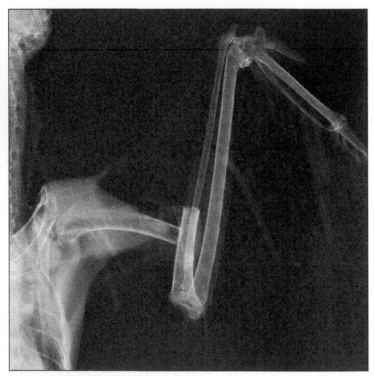

Figure 6-1. Radiograph showing the typical displacement of fragments associated with a midshaft diaphyseal fracture of the humerus.

The radial nerve passes from its caudal location at the insertion of the deltoideus major muscle across the dorsal aspect of the humerus to its cranial and superficial location as it dives into the dorsal forelimb musculature **(Figure 6-2)**. This is a particularly vulnerable location and the nerve must be identified and preserved.

Manipulation and preservation of this nerve is a constant feature of managing diaphyseal fractures. The triceps tendon courses distally on the caudal aspect of the humerus, wrapping around the distal end between the condyles and attaching to the caudal aspect of the ulna. The triceps is a very strong muscle and the bending moment it applies to the humerus is a force that must be counteracted by the fixation device.

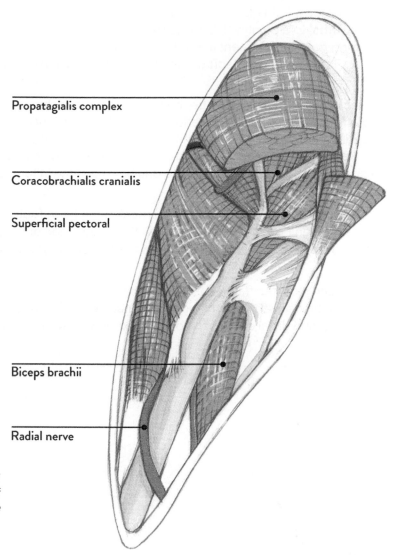

Propatagialis complex

Coracobrachialis cranialis

Superficial pectoral

Biceps brachii

Radial nerve

Figure 6-2. Dorsal view. Drawing of the musculature of the proximal humeral anatomy following transection of the propatagialis complex of muscles. The radial nerve emerges just distal to the insertion of the deltoideus major muscle to cross the humeral shaft, making it vulnerable to trauma.

Surgical Approach to the Diaphyseal Zone of the Humerus

The intramedullary pin component of the tie-in fixator may be applied in one of two ways, normograde or retrograde. For either, the patient is placed in ventral recumbency and the wing is prepped from shoulder to just distal to the elbow by removal of all feathers including the long scapulars to provide clean exposure for aseptic surgery **(Figure 6-3)**.

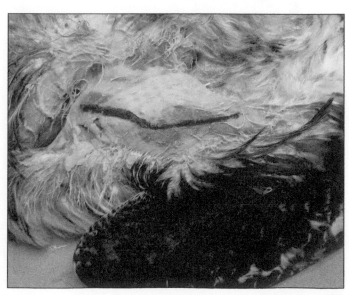

Figure 6-3. Clean exposure is accomplished by removal of all feathers from the shoulder to just distal to the elbow. Black line indicates location of the incision line.

For retrograde IM pin placement, a linear incision is made generally extending from the area of the distal pectoral crest to a point well beyond the fracture site, passing through any opening in the skin made by a projecting fracture fragment and taking care to identify and preserve the radial nerve. The skin is reflected laterally. There is no other soft tissue covering this section of bone so there is no further dissection.

The fracture fragments should be rongeured to remove sharp points and dead bone. If needed, affix bone clamps to both fragments and attempt reduction; conduct additional dissection of fibrous soft tissue around the fracture as needed to obtain reduction. If the medullary cavity, which is normally filled with air as a natural extension of the clavicular air sac, on either side of the fracture site has an internal callus, this should be removed by drilling with an oversized Steinman pin or appropriate drill bit so that the intramedullary pin is not deviated during insertion.

The specific steps involved in the placement of the tie-in fixator on the humerus by retrograde IM pin placement are illustrated in Figures 6-4 through 6-6. First is insertion of the pin at the fracture site and driving it retrograde until the distal end of the pin is flush with the end of the proximal fracture fragment **(Figure 6-4A & B)**.

In the second step, the fracture is reduced, and the pin is driven into the distal fragment. This is followed by placement of positive profile threaded external skeletal fixator pins (IMEX® Veterinary, Inc., Longview, TX, USA) in the proximal and distal ends of the bone **(Figures 6-5A-C)**. Carefully note the locations of these pins in the diagram.

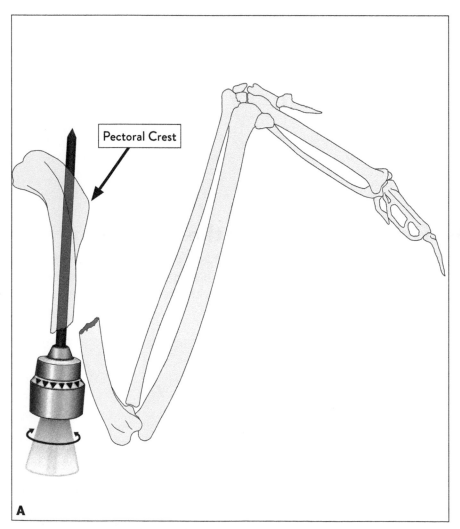

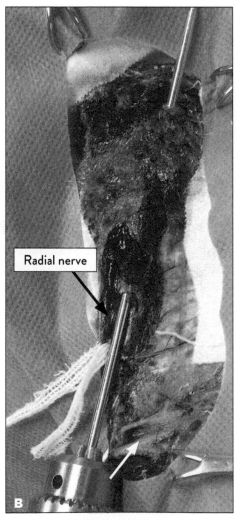

Figure 6-4A & B. Placement of IM pin by retrograde insertion into the proximal humeral fragment. This method is used when there is a pre-existing opening in the skin, which is often the case. A non-threaded Steinmann pin is used. The IM pin was inserted into the proximal fragment at the fracture site and driven retrograde exiting near the pectoral crest **(A)**. Note the location of the radial nerve *(black arrow)* retracted caudally with a strip of gauze **(B)**. Note elbow and tendons of origin of the supinator and common digital extensor *(white arrow)*. Schematic drawing courtesy of Frank Taylor. Color photo used with permission from Samour J, ed. Avian Medicine. 3rd ed. St. Louis: Elsevier; 2016. Figure 12-2b.

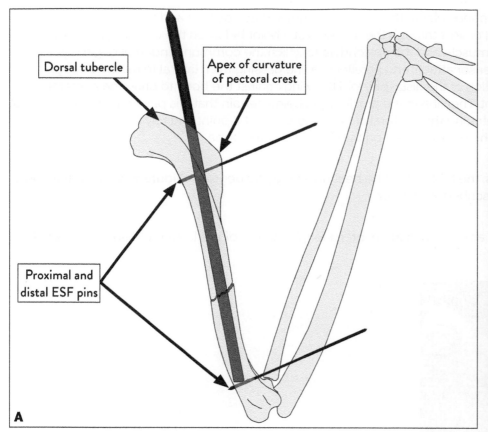

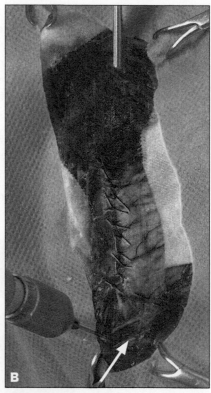

Dorsal tubercle

Apex of curvature of pectoral crest

Proximal and distal ESF pins

A

B

Figure 6-5A. Insertion of ESF Pins: In this illustration of the complete TIF on the humerus, the relationships of the ESF pin locations and the IM pin relative to landmarks on the bone can be visualized. These pins have very sharp trocars and it is not necessary to pre-drill a hole prior to insertion. After seating the trocar in the bone, use firm back and forth rotation to cut a hole in the bone until the pin threads contact the cortical surface – this is done by feel. Then apply gentle downward pressure and screw the pin into the bone turning it clockwise, letting the threads draw the pin through the bone. When the tip of the pin strikes the opposite cortex, apply additional downward pressure to drill a hole in the opposite cortex and continue to thread the pin through. Avoid backing the pin out at any point as this will degrade the engagement of the threads. Image courtesy of Frank Taylor.

Figure 6-5B. The first ESF pin is placed in the diaphysis just proximal to the humeral condyles between the origins of the extensor metacarpi radialis and the common tendon of origin of the supinator and common digital extensor *(arrow)*. Color photo used with permission from Samour J, ed. *Avian Medicine.* 3rd ed. St. Louis: Elsevier; 2016. Figure 12-2c.

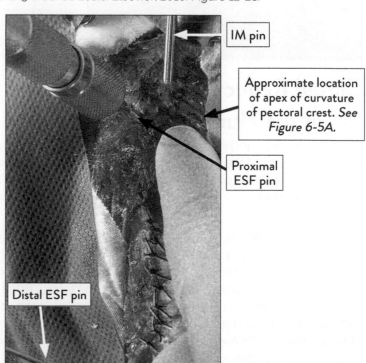

IM pin

Approximate location of apex of curvature of pectoral crest. *See Figure 6-5A.*

Proximal ESF pin

Distal ESF pin

C

Figure 6-5C. Insertion of the proximal ESF pin. The second ESF pin is placed in the diaphysis of the proximal humerus at a point medial to the apex of the curvature of the pectoral crest, a point that can be palpated for reference. To protect the soft tissues from damage by the pin threads, a tissue tunnel may be created by blunt dissection and the muscles held in retraction with a small hemostat. The wing should be folded against the body as this pin is drilled into the bone to ensure rotational alignment of the wing. Color photo used with permission from Samour J, ed. *Avian Medicine.* 3rd ed. St. Louis: Elsevier; 2016. Figure 12-2d.

They should be driven as near perpendicular to the axis of the humerus as possible and nearly parallel to each other. Begin with the distal pin and drive it through the humerus at a point between the epicondyle of origin of the extensor metacarpi radialis muscle and the epicondyle to which the common tendon of origin of the supinator and common digital extensor attach, and parallel to a line passing from lateral to medial through the humeral condyles. Upon insertion of the distal pin, fold the wing against the body to bring the humeral fragments into rotational alignment. Then insert the proximal pin being certain that it is placed in the diaphysis of the humerus and not merely penetrating the pectoral crest. It should be at a point midway between the dorsal tubercle and the highest point of the pectoral crest on the diaphysis of the bone.

Following insertion of the ESF pins, the IM pin must be bent upward by 90 degrees **(Figure 6-6)** and rotated into alignment with the ESF pins as described in Chapter 4.

At this point, attach the acrylic bar as described in Chapter 4 for placement of the latex mold and handling of the acrylic material.

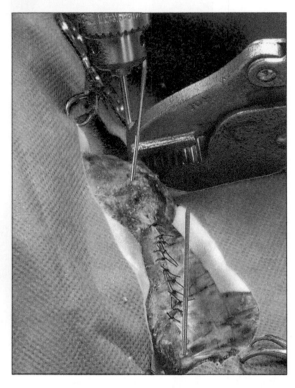

Figure 6-6. Bending of the IM pin: In order to tie the IM pin to the ESF, the exposed end of the IM pin is bent 90°. It is imperative to stabilize the pin with locking pliers (e.g., Vice-Grip™, Malco Products, DeWitt, NE, USA) to prevent transfer of bending forces to the bone and causing fracture of the bone. Color photo used with permission from Samour J, ed. *Avian Medicine*. 3rd ed. St. Louis: Elsevier; 2016. Figure 12-2e.

Closed Reduction and Normograde Placement of an Intramedullary Pin in the Humerus

Closed reduction and normograde placement of the intramedullary pin is a good choice for mid-diaphyseal closed fractures of the humerus where there is no comminution and the fragments can be easily manipulated into alignment. Once the IM pin is in place, further implantation of ESF pins and completion of a tie-in fixator is as described above.

The following illustrations (courtesy of Frank Taylor of White Bear Lake, MN, USA) show closed reduction by normograde driving of the IM pin into the humerus beginning at the distal end of the humerus **(Figures 6-7A-C)**. This method is recommended for closed fractures and avoids exposure of the fracture site while protecting the elbow joint from iatrogenic injury. To begin, the lateral edge of the triceps tendon is located (A). A small incision is made in the skin at this location and the triceps loosened from the humerus. The triceps tendon is retracted, and the tip of the IM pin is inserted under the triceps and brought perpendicular to the bone (B). The insertion site is on the caudal aspect of the humerus, midway between and proximal to the condyles at approximately the point of peak curvature of the distal humerus (B). The pin is now rotated back and forth to start drilling a hole in the bone. Once the trocar is engaged, but before the blades have penetrated through the bone cortex, the angle of the pin is reduced until it is longitudinally aligned with the long axis of the humerus. With continuing rotations, the pin is driven the remainder of the way through the cortex continuing up the medullary cavity until it arrives at the fracture site. The fracture is manually reduced, and the pin driven into the proximal fragment until it is seated at the end of the bone, but without penetrating the cortex of the proximal humerus (C). In some cases, it is necessary to make a small incision in the vicinity of the fracture site to allow visualization of the fragments and proper insertion of the intramedullary pin into the proximal fragment. The positive profile ESF pins are inserted at the points indicated (C) and the fixator is completed as described above.

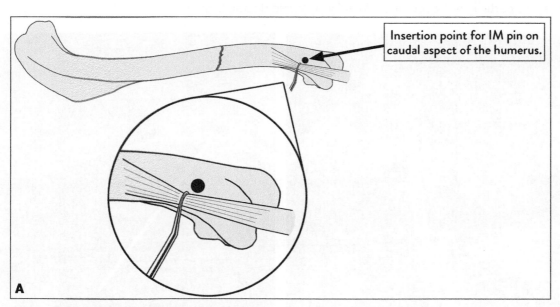

Insertion point for IM pin on caudal aspect of the humerus.

A

Figure 6-7A. This figure illustrates the insertion point of the IM pin on the caudal aspect of the humerus when conducting a normograde procedure. The tendon of the triceps muscle is retracted as shown to avoid skewering it with the IM pin..

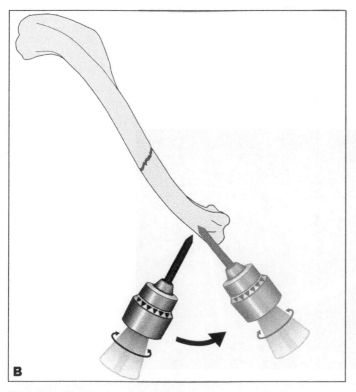

B

Figure 6-7B. The IM pin is initially held perpendicular to the bone to engage the trocar into the cortex. Once the trocar is about half-way embedded into the cortex, the angle of the pin is reduced until the pin is aligned with the bone. It is important to continue rotating the pin. This is done so that the hole is enlarged with the trocar.

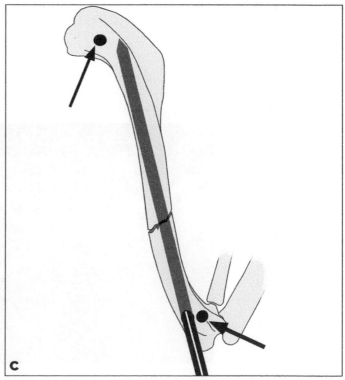

C

Figure 6-7C. This illustration shows the seated IM pin and the approximate locations of the ESF pin insertion sites *(arrows)*.

Case 1.

Radiographic Series Illustrating Humeral Fracture Repair with a Tie-In Fixator Including Retrograde IM Pin Placement (Figures 6-8A-G): This red-tailed hawk *(Buteo jamaicensis)* had a closed, transverse, midshaft diaphyseal fracture. A temporary fixator comprised of ESF pins placed proximally and distally and secured with a conventional Kirschner bar and clamp system was applied to the fracture. This device was applied at admission to hold the bone ends apart, improve circulation, and prevent exteriorization of bone fragments. At the time of application of the full fixator several days later, the proximal ESF pin was replaced. This fracture healed in 4 weeks; the fixator device was partially removed at 21 days for dynamic destabilization.

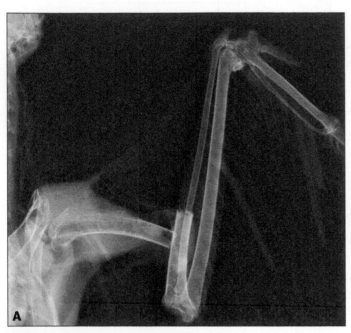

Figure 6-8A. Admission radiograph of a mid-shaft, transverse diaphyseal humeral fracture in a red-tailed hawk *(Buteo jamaicensis)*. The basic tie-in fixator is the ideal mode of fixation for this kind of fracture.

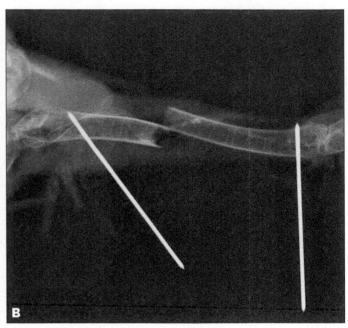

Figure 6-8B. Application of ESF pins for a temporary fixator at time of admission (caudal-cranial view). 0.062-inch (1.6-mm) interface pins were placed proximally and distally. A 1/8-inch (3.2-mm) stainless steel rod and conventional K-E clamps (not shown) were used to stabilize the construct. The remainder of the fixator was applied 3 days later.

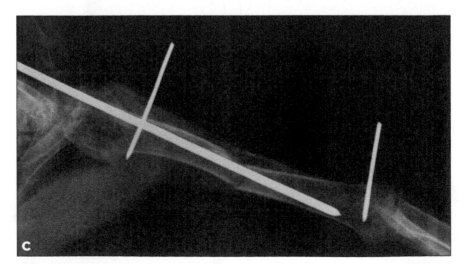

Figure 6-8C. Intra-operative radiograph taken during application of the tie-in fixator (caudal-cranial view). The IM pin was driven retrograde into the proximal fragment, exiting between the proximal humeral tubercles. The fracture was reduced, and the pin was then driven into the distal fragment as shown.

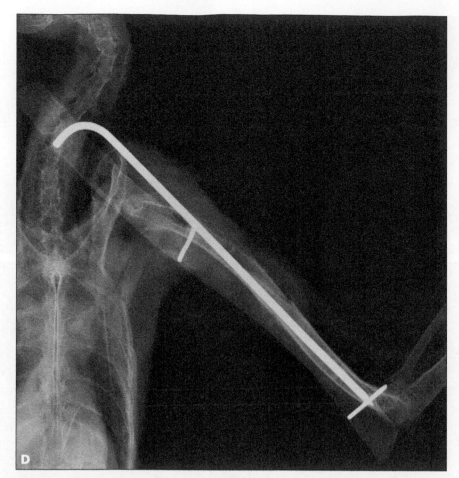

Figure 6-8D. Post-operative radiograph (dorso-ventral view) taken 1.5 weeks after completion of tie-in fixator. Soft callus formation is evident at the fracture site. The shadow of the acrylic connector bar is visible.

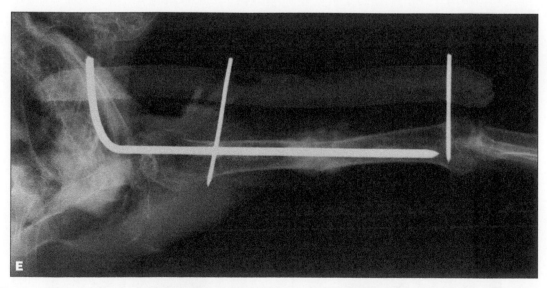

Figure 6-8E. Post-operative radiograph (dorso-ventral view) taken at 2.5 weeks. Note near complete callus formation and limited remodeling.

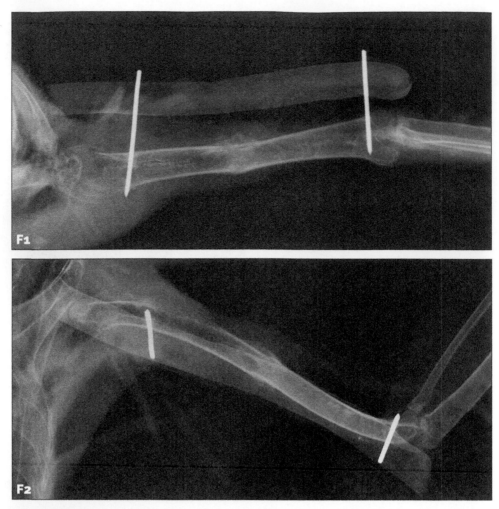

Figure 6-8F1,2. Post-operative caudal-cranial (1) and dorso-ventral (2) views on day 28 after removal of IM pin at 21 days; external fixator bar was left in place for an additional week to provide support.

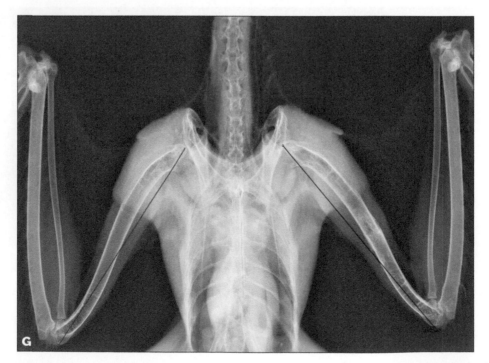

Figure 6-8G. Radiograph after removal of fixator (ventro-dorsal view); healing complete in 35 days—repaired humerus was 0.05 cm longer than opposite limb; this had no impact on the bird's ability to fly.

Proximal Humeral Zone Fractures
Tension Band – Tie-In for Fixation of Proximal Humeral Fractures:

Fractures that occur in the proximal zone of the humerus are most often transverse. A complicating factor for fixation is the curvature of this segment of bone. It is often difficult to gain enough purchase on the proximal fragment with an intramedullary pin as would be used in a conventional tie-in fixator; and there is often insufficient bone surface to accept an ESF pin proximal to the fracture site. A technique to solve this orthopedic problem is the use of a tension band **(Figures 6-9A1-3)**,, illustrated by Frank Taylor. This device can stand alone or be incorporated into a Tie-in fixator.

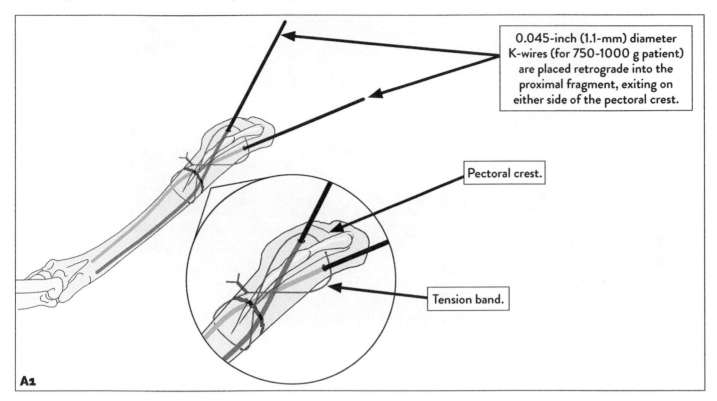

0.045-inch (1.1-mm) diameter K-wires (for 750-1000 g patient) are placed retrograde into the proximal fragment, exiting on either side of the pectoral crest.

Pectoral crest.

Tension band.

A1

Figure 6-9A1. Illustration of key elements of the tension band fixator. Smaller diameter pins may be used in smaller birds and up to 0.062-inch (1.6 mm) in larger birds (~ 1600 g); beyond 0.062 inches, the pins will not flex sufficiently to be useful in this application.

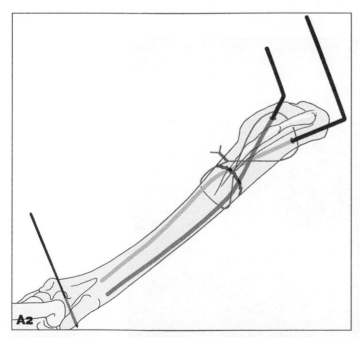

A2

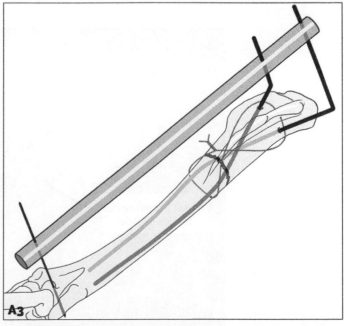

A3

Figure 6-9A2. Intermediate stage of application of the tension-band fixator showing the distal ESF pin and the bent-up ends of the IM pins.

Figure 6-9A3. The completed tension-band fixator after application of the acrylic bar.

The method resembles one used for repair of proximal humeral fractures in humans. The procedure is presented in stepwise fashion **(Figures 6-9B1-11)** and includes incorporation of the tension band into a tie-in fixator.

Step 1

The patient **(Figure 6-9B1)** is placed in ventral recumbency and the dorsal surgical site from shoulder to elbow is plucked and prepped for surgery. Be certain to remove feathers from a large enough area around the shoulder to allow access for manipulating the intramedullary K-wires. The intended incision line is indicated.

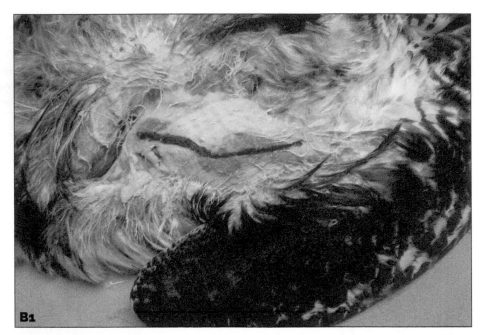

Figure 6-9B1. Cadaver of red-tailed hawk *(Buteo jamaicensis)* with incision line indicated for surgical approach to a proximal humeral fracture.

Step 2

Subperiosteally elevate the deltoideus major muscle from the pectoral crest **(Figure 6-8B2)**.

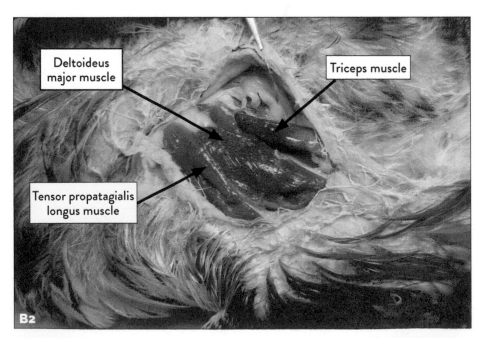

Figure 6-9B2. Muscle identification of the lateral proximal humerus of a red-tailed hawk *(Buteo jamaicensis)*. Elevate the deltoideus major muscle on the dorsal surface and the propatagialis complex ventrally from the pectoral crest.

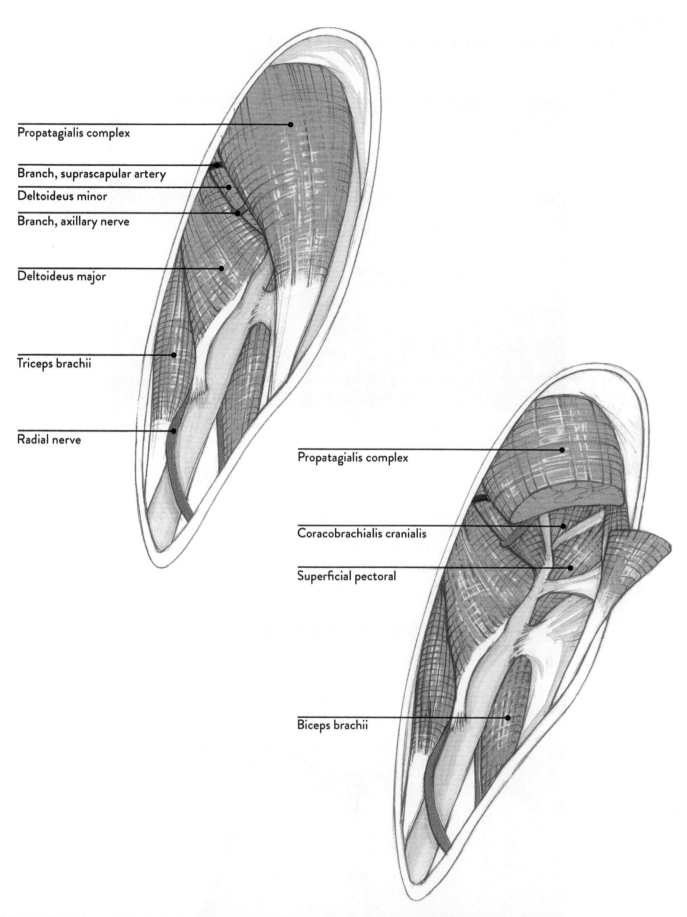

Propatagialis complex

Branch, suprascapular artery

Deltoideus minor

Branch, axillary nerve

Deltoideus major

Triceps brachii

Radial nerve

Propatagialis complex

Coracobrachialis cranialis

Superficial pectoral

Biceps brachii

Figure 6-9B3. Anatomical drawings of the approach to the proximal humerus. Normally the propatagialis complex of muscles is not transected.

Step 3

Dissect and elevate fracture fragments as necessary **(Figure 6-9B4)**.

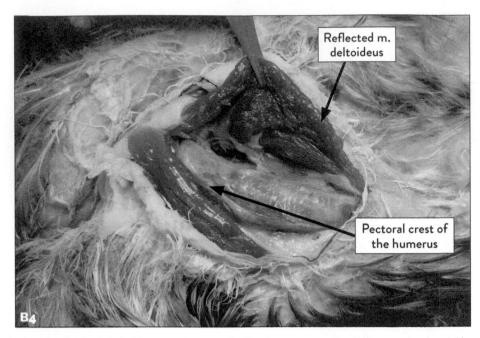

Figure 6-9B4. Elevated and reflected deltoideus major muscle; the tensor propatagialis muscle should be similarly reflected from the ventral portion of the crest.

Step 4

Two small diameter K-wires (typically 0.045 inch [1.1 mm]) are inserted at the fracture site and driven retrograde until their distal tips are flush with the fracture site **(Figure 6-9B5)**. They are placed at small angles (10-15 degrees) to the axis of the bone so that they cross each other inside the medullary cavity to exit the bone on the opposite side of entry on either side of the pectoral crest.

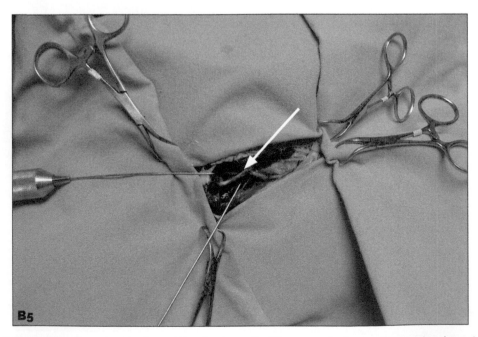

Figure 6-9B5. Insertion of small diameter K-wires at the fracture site. The arrow indicates the pectoral crest as a landmark.

Step 5

The fracture is reduced **(Figure 6-9B6)** and the pins advanced into the distal fragment, incrementally and alternately.

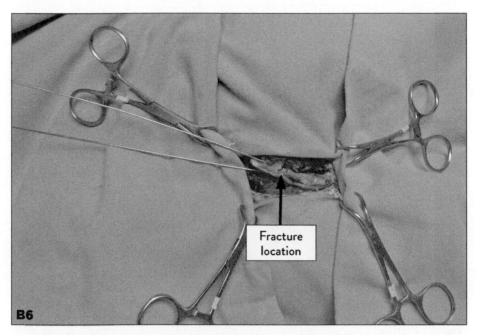

Figure 6-9B6. Reduction of the fracture, with the pins advanced into the distal fragment.

Step 6

A small diameter wire (26 gauge) is passed through a hole drilled transversely in the distal fragment about 1 bone diameter distad to the fracture site and another drilled through the proximal fragment caudad to the exit point of the K wires **(Figure 6-9B7)**; to form a figure-of-8 pattern.

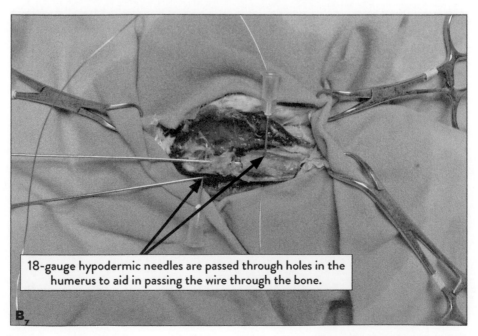

Figure 6-9B7. Procedures for placement of a small diameter wire through the distal and proximal fragments of the fracture site.

Step 7

Once the wire is placed, it is tightened thereby completing a tension band **(Figure 6-9B8)**. The K-wires are left projecting at the head of the humerus for future retrieval or may be bent at 90 degrees to be incorporated with ESF pins placed along the diaphysis of the humerus and incorporated into a tie-in fixator. In smaller birds (less than 300 g) it is enough to simply place the K wires.

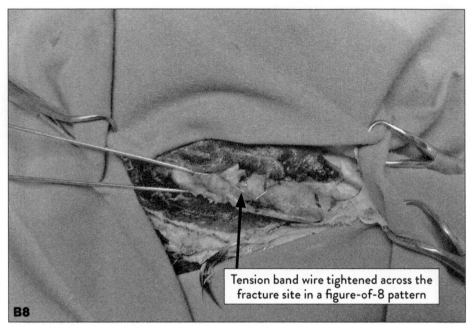

Tension band wire tightened across the fracture site in a figure-of-8 pattern

Figure 6-9B8. Completion of a tension band in a figure-of-8 pattern.

Step 8

The muscles are sutured back to the pectoral crest using monofilament absorbable suture in a simple interrupted pattern and the skin is closed over the top **(Figure 6-9B9)**. One or two ESF pins are then placed in the distal fragment.

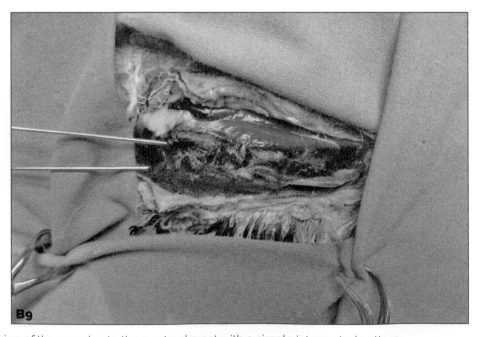

Figure 6-9B9. Suturing of the muscles to the pectoral crest with a simple interrupted pattern.

Step 9

The K-wires protruding from the proximal fragment are bent at 90° **(Figure 6-9B10)**.

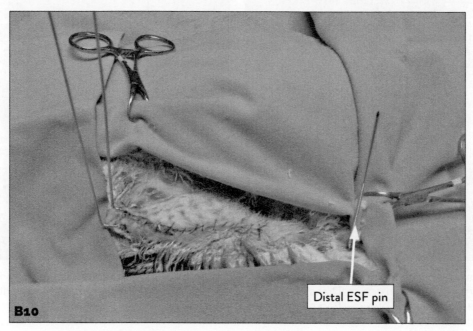

Distal ESF pin

B10

Figure 6-9B10. K-wires protruding from the proximal fragment are bent at 90°.

Step 10

A methacrylate bar is used to connect all elements together in a tie-in **(Figure 6-9B11)**. 2-inch x 2-inch (5-cm x 5-cm) gauze sponges are placed loosely beneath the bar (AKA "fluff") to provide soft tissue protection and to absorb fluids emanating from the pin tracts in the post-operative period.

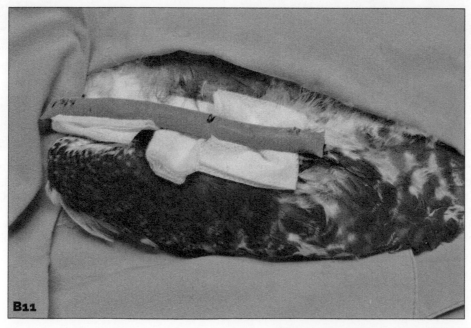

B11

Figure 6-9B11. Placement of a methacrylate bar in a tie-in procedure, with gauze sponges loosely placed beneath for soft tissue protection and absorption of fluids post-operatively.

Radiographic Series Demonstration

A radiographic series demonstrating hardware placement for the tension-band tie-in (**Figures 6-10A-D**).

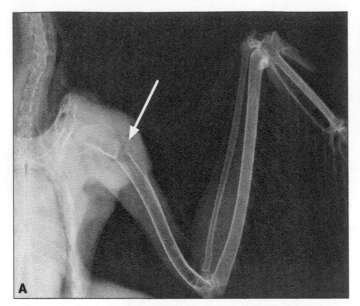

Figure 6-10A. Admission ventro-dorsal view. This red-tailed hawk *(Buteo jamaicensis)* sustained a proximal transverse fracture *(arrow)* of the humerus. The proximal fragment is too short to obtain adequate fixation with a single intramedullary pin placed in the medullary cavity. A two-pin tension band-type fixator is an appropriate choice of fixation.

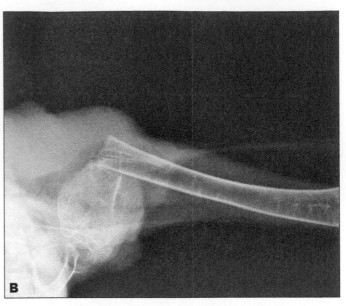

Figure 6-10B. Admission caudal-cranial view. In this view, the angular displacement of the fragments of this transverse fracture is clear.

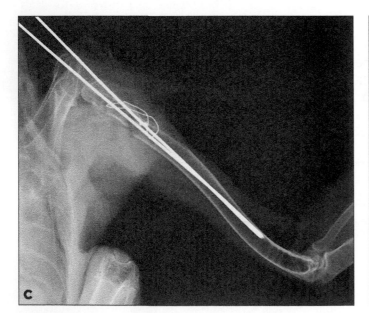

Figure 6-10C. This intra-operative ventro-dorsal image was taken to check the placement of the two K-wires after retrograde insertion into the proximal fragment, reduction of the fracture, and seating of the pins in the distal fragment. Note the 26-gauge interfragmentary cerclage wire holding the fragments in alignment.

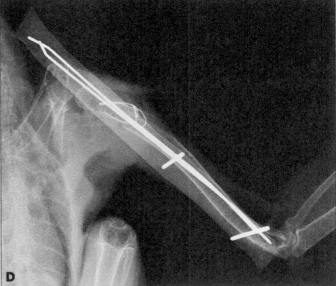

Figure 6-10D. Post-operative dorso-ventral view. The completed fixator can be seen. Two 0.045-inch (1.1-mm) ESF pins were inserted into the distal fragment; a pin in the proximal fragment was intentionally omitted owing to the purchase of the two K-wires on the proximal fragment. An acrylic bar was affixed to the pins as described above. Note the two bent up ends of the K-wires included in the acrylic bar.

Distal Humeral Zone
The Cross-Pin Tie-In Fixator for Fixation of Subcondylar Humeral Fractures

An important variation on the theme of the tie-in fixator is a cross-pinning technique to repair peri-articular and sub-condylar fractures, especially of the distal humerus and distal femur **(Figure 6-11)**.

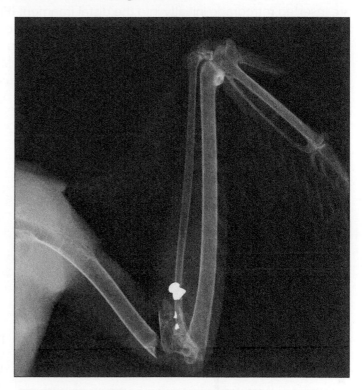

Figure 6-11. Distal humeral sub-condylar fracture for which cross-pin tie-in fixation is a suitable choice. More proximally located fractures may be repaired with a standard tie-in fixator.

This method of repairing distal fractures is a variation of the "Tie-In" procedure, using K-wires in a "Rush pin" style instead of a conventional intramedullary pin. Part of the stability achieved is due to lateral pressure of the pins on the walls of the pneumatic cavity of the bone. The method involves insertion of two small IM pins (K-wires: typically 0.035 [0.9 mm] - 0.045 inch [1.1 mm]); sized for the patient); that pass through the condyles, cross each other in the medullary cavity of the bone, and are driven alternately and incrementally into the proximal fragment, curving along the wall and placing lateral pressure on it. These wires are then bent at right angles and incorporated into the connecting bar placed on the ESF pins that are part of this construct.

Step 1
Place patient in ventral recumbency and liberally remove feathers between the shoulder joint and elbow joint, extending about one-third of the way distally along the dorsal forewing.

Step 2
Incise the skin dorsally over the distal humerus and the elbow joint beginning at the midsection of the humerus and extending just distal to the elbow joint.

Step 3
Dissect any soft tissues away to expose the fragment ends; reflect the triceps as necessary.

Step 4
Select two K-wires that are appropriately sized for the bone. In most cases this will be either, 0.035 inch (0.9 mm)

or 0.045 inch (1.1 mm); in small birds (200 g), an even smaller 0.028-inch (0.7mm) size is available. 0.045-inch pins can be used in birds as large as 1.5 kg; and 0.062-inch pins may be suitable in larger birds (e.g., 1.5-2 kg or more in weight). The pins must be sufficiently small so that they can be easily flexed when being placed.

Step 5

Pin insertion **(Figures 6-12 A-C)**. The two K-wires are worked simultaneously into the bone fragments. Pins are inserted retrograde initially into the distal fragment **(Figure 6-12A)**. Insert the first pin diagonally into the medullary cavity, aiming for the condyle opposite the side of entry. The pin should be driven retrograde through the condyle while being maintained at about a 20° angle relative to the longitudinal axis of the bone. They should be retrograded until the ends are flush with or just slightly beyond the edge of the fracture site, then worked into the open end of the proximal fragment (*Figures 6-12 A-C courtesy of Frank Taylor*).

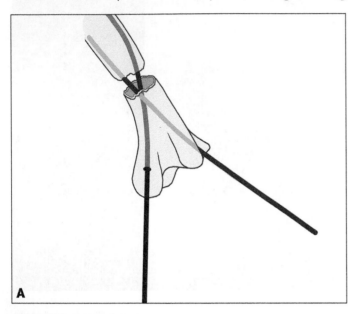

Figure 6-12A. Initial stages of insertion of K-wires for the cross-pin fixator. The angle between the pins should not exceed 15-20° or it will not be possible to bend the wires sufficiently to advance into the proximal fragment.

Step 6

Driving pins into the proximal fragment **(Figure 6-12B)**. The fracture is reduced, and the pins driven into the proximal fragment. Pins are driven 0.5-1 cm at a time, alternately, until seated in the proximal fragment. The most common mistake at this point is to insert one pin too far in advance of the other. It is necessary for the pins to flex and deflect off the opposite cortex of the proximal fragment in order to gain purchase. Continue to drive the pins into the proximal fragment for about two-thirds of the length of that fragment.

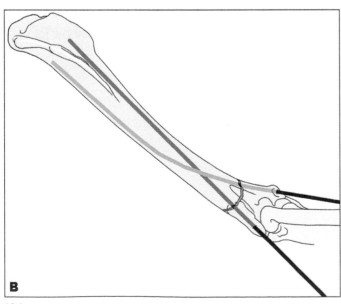

Figure 6-12B. Insertion of the K-wires into the proximal fragment. The fracture is partially reduced, and the pins are alternately driven into the proximal fragment, about 0.5-1 cm at a time, until seated in the proximal fragment.

Step 7

Completion of the "tie-in" configuration **(Figure 6-12C)**. Both K-wires are bent dorsally at roughly 90 degrees. An interface half pin may be placed, at the surgeon's discretion, into the distal fragment near the elbow. Another pin may be placed in the proximal fragment to provide additional strength, as deemed necessary. Latex tubing (penrose drain) is placed over the interface pins and the two K-wires and the fixator is completed as above. **Important:** Fold the wing against the body in a normal resting position and hold until the acrylic cures. This is necessary to assure proper rotational alignment.

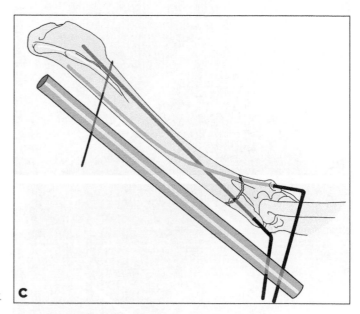

Figure 6-12C. Illustration of the completed cross-pin tie-in fixator.

Radiographic Series Demonstrating the Application of a Cross-Pin Tie-In Fixator to a Distal Humeral Fracture
Case 2.

Use of a cross-pin tie-in fixator in a distal humeral fracture of a red-tailed hawk *(Buteo jamaicensis)* caused by a projectile from a pellet gun (Figures 6-13A-F):

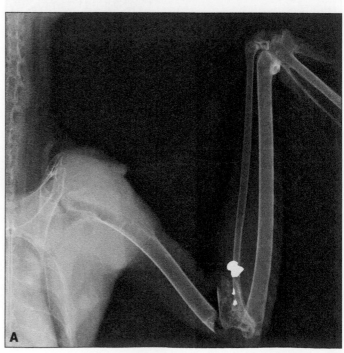

Figure 6-13A. Admission ventro-dorsal view. The distal fragment is too short (i.e., less than two bone diameters) to accommodate an intramedullary pin.

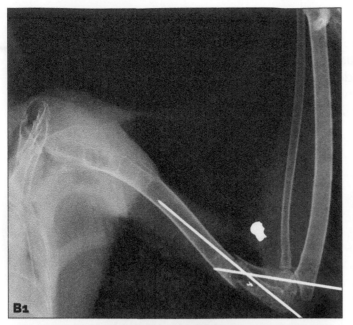

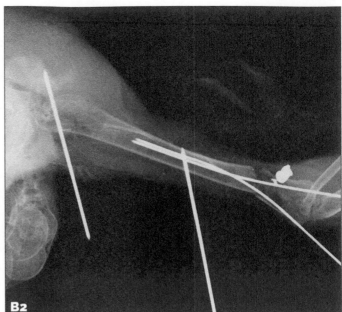

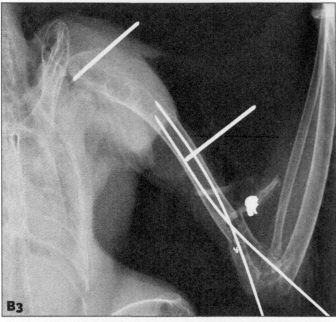

Figure 6-13B1-3. Intra-operative images. Ventro-dorsal view showing placement of IM pins, caudal-cranial, and ventro-dorsal views after addition of ESF pins. In the upper image **(B1)**, both K-wires have been driven retrograde through the condyles, the fracture has been reduced, and one pin has been advanced into the proximal fragment. In the lower caudal-ventral view **(B3)**, both K-wires have been advanced into the proximal fragment and two ESF pins have been placed in the proximal fragment.

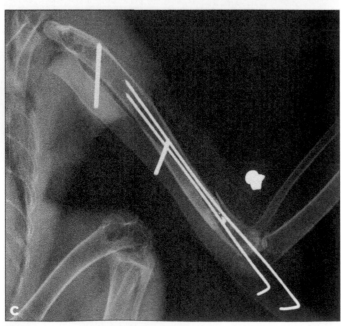

Figure 6-13C. Radiograph taken 10 days post-operatively. Ventro-dorsal view: Shadow of the acrylic bar is visible.

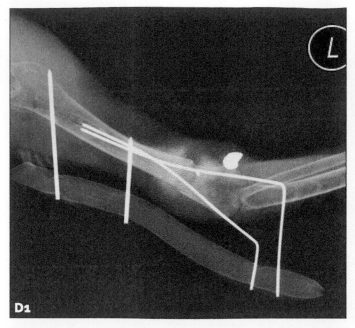

Figure 6-13D1. 20 days post-operative caudal-cranial view. Note callus formation.

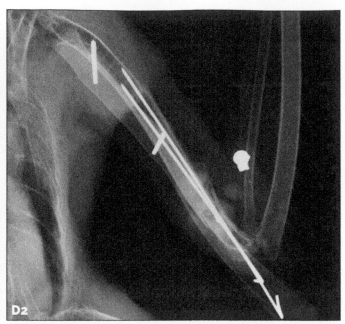

Figure 6-13D2. 20 days post-operative ventro-dorsal view. Note callus formation.

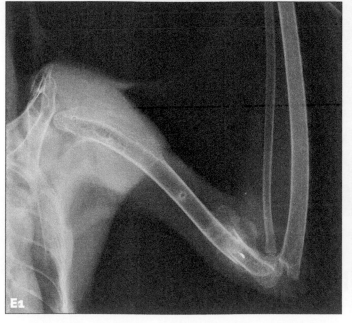

Figure 6-13E1. 46 days post-operative ventro-dorsal view. Fixator removed at day 35; projectile had exteriorized and was removed.

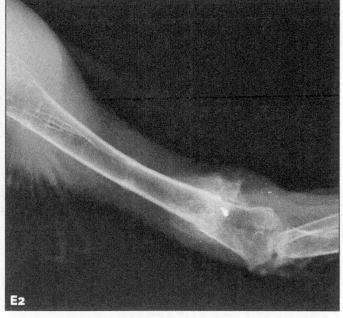

Figure 6-13E2. 46 days post-operative dorsal-oblique view. Note full extension at elbow. The fixator was removed at day 35.

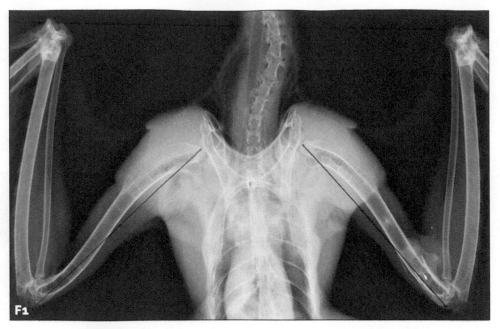

Figure 6-13F1. 129 days post-operatively: Pre-release. Ventro-dorsal view. Repaired humerus was 0.6 cm shorter; this did not impair flight and the bird was released.

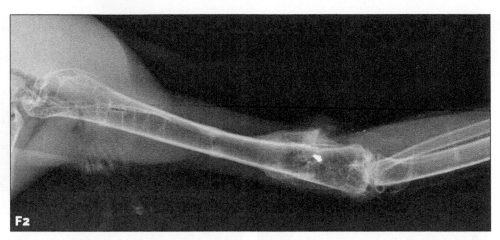

Figure 6-13F2. 129 days post-operatively: Pre-release. Caudal-cranial view. Note remodeling of callus and integrity of joint elements at the elbow.

Fixation of Fractures of the Ulna and/or Radius

General Considerations

Mid-shaft fractures of the ulna are most common, followed by distal and proximal, with or without concomitant radial fracture. Contrary to what is often stated, simple splinting or bandaging of the wing will not reliably result in a functional union of either bone regardless of whether the other is still intact and acting as an "internal splint." Such management invites the formation of a synostosis. Further, the prolonged immobilization of the wing needed for healing with coaptive management may lead to dysfunctional joints and contraction of the propatagium in many cases. Nonetheless, there are circumstances where owing to a need to preserve soft tissue or manage a severely comminuted fracture near a joint, coaptation may still be a good choice. In general, however, a tie-in fixator applied to the ulna will provide the stabilization needed to assure problem-free healing with minimal need for additional bandaging. All radial fractures, regardless of whether the ulna is intact or not should be stabilized with an intramedullary pin. This is necessary to reduce the risk of it developing a synostosis with the ulna. If both bones are fractured the radius should be pinned first, and the tie-in subsequently applied to the ulna **(Figures 6-14A & B)**.

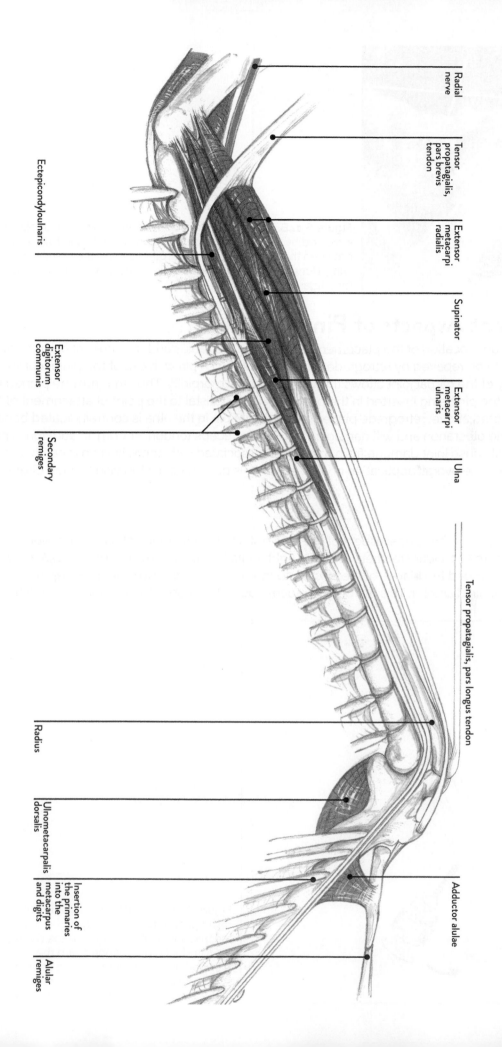

Figure 6-14A. Dorsal drawing of the radius and ulna showing landmarks. The secondary flight feathers insert, along the caudal margin of the ulna. The tensor propatagialis pars longus is a tendon in the propatagium, supporting the leading edge of the wing.

Radial nerve

Tensor propatagialis, pars brevis tendon

Extensor metacarpi radialis

Supinator

Extensor metacarpi ulnaris

Ulna

Tensor propatagialis, pars longus tendon

Adductor alulae

Insertion of the primaries into the metacarpus and digits

Alular remiges

Ulnometacarpalis dorsalis

Radius

Secondary remiges

Extensor digitorum communis

Ectepicondyloulnaris

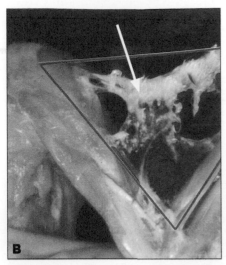

Figure 6-14B. The propatagium corresponds to the white elastic connective tissue indicated by the arrow. The propatagium is the broad fold of skin, filling in the angle between the shoulder and the carpus, forming the cranial or leading edge of the wing. Between the two layers of skin of the propatagium are elastic fibers which form ligaments.

Important Aspects of Pin Placement

The method and location of the placement of IM pins in the radius and ulna are critical in minimizing morbidity. The radius can be repaired by retrograde placement of the IM pin with exit of the pin occurring at the carpus. The anatomy of the carpal joint allows this without undue morbidity. The ulna must be pinned in normograde fashion with the pin being inserted in the proximal end just distal to the point of attachment of the triceps tendon. As noted above, retrograde placement of the IM pin in the ulna is contraindicated because the pin exits the ulna at the olecranon and will damage the joint, the triceps tendon, or both. In addition, a pin exiting at the olecranon will cause joint damage from movement associated with controlled physical therapy in the post-operative period. The overall application of a tie-in fixator is presented in stepwise fashion **(Figures 6-15A-E)**.

Step 1

Introduce the pin on the caudal aspect of the ulna distal to the olecranon at a point between the bases of the second and third secondary feathers at a near right angle to the long axis **(Figures 6-15A, B)**. With a back-and-forth rotation, embed the blades of the trocar into the cortex to about two-thirds its depth; do not penetrate the cortex to a full pin diameter. This mirrors the process described above for normograde insertion into the humerus.

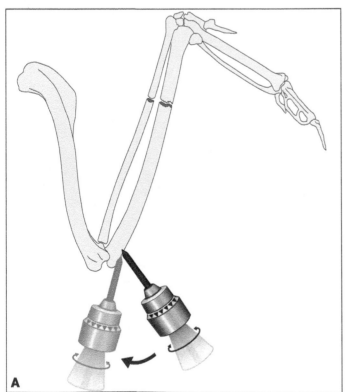

Figure 6-15A. The IM pin is initially drilled into the bone at a near right angle to the long axis of the bone. Once the tip of the trocar is firmly engaged in the cortex, the angle of the pin is reduced until aligned with the long axis of the bone. It is important to continue rotating the pin so the trocar cuts a suitable elongated hole in the bone; otherwise the bone will break out. Image courtesy of Frank Taylor.

Step 2

Reduce the angle of the pin so that it aligns with the long axis while continuing the rotations of the chuck so that an elongated hole is cut in the bone. Once aligned, advance the pin to the level of the fracture **(Figure 6-15B)**. Using another pin of the same length as a measuring stick is useful for precise pin placement.

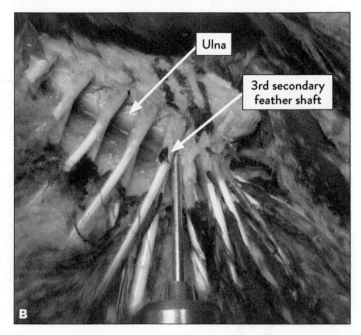

Figure 6-15B. In this figure, the trocar of the IM pin is placed at a near right angle with the ulna at a point between the attachments of the second and third secondary feathers. Once the trocar blades are engaged, rotation of the pin is continued as the angle is reduced until the pin aligns with the bone.

Step 3

The fracture is reduced and the pin is driven towards the distal end of the bone **(Figure 6-15C)**. Driving of the IM pin should stop short of the end of the ulna to leave space for the distal ESF pin. Following placement of the latter, the IM pin can be gently tapped into place, wedging the trocar between the ESF pin and the cortex of the ulna.

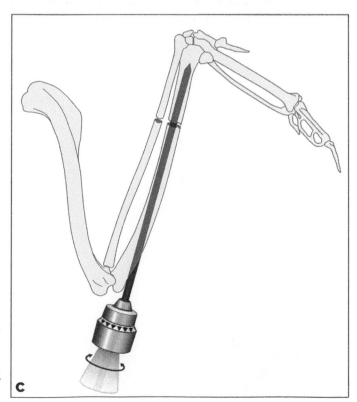

Figure 6-15C. In this figure, the normograde placement of the IM pin is seen fully seated into the ulna. Note the entry point of the IM pin slightly distal to the proximal end of the bone. The pin stops short of the distal end of the ulna to allow room for the insertion of an ESF pin for the remainder of the tie-in fixator. Image courtesy of Frank Taylor.

Step 4

An ESF pin is inserted in the proximal fragment of the ulna between the olecranon and the point of entry of the IM pin **(Figure 6-15D)**, taking advantage of the curvature of the proximal portion of the ulna so that the ESF pin does not have to share the marrow cavity space with the IM pin.

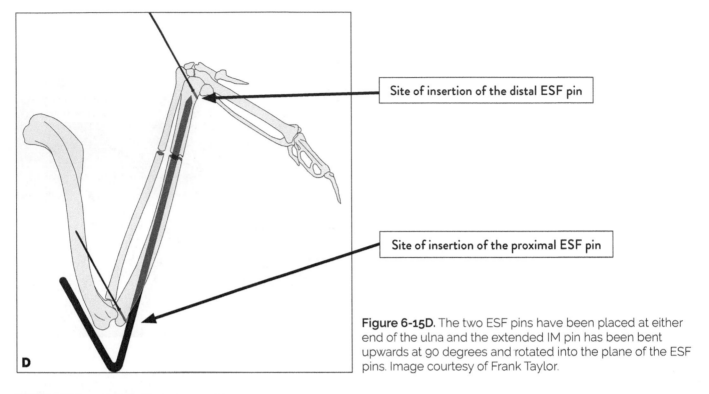

Site of insertion of the distal ESF pin

Site of insertion of the proximal ESF pin

Figure 6-15D. The two ESF pins have been placed at either end of the ulna and the extended IM pin has been bent upwards at 90 degrees and rotated into the plane of the ESF pins. Image courtesy of Frank Taylor.

Step 5

The remaining steps follow the procedure detailed above for other applications of the tie-in fixator. The IM pin is bent at 90° at its point of exit from the ulna and latex tubing is placed over the pins. Additional ESF pins can be installed in either or both ulnar fragments for additional strength prior to injecting the acrylic. **(After injecting the acrylic, but before it cures, the wing must be folded against the body to establish rotational alignment).** Fluff (2-in x 2-in [5-cm x 5-cm] gauze sponges) may be placed underneath the fixator bar **(Figure 6-15E)**.

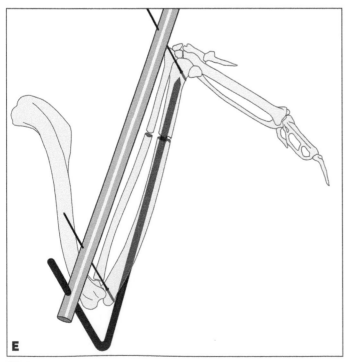

Figure 6-15E. The completed tie-in fixator is affixed to the ulna. Image courtesy of Frank Taylor.

Recommendations and examples for fixation of various types and locations of forearm fractures are illustrated in the following series of radiographs.

Basic Tie-In Fixator Case Applied to an Ulnar Fracture
Case 3.

A Simple midshaft fracture of the Radius and Ulna: The following series illustrates a simple midshaft fracture of the radius and ulna in a red-tailed hawk *(Buteo jamaicensis)* **(Figures 6-16A-F)**. The series includes radiographs on admission and post-operatively on days 1, 12, 20, 37, and 57. An IM pin was placed into the radius – this is essential to prevent excess callus formation and development of a synostosis due to instability.

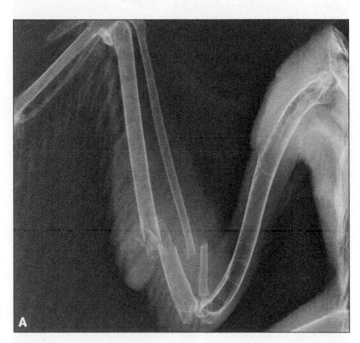

Figure 6-16A. Admission ventro-dorsal view. Note extensive soft tissue swelling that must be given 2-3 days to resolve before surgery is attempted. In this case, both bones will need surgical implants to effect stabilization.

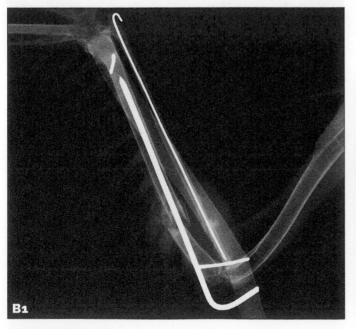

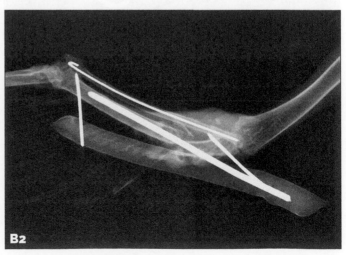

Figure 6-16B1, 2. Post-operative ventro-dorsal **(1)** and caudal-cranial **(2)** views. Note hook at end of IM pin in radius that provides an anchor point that can be taped to the main fixator to prevent the patient from pulling it out.

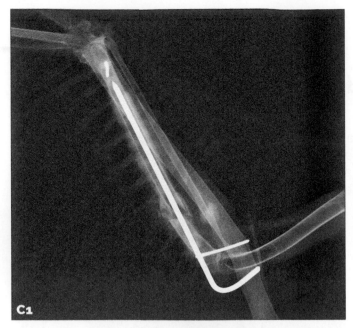

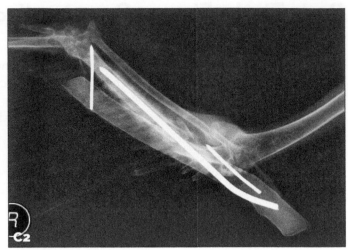

Figure 6-16C1, 2. Day 12 post-operative ventro-dorsal **(1)** and caudal-cranial **(2)** views. The IM pin was removed from radius owing to evidence of enough soft callus formation to stabilize radial fragments and to reduce chance of injury to metacarpal joint.

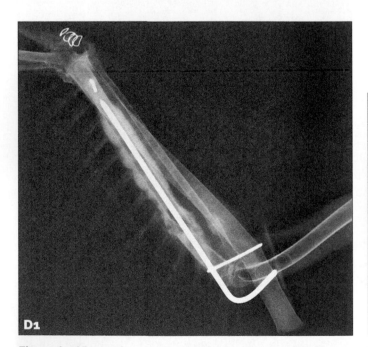

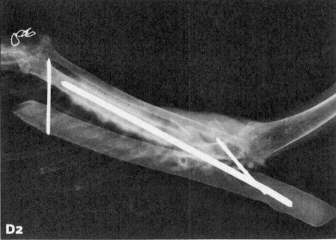

Figure 6-16D1. 20 days post-operative ventro-dorsal view. Callus can be seen forming in the radius; notable osteomyelitis is present in ulna.

Figure 6-16D2. 20 days post-operative caudal-cranial view. Callus forming, osteomyelitis present in ulna. The osteomyelitis was treated with clindamycin – 100 mg/kg q12h until WBC normalized (approx. 3 weeks).

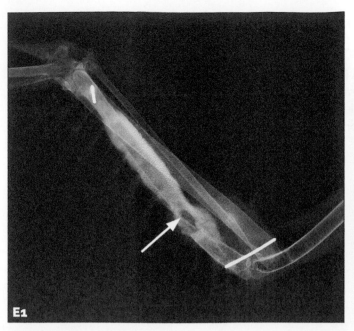

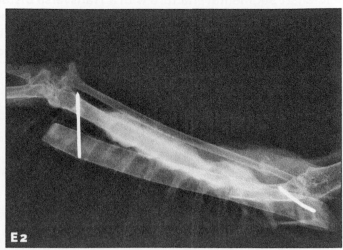

Figure 6-16E1, 2. 37 days post-operative ventro-dorsal & oblique views. Radial fracture healed; ulnar fracture joined by external callus, small sequestrum *(arrow)* forming in ulna, osteomyelitis partially resolved.

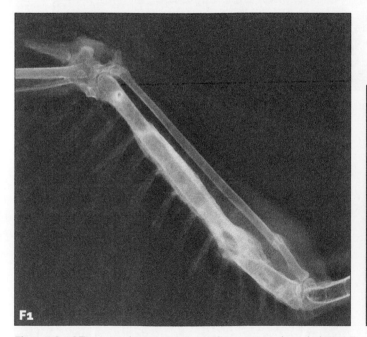

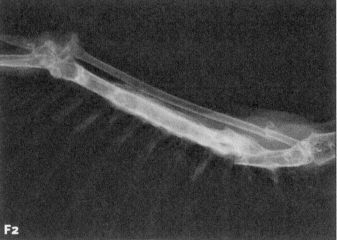

Figure 6-16F1, 2. 57 days post-operative ventro-dorsal views. Fractures healed in both bones and osteomyelitis resolved. Patient was capable of near normal flight at this point and was ultimately released.

Use of Temporary Stabilization for Radius and Ulna Fractures
Case 4.

Mid-shaft Segmental Fracture with a Transverse Distal Radius Fracture in a Bald Eagle *(Haliaeetus leucocephalus)*: This case demonstrates the utility of a temporary fixator in a situation where a) there was a highly unstable fracture and b) the trauma sustained by the patient mandated several days of recovery before definitive fixation could be applied. The use of the temporary fixator is illustrated **(Figures 6-17A & B)**.

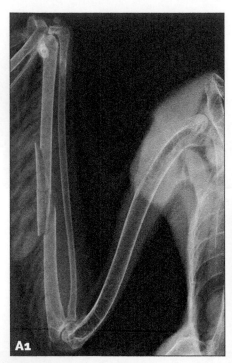

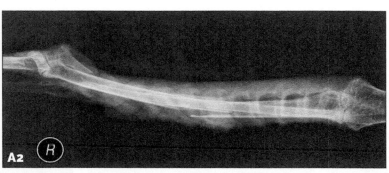

Figure 6-17A1, 2. Admission ventro-dorsal (l) and caudal-cranial (r) views.

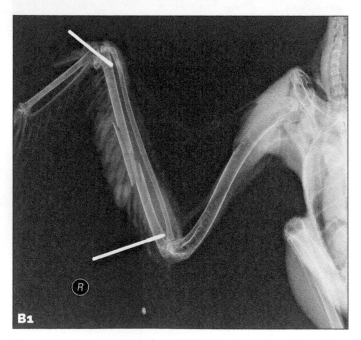

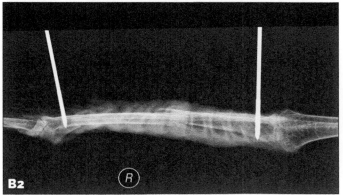

Figure 6-17B1, 2. Application of ESF interface pins at locations in the proximal and distal ulna during admission procedure as a temporary stabilizer (ventro-dorsal and caudal-cranial views; a 3/16-inch (4.8-mm) diameter stainless steel bar and Kirschner clamps (not shown) were applied to hold the construct in place). The wing was taped to the body pending surgical repair.

Management of Fractures of the Radius and Ulna with an IM Pin in the Radius and a Hybrid Fixator on the Ulna

Case 5.

Segmental Mid-Shaft Fracture of the Radius and Ulna in a Great Horned Owl (*Bubo virginianus*): The following series illustrates a segmental mid-shaft fracture of the radius and ulna. Note the placement of an IM pin into the radius **(Figures 6-18A-F)**.

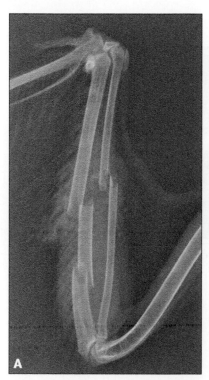

Figure 6-18A. Admission radiograph ventro-dorsal view.

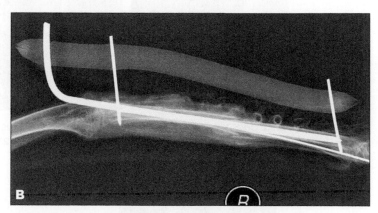

Figure 6-18B. Post-operative radiograph (cranial-caudal view) after placement of a 1/16-inch (1.6-mm) diameter pin in the radius and a tie-in fixator on the ulna. A 7/64-inch (2.8-mm) diameter IM pin was placed in the ulna.

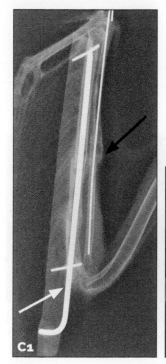

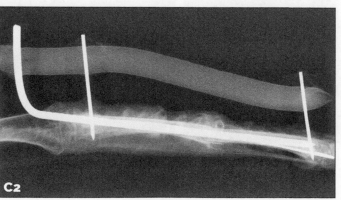

Figure 6-18C1, 2. 14 days post-operative ventro-dorsal **(1)** and caudal-cranial **(2)** views. Callus evident on both radius and ulna; however, lucency *(black arrow)* at the radial fracture suggests a sequestrum is forming around dead bone. On the VD projection, note the point where the IM pin enters the ulna at the apex of its proximal curvature *(white arrow)*.

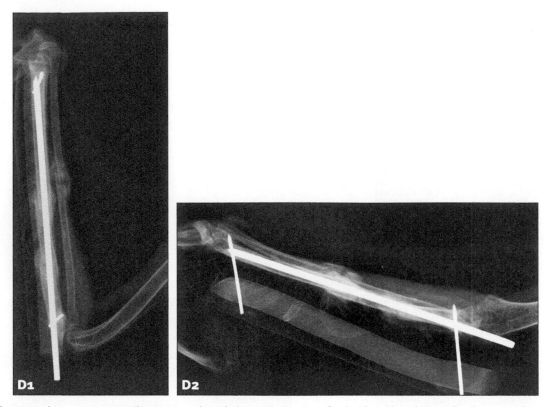

Figure 6-18D1, 2. 42 days post-operative ventro-dorsal views. Callus has formed on the ulna; radius has enveloped sequestrum with callus and is stable; IM pin removed from radius **(2)**.

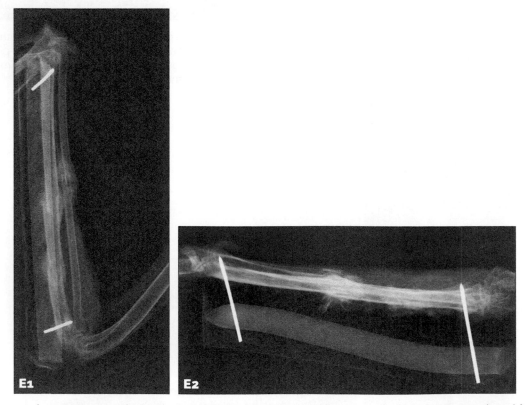

Figure 6-18E1, 2. 50 days post-operatively. Fixator partially deconstructed by removal of IM pin. Ventro-dorsal **(1)** and caudal-cranial **(2)** views. There was concern about the state of the callus on the radius, but no intervention was undertaken.

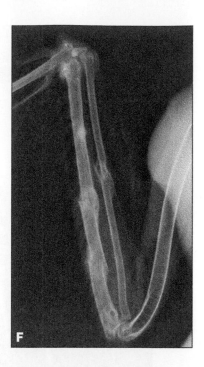

Figure 6-18F. 66 days post-operative ventro-dorsal view. Pre-release radiographs. Note complete union of radius.

Case 6.

A Highly Comminuted Fracture of the Distal Ulna with a Radial Fracture in a Great Horned Owl *(Bubo virginianus)*: A tie-in fixator was applied to the ulna and an intramedullary pin retrograded into the radius, exteriorizing at the distal end **(Figures 6-19A-D)**. Because of the paucity of soft tissue at the distal end of the radius and ulna, no attempt was made to manipulate the ulnar fragments into alignment with the remainder of the bone. Note the new fracture in the proximal ulna that formed during recovery and subsequently healed without incident.

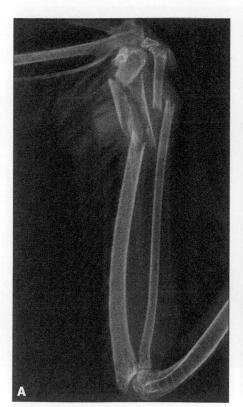
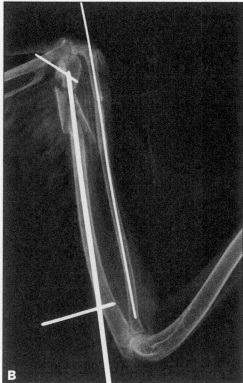

Figure 6-19A. Admission ventro-dorsal view.
Figure 6-19B. Intra-operative ventro-dorsal view.

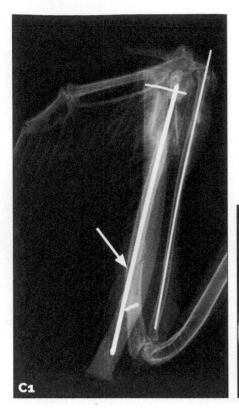
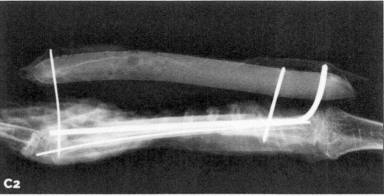

Figure 6-19C1, 2. 10 days post-operative ventro-dorsal and caudal-cranial views. Abundant callus is evident at fracture sites in both bones. Note iatrogenic fracture at the site of pin entry in the ulna *(arrow)*.

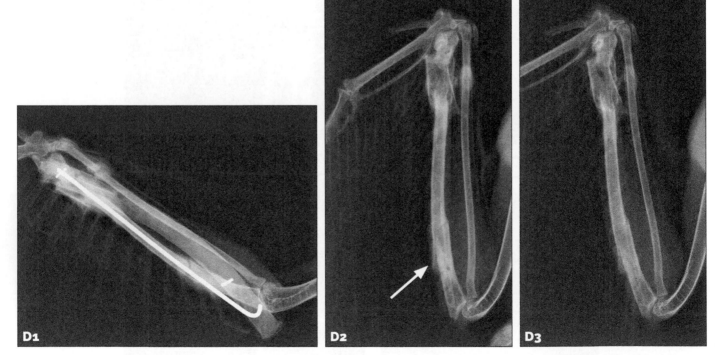

Figure 6-19D1, 2, 3. Days 16, 51, and 105 post-operative ventro-dorsal views from left to right. Fixation removed at 6 weeks post-operatively. Iatrogenic fracture healed without any further attention *(arrow)*.

Management of Gunshot Fractures (2 Cases)
Case 7.

High Energy Gun Shot Injury in a Bald Eagle *(Halianeetus leucocephalus)*: With extensive soft tissue damage, minimal manipulation of soft tissues at the fracture site is essential. Fixation was accomplished with a type I fixator **(Figures 6-20A-E)**.

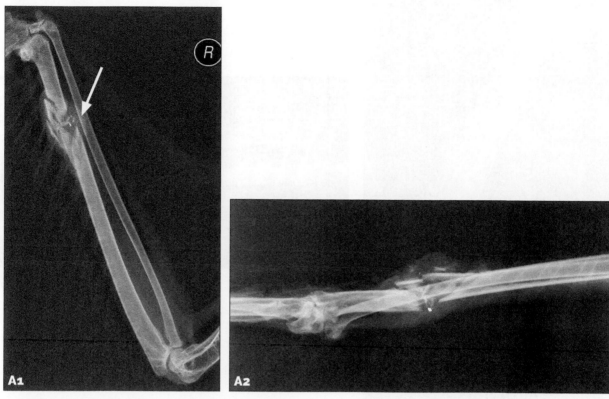

Figure 6-20A1, 2. Admission ventro-dorsal and caudal-cranial views. This was a comminuted fracture of the ulna with an intact radius. Note slight reactivity on the cortex of the radius *(arrow)*.

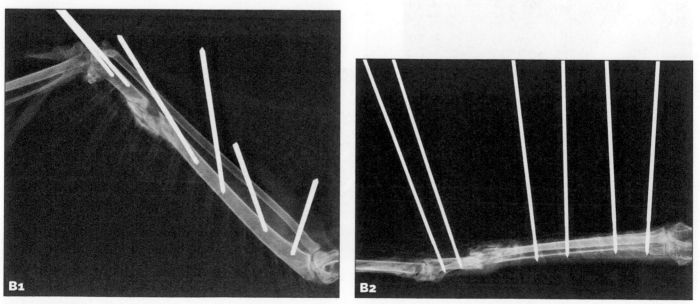

Figure 6-20B1, 2. Intra-operative ventro-dorsal **(1)** and caudal-cranial **(2)** views. ESF pins have been placed on either side of the fracture for a Type I fixator.

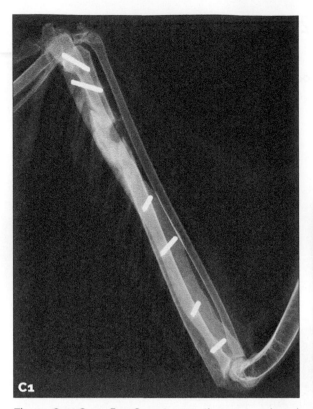

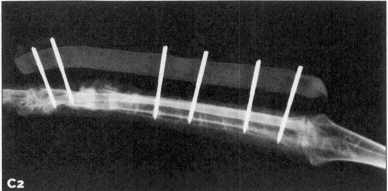

Figure 6-20C1, 2. Day 8 post-operative ventro-dorsal and cranial-caudal views. Note the number of pins on either side of the construct that contribute to the strength of the construct.

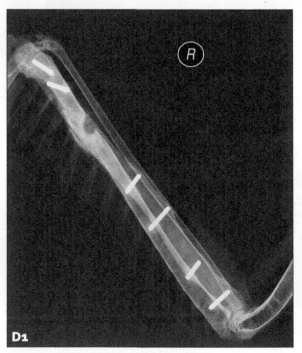

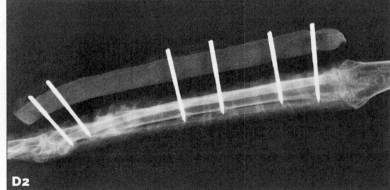

Figure 6-20D1, 2. Day 20 post-operative ventro-dorsal and cranial-caudal views. Remodeling callus is evident and there is no evidence of reactivity in the radial cortex.

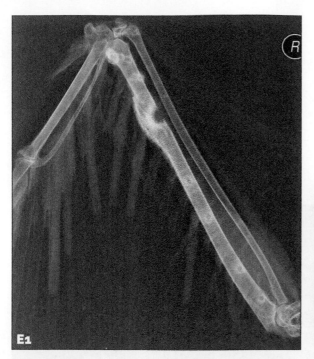

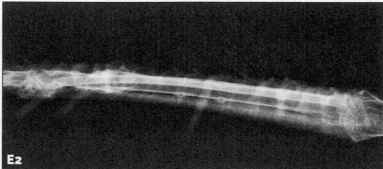

Figure 6-20E1, 2. Day 47 post-operative ventro-dorsal and cranial-caudal views. Pre-release x-ray. Callus is remodeled, new feathers are growing in and radio-dense blood shafts can be seen.

Case 8.

Midshaft Ulna Fracture in a Bald Eagle (*Haliaeetus leucocephalus*): A gunshot injury caused a midshaft ulna fracture with comminution and modest soft tissue damage. Options for fixation include a type I ESF or coaptation; coaptation (figure-of-eight plus body wrap) was chosen **(Figures 6-21A-D)** owing to the minimal displacement of fragments and an expected reduction in morbidity compared with a surgical management option *(See Figures 6-20A-E)* where a Type I fixator was used. A hybrid fixator would have been a less desirable choice. As seen in some other cases, the use of coaptation alone did invite the possibility of a synostosis, however, that did not occur in this case.

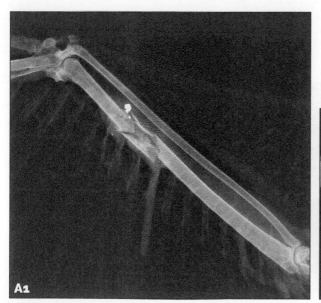

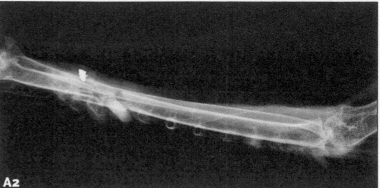

Figure 6-21A1, 2. Admission ventro-dorsal and caudal-cranial views. Note butterfly fragment and the minimal displacement of the fracture fragments.

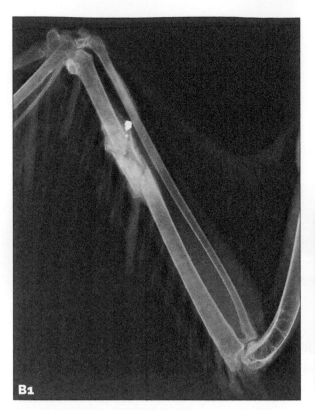

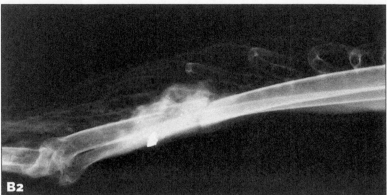

Figure 6-21B1, 2. Day 17 ventro-dorsal and caudal-cranial views. The ulna is well healed, and the butterfly fragment has migrated into a satisfactory location to be incorporated into the callus. Note the mild reaction in the radius that did not advance to a synostosis.

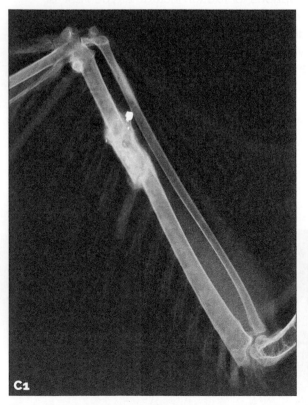

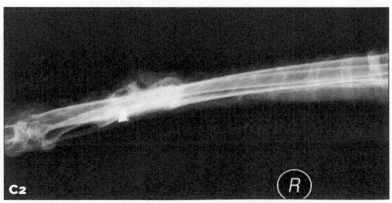

Figure 6-21C1, 2. Day 30 ventro-dorsal and caudal-cranial views. Evidence of remodeled callus is apparent in both views. There is no evidence of a synostosis.

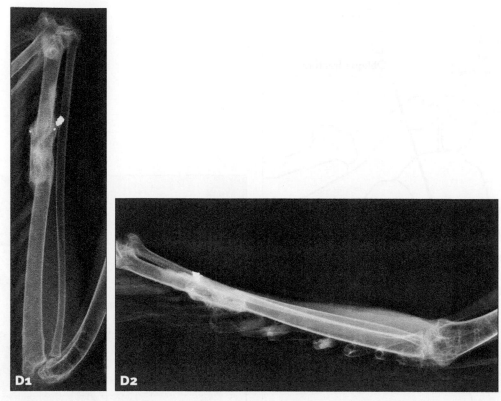

Figure 6-21D1, 2. Day 50 ventro-dorsal and caudal-cranial views. This figure is a set of radiographs taken as part of the pre-release evaluation for this eagle.

Interfragmentary Pins and Wires for Management of Oblique Fractures and Butterfly Fragments

Another method of repair of oblique fractures, especially those occurring in the distal ulna consists of small K-wires placed perpendicularly to the reduced oblique fracture line with a figure-of-8 surgical wire retainer wrapped around them thus pulling the oblique fragments together **(Figures 6-22A & B)**. Ventro-dorsal and caudal-cranial views.

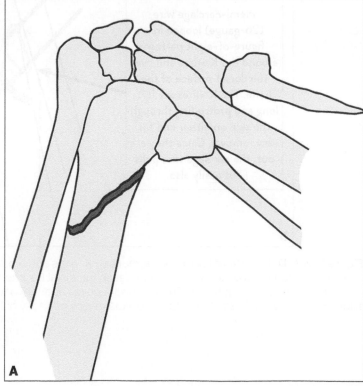

Figure 6-22A. Typical fracture for which this interfragmentary wire and pin method is effective. The distal fragment is too short to gain purchase with an IM pin.

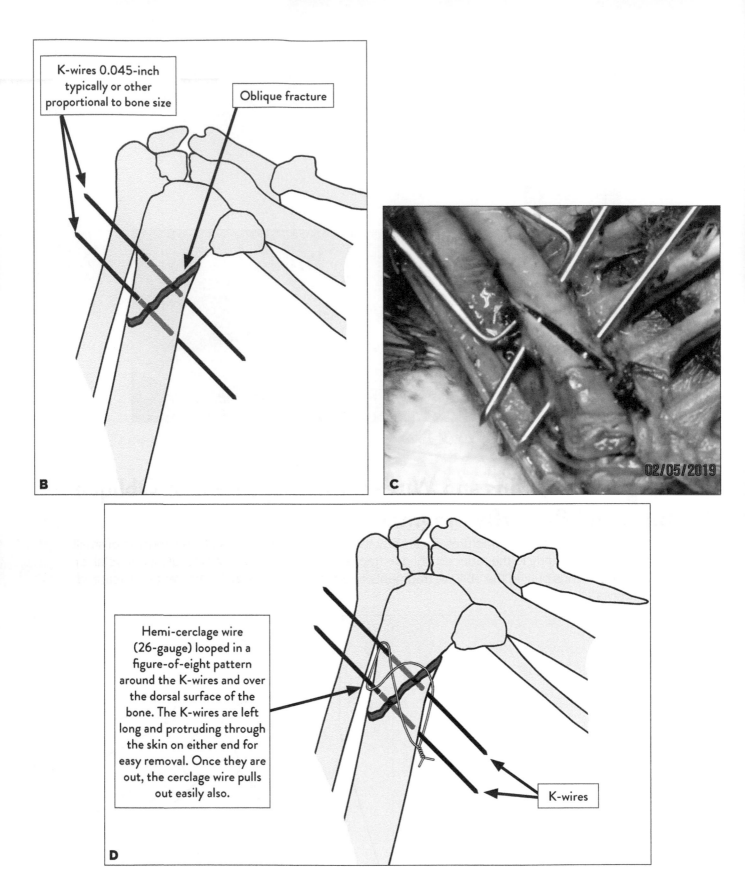

Figure 6-22A-D. The use of two-interfragmentary K-wires and a hemi-cerclage for the stabilization of an oblique fracture is shown. The method is used in this case because the distal fragment of the ulna is too short to allow purchase with an IM pin as would be used on a tie-in fixator. This method requires about two weeks of post-operative coaptation (body wrap) to provide additional support until a callus is forming. Illustrations courtesy of Frank Taylor.

Case 9.

Distal Oblique Fracture of the Ulna in a Barred Owl *(Strix varia)*: This radiographic series illustrates a distal oblique fracture of the ulna in which the distal fragment was too short to permit installation of a tie-in fixator. Two 0.04-inch (1.1-mm) K-wires were placed through the bone cortices perpendicular to the fracture line and used as anchor points for a hemi-cerclage wire placed in a figure-of-8 pattern over the dorsal surface of the ulna **(Figures 6-23A-D)**.

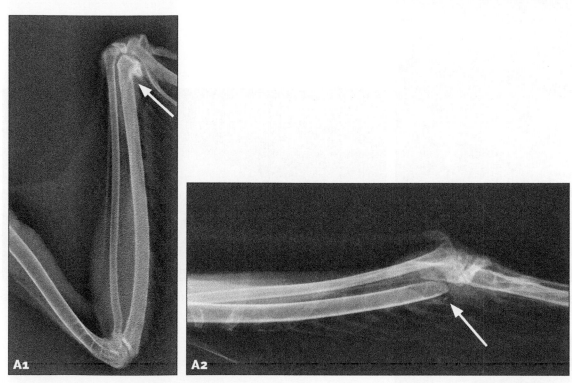

Figure 6-23A1, 2. Admission ventro-dorsal and caudal-cranial views. Displacement and obliquity of the fragments is especially apparent in the caudal-cranial view *(arrows)*. The fracture is difficult to appreciate in the ventro-dorsal view **(1)**.

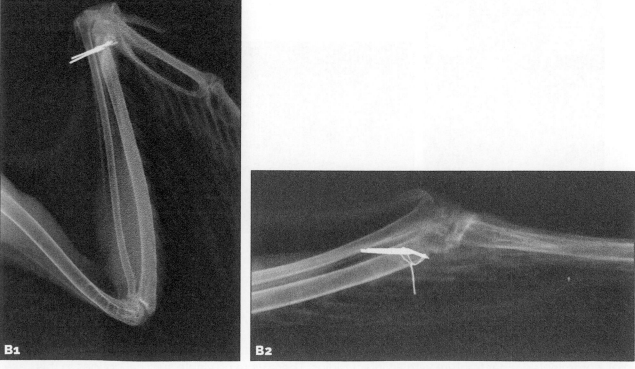

Figure 6-23B1, 2. Ventro-dorsal and caudal-cranial views taken on day 23 post-operatively; fixation was removed on day 23. Note that the interfragmentary wires were well extended beyond the skin edge to allow easy removal.

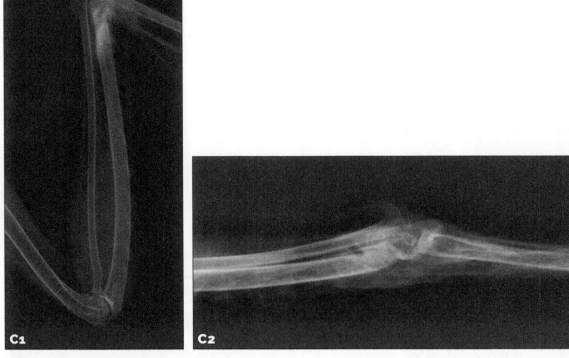

Figure 6-23C1, 2. 37 days post-operative ventro-dorsal and caudal-cranial views. The fixation has been removed in its entirety. Remodeled callus is evident and there is no synostosis.

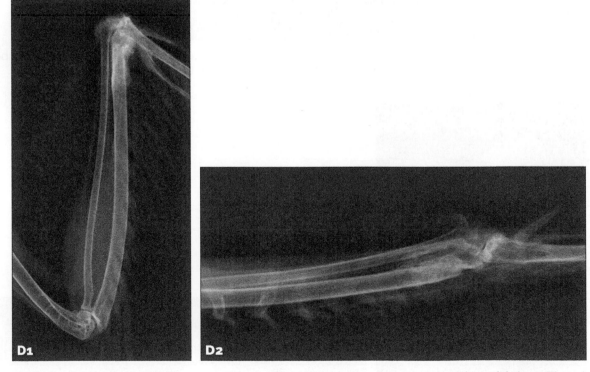

Figure 6-23D1, 2. 77 days post-operatively – pre-release radiographs. Ventro-dorsal and caudal-cranial views. There is further evidence of remodeling.

A Difficult Ulnar Fracture Case

Case 10.

Proximal Ulna Fracture (Figures 6-22A-F): This bald eagle *(Haliaeetus leucocephalus)* presented with a proximal, comminuted ulnar fracture with an intact radius. There were no viable surgical options in this case. Careful management of the soft tissues and immobilization of the wing with a well-padded figure-of-eight bandage and taping to the body was effective. Note in this case the ulna fractured a second time during the healing process for unknown reasons at a point distal to the original fracture. Both fractures healed over a 6-week period. One attempt to manage a similar fracture in another case with a small plate failed owing to necrosis of the traumatized soft tissue that was sutured over the plate.

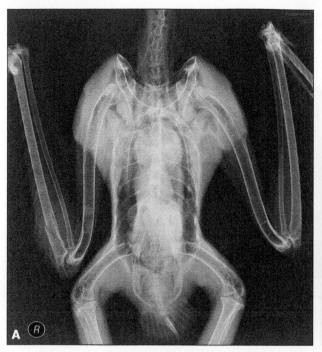

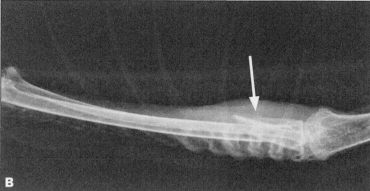

Figure 6-24A, B. Admission radiograph of an oblique proximal ulnar fracture. Ventro-dorsal and caudal-cranial views. There are no options for internal or external fixation, hence coaptation (figure-of-8 with taping to the body) was used for stabilization. Note slight misalignment of proximal ulnar fragment *(arrow)*. Physical therapy other than massage of the patagium was delayed until callus was well-formed.

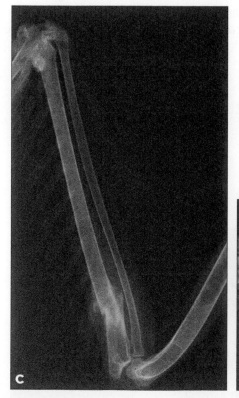

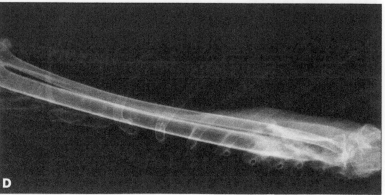

Figure 6-24C, D. Radiographs taken after 3 weeks of coaptation. Ventro-dorsal and caudal-cranial views showing progress of healing and remodeling. Note the formerly misaligned proximal fragment (posterior-anterior view) is aligning with the distal fragment. Coaptation was discontinued; however, the bird was given another 3 weeks of cage confinement to prevent use of the wing.

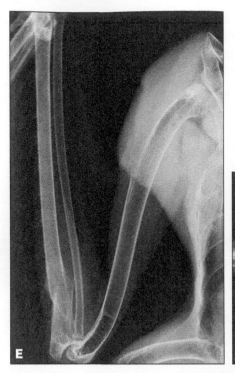

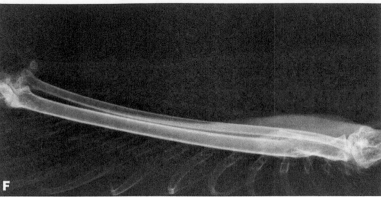

Figure 6-24E, F. Ventro-dorsal and caudal-cranial views. Radiographs taken at 5 months after initiation of treatment. This was a pre-release x-ray following 4 weeks of active flight conditioning. Remodeling is evident in both views. Note the alignment of the fragments in the caudal-cranial view. Displaced fragments often realign during healing and subsequent use of the limb as ordinary forces are applied to the bone.

Some Problems Encountered in Repair of Radius and Ulna Fractures
Case 11.

Misplacement of the IM Pin During an Attempt at Closed Reduction and Stabilization in a Bald Eagle (*Haliaeetus leucocephalus*): This case **(Figures 6-25 A-H)** demonstrates the importance of intra-operative radiographs when attempting closed pin placement. This case also demonstrates complications from synostosis at a radial fracture site despite the placement of an intramedullary pin in the radius.

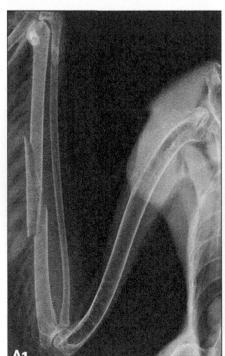

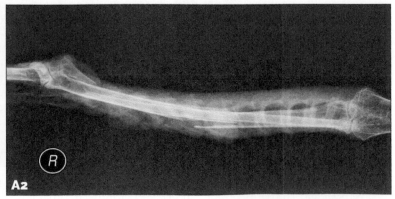

Figure 6-25A1, 2. Admission ventro-dorsal and caudal-cranial views. This was a closed fracture of the ulna with a large butterfly fragment.

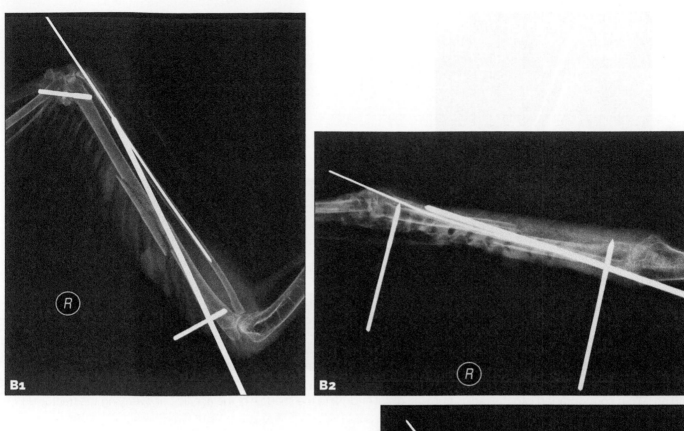

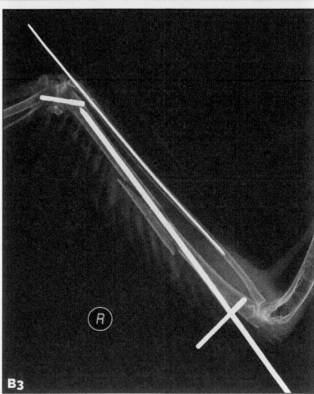

Figure 6-25B1-3. Misplacement of IM pin in the ulna. Intra-operative radiograph reveals that IM pin did not enter the marrow cavity of the distal ulna. Ventro-dorsal and caudal-cranial views. Corrected pin placement. Ventro-dorsal view **(3)**.

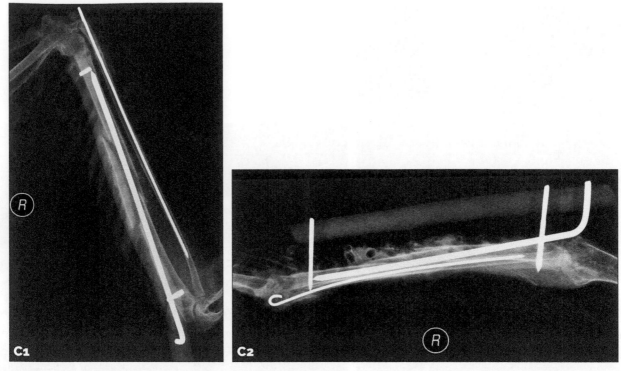

Figure 6-25C1, 2. Day 8 post-operative: Ventro-dorsal and caudal-cranial views. A tie-in fixator has been applied to the ulna and an IM pin normograded into the radius from the distal end. Note the shadow of the acrylic bar overlying the fracture in the ulna in the VD projection.

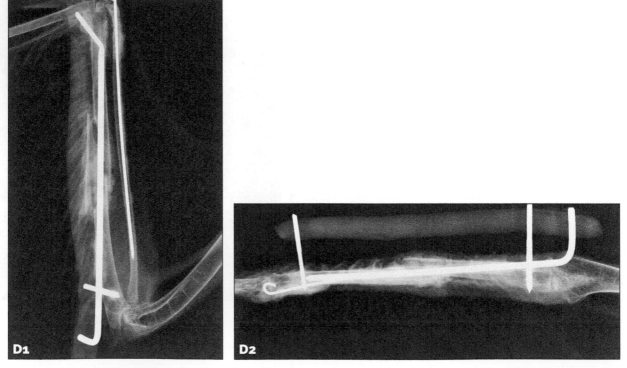

Figure 6-25D1, 2. Day 18 post-operative ventro-dorsal and caudal-cranial views. Note reactivity of cortices at fracture sites in both the radius and the ulna. Such reactivity can be difficult to distinguish from osteomyelitis. The CBC can be useful in detecting if there is an inflammatory process ongoing. There was no white cell elevation and no morphologic changes indicative of a problem. No further action was taken.

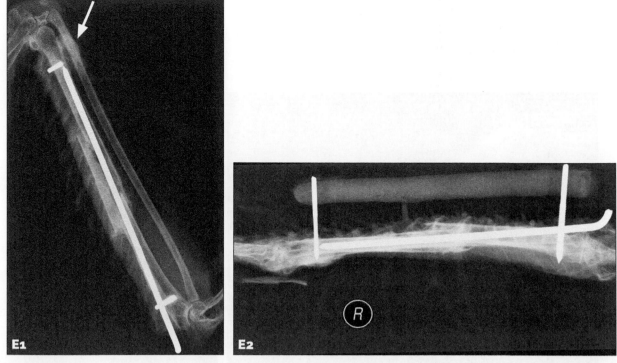

Figure 6-25E1, 2. Day 34 post-operative ventro-dorsal and caudal-cranial views. Fractures nearly healed; note increased bone density in distal radius at site of forming synostosis *(arrow)*. Fixation was removed. There was no longer any concern about possible osteomyelitis.

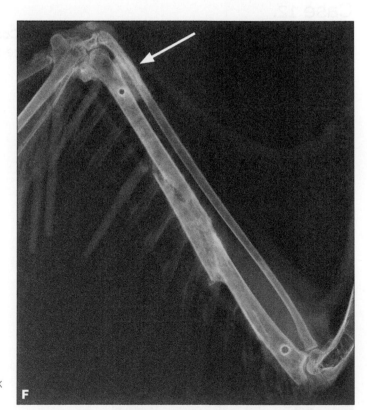

Figure 6-25F. Day 43 post-operative ventro-dorsal view. Fixation removed, fractures healed; note synostosis *(arrow)* and new feather growth. Further surgery was required to break down synostosis.

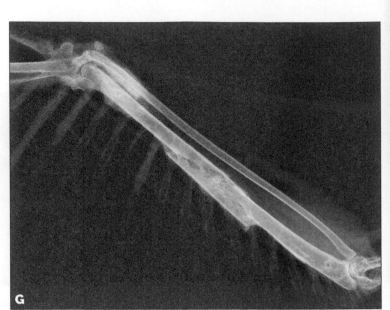

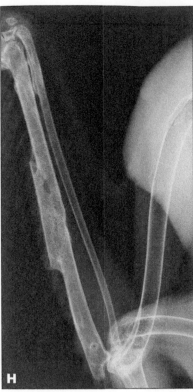

Figure 6-25G. Ventro-dorsal view. Day 86: Synostosis surgically removed, separating the radius and the ulna.

Figure 6-25H. Ventro-dorsal view on day 102. Healing and remodeling of the callus is complete, and synostosis is resolved.

Case 12.

Synostosis in a Simple Ulnar Fracture Managed with Coaptation in a Red-tailed Hawk *(Buteo jamaicensis)*:
A simple ulnar fracture with an intact radius was managed with coaptation **(Figures 6-26A-E)**. It subsequently developed a synostosis that required resection.

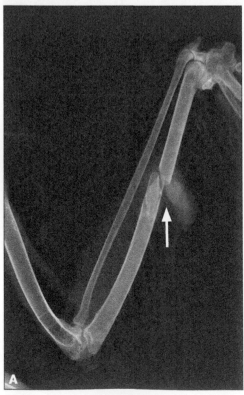

Figure 6-26A. Admission ventro-dorsal view: Note radio-dense area that is a hematoma *(arrow)*. These should be opened and debrided of clotted blood at the time of admission; treat as an open wound.

226

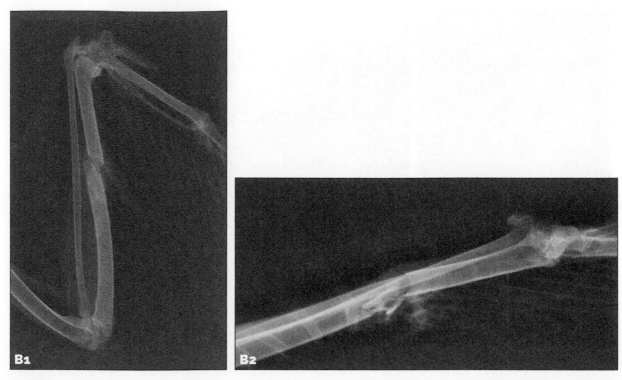

Figure 6-26B1, 2. Ventro-dorsal and caudal-cranial views after 4 days of treatment with bandaging only.

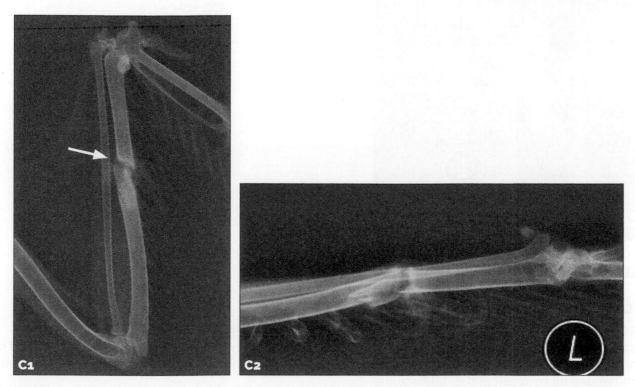

Figure 6-26C1, 2. Day 14: Ventro-dorsal and caudal-cranial views. First signs of a reaction between the ulna and radius occurring at the fracture site *(arrow)* are visible. Note increased density in the radius and the ulna.

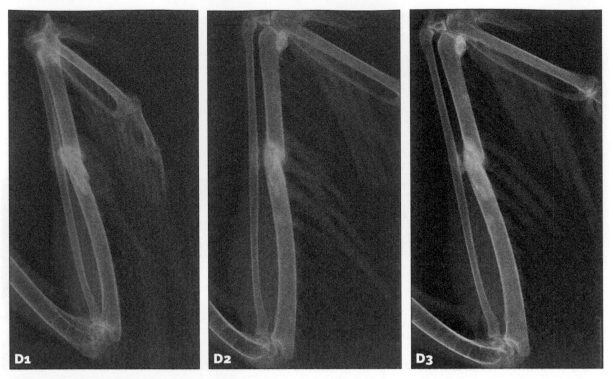

Figure 6-26D1-3. Ventro-dorsal views. Progression of formation of synostosis: days 28, 38, 65, from left to right.

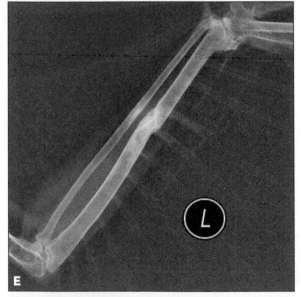

Figure 6-26E. Day 75 following resection of synostosis and insertion of abdominal fat between the bones to prevent the bridge from reforming. Ventro-dorsal view.

Management of Radial Fractures

Radial Fractures with an Intact Ulna

Management options for situations where the radius is fractured and the ulna is intact include 1) no fixation and coaptation - recommended only for very proximal radial fractures; and 2) an intramedullary pin installed by normograde or retrograde placement, exiting at the distal end of the radius for diaphyseal and distal fractures – recommended for midshaft and distal fractures.

Proximal Radial Fractures

Proximal radial fractures (within 2-3 bone diameters of the elbow) occur commonly in falcons and occasionally in other raptors, presumably from collisions with overhead wires. Fractures are usually transverse, and they may or may not be accompanied by varying degrees of elbow luxation. While proximal radial fractures are difficult to approach surgically owing to soft tissue issues, they are generally held in place by overlying muscle and not inclined toward synostosis because of the distance between the radius and ulna. In most cases the proximal fragment is too short for pinning. Coaptation applied for 3-4 weeks with intermittent physical therapy beginning after the second week is commonly utilized. If the ulna is luxated from the humerus, imbrication of the edges of the triceps tendon and the common digital extensor tendon will aid in stabilization of the joint. Undesired outcomes include arthritis at the elbow and non-union. The case below illustrates this management approach.

Case 13.

Closed, Transverse Fracture of the Radius in a Merlin *(Falco columbarius)*: The following radiographic series **(Figures 6-27A-F)** illustrates a low energy, closed, transverse fracture of the proximal radius (arrow). The ulna was intact, and the elements of the elbow joint were luxated. In this location the radius was protected and contained by soft tissue, which also increased the difficulty of access, further discouraging a surgical intervention. This fracture was adequately managed with coaptation — a figure-of-eight bandage and body wrap with regular physical therapy under isoflurane anesthesia starting the second week after onset of treatment.

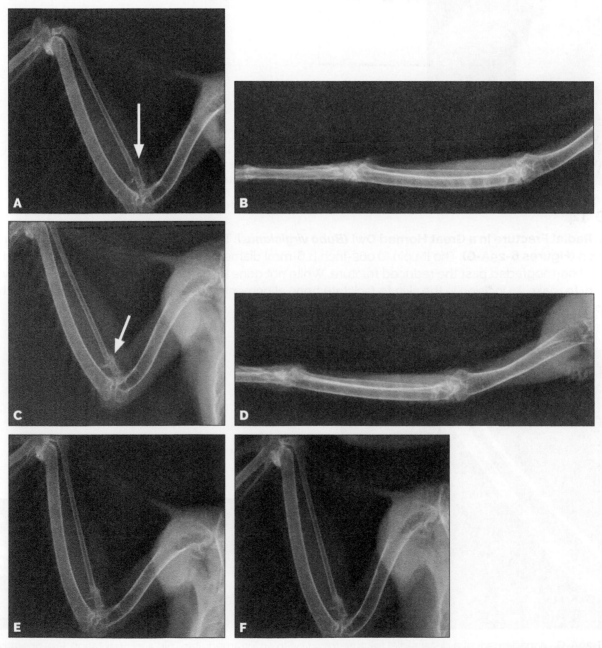

Figure 6-27A-F. This series follows the healing of a proximal radial fracture that was managed by coaptation (figure-of-8 with taping to the body) for 6 weeks. Coaptation was applied through day 21 only, followed by cage rest/confinement for the remainder. Admission. Ventro-dorsal **(A)** and caudal-cranial **(B)** views; Day 21 ventro-dorsal **(C)** and caudal-cranial **(D)**; day 38 ventro-dorsal **(E)** and day 46 ventro-dorsal **(F)**.

Distal Radial Fractures

Radial fractures in the distal three-fourths of the bone are best managed by intramedullary pinning. The radius is a very mobile bone and even when the ulna is intact and the wing is stabilized with a figure-of-eight bandage, the radius tends to move, leading to formation of a large external callus. Further, there is a high probability of the formation of a synostosis, a bony bridge between the two bones, especially with more distally located fractures if the radius is not stabilized. The radial pin may be placed by introduction at the fracture site of the radius and retrograded toward the metacarpus, or, with good technique, it may be drilled into the distal end of the radius and normograded into the proximal fragment after fracture reduction **(Figure 6-28)**.

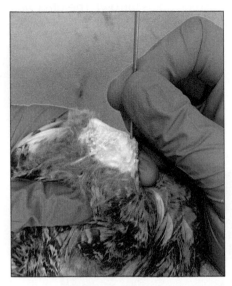

Figure 6-28. Demonstration of the insertion of an IM pin at the distal end of the radius in a cadaver specimen of a great horned owl *(Bubo virginianus)*.

Case 14.

A Distal Radial Fracture in a Great Horned Owl *(Bubo virginianus)*: The injury was repaired with an IM pin and coaptation **(Figures 6-29A-G)**. The IM pin (0.062-inch [1.6-mm] diameter) was introduced at the distal end of the radius and normograded past the reduced fracture. While not done in this case, in some instances it may be necessary to make an incision in the skin to facilitate bone alignment. This radiographic series begins with the post-operative radiograph.

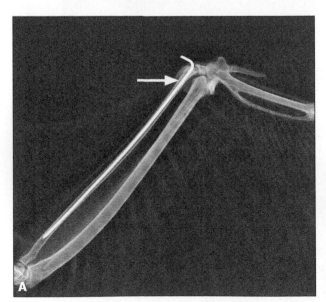

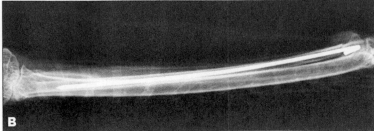

Figure 6-29A-G. Management of a distal radial fracture *(arrow)* with an intramedullary pin and coaptation. Pre-operative radiographs not available. Post-operative ventro-dorsal and caudal-cranial views. The IM pin was inserted at the distal end of the radius and driven normograde. The wing was taped to the body for further restriction of movement.

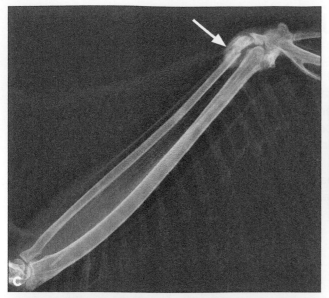

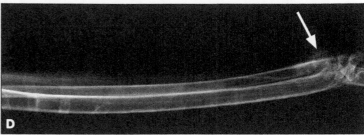

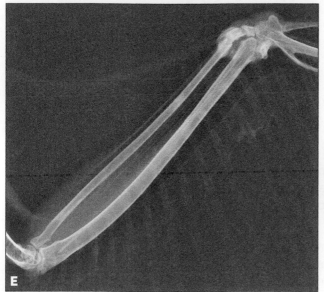

Figure 6-29C,D. Radiographs taken at 10 days post-op.. Ventro-dorsal (and caudal-cranial views. The IM pin was removed just prior to the radiograph. There was enough soft callus *(arrows)* to stabilize the fragments. Coaptation was continued for another week.

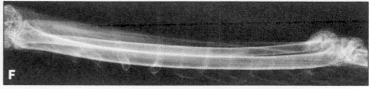

Figure 6-29E,F. Radiographs taken at 17 days post-op. Ventro-dorsal **(E)** and caudal-cranial **(F)** views. Enough callus was present to maintain fragment alignment without need for further coaptation. Twice weekly PT followed.

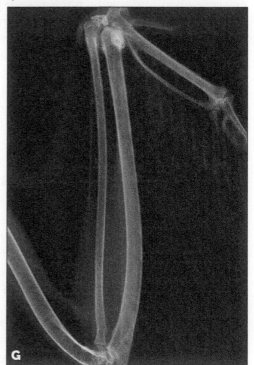

Figure 6-29G. Radiograph taken at 4 months post-admission. Ventro-dorsal view. This was a pre-release radiograph. There is a complete bony union and the callus is remodeled.

Methods of Fixation for The Major Metacarpal
General Considerations
Fractures of the major metacarpal bone are among the most challenging to manage, either surgically or non-surgically. Most metacarpal fractures are high-energy fractures. The energy of the fracturing agent, be it a fence wire, power line or projectile, is concentrated over a very small area that has little soft tissue protection. Indeed, the small amount of soft tissue present absorbs a good portion of that energy and is generally damaged in the process. Metacarpal fractures typically present as open and/or comminuted. Additionally, there is most often a significant degree of swelling and edema associated with metacarpal injuries **(Figure 6-30)**, especially in falcons (so-called wing-tip edema) that must be managed before determinative fixation is applied; all the while, however, the metacarpus must be immobilized with a soft bandage and taping of the wing to the body.

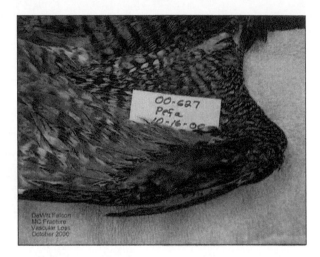

Figure 6-30. Wing-tip edema associated with a major metacarpal fracture in a peregrine falcon *(Falco peregrinus)*. Used by permission from Samour J, ed. *Avian Medicine*. 3rd ed. St. Louis: Elsevier; 2016.

The minor metacarpal bone capable of providing internal support and load-sharing if it is not fractured, thereby improving the prognosis **(Figure 6-31)**. No other bone in the avian appendicular skeleton requires more attention to careful assessment and selection of a proper fixation device to maximize the healing potential of a fracture.

Successful treatment options include coaptation using a reinforced splint (aka curved-edge splint) and figure-of-eight bandage, Type I ESFs, and IM pins supported by coaptation. Experience has shown the hybrid fixator to have a lower success rate owing most likely to the additional amount of soft tissue handling associated with its application. Metacarpal fractures are highly unstable, and re-establishment of load-sharing is not possible, hence the fixator or coaptation device must bear the entire load during healing. Coaptation alone is suitable for the low-energy, transverse, reducible fracture, especially if the minor metacarpal is intact. Because the wing must be bound in a splint for up to 3 weeks, the potential for immobilization-related morbidity is substantial. Healing times are lengthened with conservative management. However, the rate of successful outcomes is comparable to surgical management. Splints made from moldable material (e.g., Sam Splint.™ SAM Medical®, Tualatin, OR, USA) a thermoplastic casting material (preferred) molded into a "curved edge splint" have been a satisfactory means of coaptively stabilizing metacarpal fractures **(Figures 6-32A-C & 6-33A-D)**.

Management of Edema and Swelling of the Wingtip
Owing to the edema of the soft tissues mentioned above, nearly all metacarpal fractures are managed initially with a semi-rigid splint held in place by a figure-of-eight bandage for up to a week. During this time treatment of the edema consists of at least once or sometimes twice daily hot packing the wing for 5-10 minutes. This is accomplished by immersing a cotton fabric surgical drape or equivalent in very warm water (120° F) and wrapping it around the tip of the wing. Hold it there until the fabric cools, then repeat the process several times for a total duration of 10 minutes. The patient is restrained, chemically sedated, or maintained under isofluorane anesthesia during treatment. Upon completion, the wing is dried with a blow dryer on low heat. Dimethylsulfoxide (DMSO) is applied over the area once or twice in the first days of treatment, and peripheral vasodilating drugs are administered orally for the duration. Keep the wing bandaged in a splint and taped to the body with white adhesive tape. Within 3-5 days, there should be notable improvement in the condition of the wing as evidenced by cessation

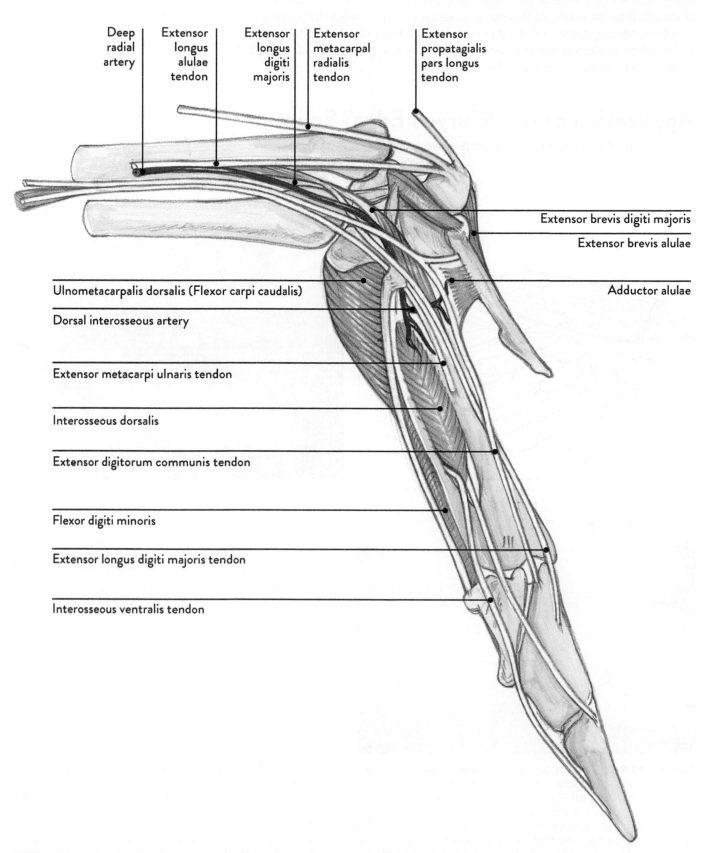

Deep radial artery

Extensor longus alulae tendon

Extensor longus digiti majoris

Extensor metacarpal radialis tendon

Extensor propatagialis pars longus tendon

Extensor brevis digiti majoris

Extensor brevis alulae

Adductor alulae

Ulnometacarpalis dorsalis (Flexor carpi caudalis)

Dorsal interosseous artery

Extensor metacarpi ulnaris tendon

Interosseous dorsalis

Extensor digitorum communis tendon

Flexor digiti minoris

Extensor longus digiti majoris tendon

Interosseous ventralis tendon

Figure 6-31. Anatomical drawing of the dorsal carpometacarpus. The major metacarpal bone has tendons of insertion along its cranial margin. **Osseous elements of the dorsal metacarpus are identified on page 135 in Chapter 5.**

of fluid leakage, reduced swelling, improved color, and a degree of warmth that persists after the cessation of applying the compresses. The treatment is continued for a few more days and should be accompanied by signs of steady improvement. At this point, a decision can be made to continue to provide immobilization with a splint or intervene surgically. The decision is based on the extent of bone damage and the alignment of the fragments with fixation preferred in cases where alignment can be improved. An added benefit of applying fixation is that it makes post-operative physical therapy easier.

Application of the "Curved Edge" Splint

Application of a "curved edge" splint **(Figures 6-32A-C & 6-33A-D)**.

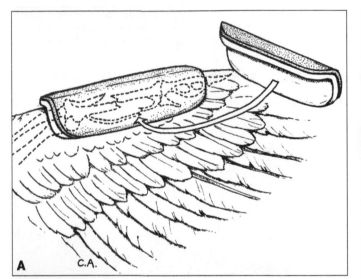

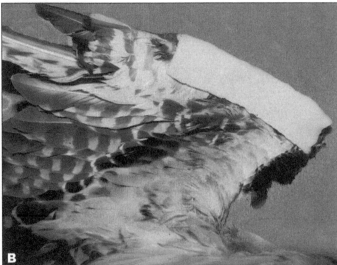

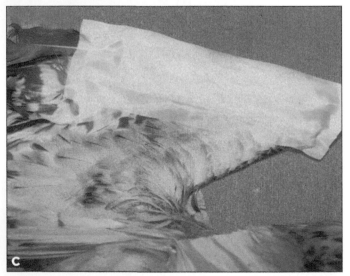

Figure 6-32 A-C. Curved edge splint schematic **(A)** and application to the ventral surface of an Osprey's wing *(Pandion haliaetus)*. The splint does not wrap around the leading edge -- it only comes from the ventral side up to be flush with the top surface of the wing **(B)**. Face-to-face tapes "pinch" it around the contours of the metacarpal bones to form a one-side cast **(C)**. To the extent possible, the opposing faces of adhesive tape are worked between the feather shafts to gain contact with each other. Cutting and removal of the outer seven primary feathers near their base will reduce the distractive forces created by the weight and leverage effect of the long feathers. They are saved and imped back in after the fracture has healed or wait for a molt. Do not pull the primary feathers from the bone as they will not repopulate with normal feathers due to follicular damage. Figures used with permission from Samour J. Avian Medicine, 2nd ed. Maryland Heights, MO: Mosby-Elsevier; 2008. P.333.

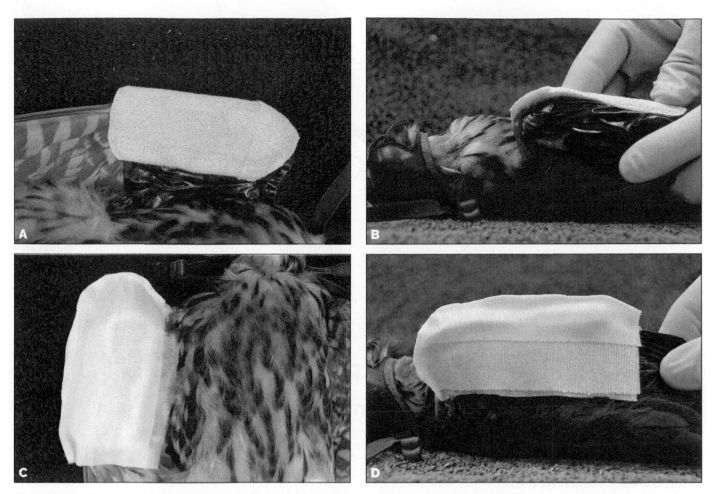

Figure 6-33 A-D. Curved-edge splint made from moldable thermoplastic applied to a merlin *(Falco columbarius)*. A piece of thermoplastic is cut to the length of the metacarpus and molded to the ventral aspect of the bone **(A)** with a right-angle bend covering the leading edge of the bone **(B)**. The splint is sandwiched in place using overlapping pieces of adhesive tape applied ventrally **(C)** and dorsally **(D)**. Figures used with permission from Ponder JB, Redig P. Surgery: Orthopedics. In: Speer BL, ed. *Current Therapy in Avian Medicine and Surgery.* St. Louis: Elsevier, 2016. p. 662.

Application of Type I External Fixation to the Metacarpus

Type I external fixation, in the authors' experience, is the surgical choice for highly comminuted metacarpal fractures with extensive soft tissue damage because reduction, alignment and stabilization can be accomplished with minimal manipulation of the soft tissue. Type I fixator application is facilitated by using a jig comprised of a conventional Kirschner external fixator bar and clamps placed along the dorsal surface to align pins prior to bonding them with the acrylic bar **(Figure 6-34)**. Radiographs are taken intra-operatively to help ensure alignment. Metacarpal fractures repaired with a Type I fixator must be further restrained by taping the wing to the body to prevent a sudden flap of the wing from dislodging the fixator.

Figure 6-34. The use of a jig in conjunction with an acrylic bar to facilitate alignment of fragments. The ESF pins are placed on either side of the fracture using the clamps on the ESF bar as drill guides. The bar and clamps are removed, and latex tubing is placed onto the pins. The bar and clamps are replaced, and radiographs are taken to check alignment. By loosening the clamps and manipulating the pins, fragments can be aligned and checked radiographically. When alignment is satisfactory in both planes, the latex is filled with acrylic and removed when cured. From Samour J. Avian Medicine. 3rd ed. St. Louis: Elsevier; 2016. p. 112.

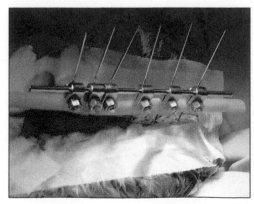

Some metacarpal fractures are displaced proximally or distally. In these cases, an "asymmetric" Type I fixator, in which there is only 1 pin in the short fragment, can be used successfully **(Figure 6-35)** when combined with taping of the wing to the body.

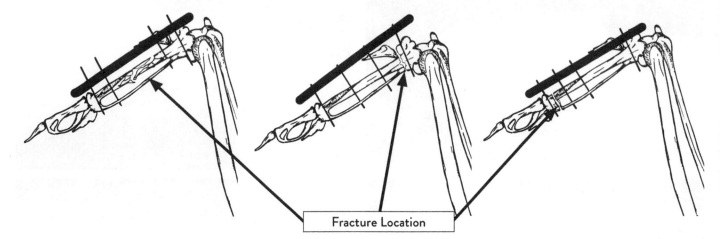

Fracture Location

Figure 6-35. Symmetric and asymmetric Type I fixators applied to metacarpal fractures in midshaft, proximal, and distal locations, respectively. Additional coaptation, usually in the form of taping the wing to the body, is necessary to provide adequate stabilization.

Procedure for Applying a Type I Fixator to the Major Metacarpal Bone Utilizing a Jig for Alignment

(Figures 6-36A-E, courtesy of Frank Taylor)

Materials Required

· Four to six positive profile threaded interface half pins appropriately sized for the specimen – approximately 25% of the bone diameter.

· A set of Kirschner external fixator bar (1/8-inch, [3.2-mm] diameter) and four clamps

· Latex tubing (Penrose drain) – typically 3/8-inch diameter, or size for patient to approximate diameter of the bone.

· Orthopedic and general surgery equipment

Step 1

Place two interface pins, one each at the proximal and distal ends of the major metacarpus, perpendicular to the dorsal surface; place four clamps on the Kirschner bar.

Step 2

Place Kirschner clamps on either end of the bar over the previously installed interface pins and tighten clamps on these pins **(Figure 6-36A)**.

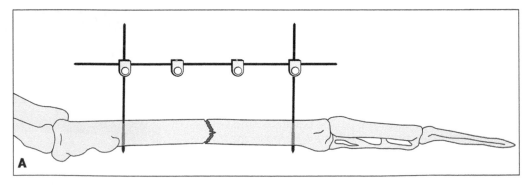

Figure 6-36A.

Step 3

Using the center clamps as drill guides, place two more interface pins into the major metacarpal fragments on either side of the fracture **(Figure 6-36B)**.

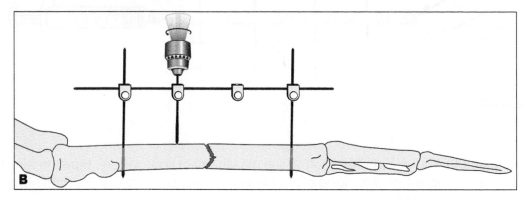

Figure 6-36B.

Step 4

Temporarily remove the jig. Place a length of latex tubing over the ends of the interface pins, sliding it down the pins to near the skin. Fold the wing against the body to obtain proper rotational alignment. Reattach the bar tightening the clamps only on the outside two pins. Reduce the fracture, aligning it in dorsal-ventral and anterior-posterior planes **(Figure 6-36C)**. When you are satisfied with the alignment, tighten the clamps on the middle pins.

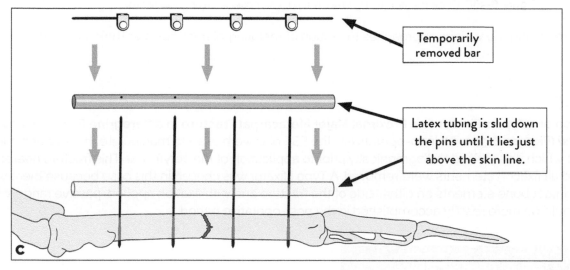

Temporarily removed bar

Latex tubing is slid down the pins until it lies just above the skin line.

Figure 6-36C.

Step 5

Take ventro-dorsal and caudal-cranial digital radiographs to check alignment. If proper alignment is not achieved, loosen clamps on pins and manipulate fragments; retighten pins and re-radiograph. Repeat as often as necessary to achieve alignment.

Step 6

Once alignment is achieved, fill latex tubing with acrylic, clamp and hold until the acrylic cures **(Figure 6-36D)**. Again, ensure that the wing is folded against the body in proper perching position.

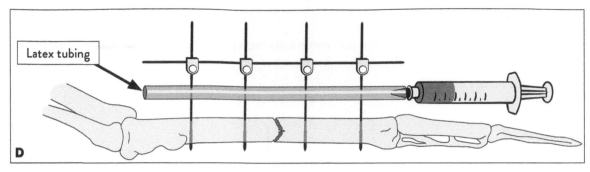

Figure 6-36D.

Step 9

Remove jig **(Figure 6-36E)**. Perform whatever soft-tissue management is necessary. Tape the wing to the body for 2-3 weeks to prevent inadvertent dislodging of the fixator by a sudden wing-flap. Perform physical therapy twice weekly under isoflurane anesthesia.

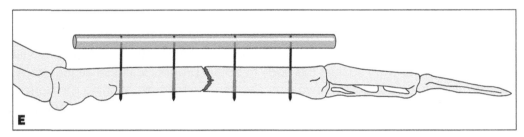

Figure 6-36E. Once the acrylic is cured, the jig is removed, leaving the fixator.

Cases representing the various approaches to fixation of metacarpal fractures and their outcomes are presented below.

Case 15.

Application of a Type 1 Fixator to a Proximal Major Metacarpal Fracture in a Peregrine Falcon *(Falco peregrinus)* (Figures 6-37A-C): Intra-operatively, the ESF pins were used to manipulate the fragments into alignment which was verified radiographically prior to application of the acrylic bar. This fracture healed in four weeks and all fixation elements were removed. A Type I fixator was chosen in this case because there was good access to intact bone elements on either side of the fracture and with fixation applied, passive range-of-motion therapy could be more readily accomplished in the post-operative period.

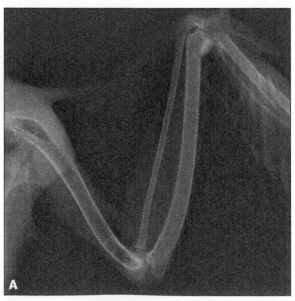

Figure 6-37A. Admission ventro-dorsal view. There is a minimally displaced oblique fracture of the major metarcarpus. Note the swollen soft tissue – wing tip edema.

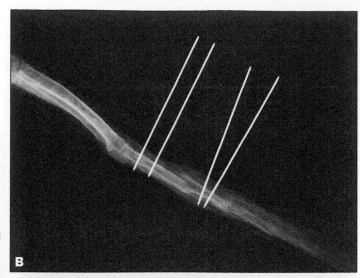

Figure 6-37B. Intra-operative caudal-cranial view. Two interface pins (.045-inch [1.1-mm] diameter) have been placed on either side of the fracture. As alignment was satisfactory, the acrylic bar was installed.

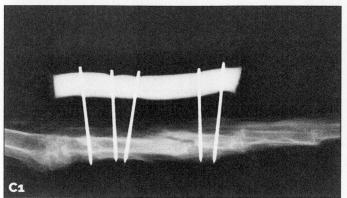

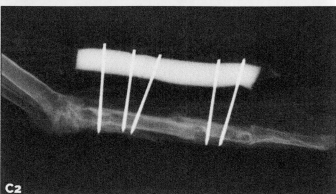

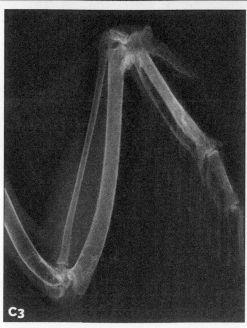

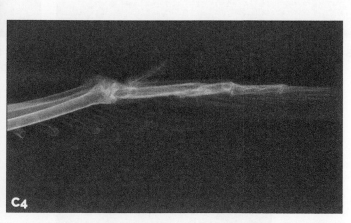

Figure 6-37C1-4. Radiographs taken at 12, 22 and 30 **(C3, 4)** days demonstrate the progression of healing. Fixation was removed at 28 days.

Case 16.

Application of an Asymmetric Fixator on the Major Metacarpal in a Red-tailed Hawk *(Buteo jamaicensis)* (Figures 6-38A-E): This method is used when the proximal or distal fragment is very short and the length of the lever arm of the remainder of the wing makes stabilizing the fragments with a splint difficult at best. In this case, two positive profile threaded interface pins (0.045 inches [1.1 mm]) were placed in the proximal fragment in a crossed manner in order to gain better purchase on the bone. In many cases, there is only enough room for one pin. While not as

239

stable as a two-pin configuration, the pins will maintain the bones in alignment while additional stabilization is provided with coaptation for the first two weeks post-operatively. After that, the fixator pins will maintain adequate stabilization for the duration of the healing period.

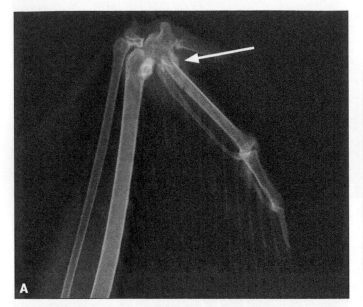

Figure 6-38A. Admission. Ventro-dorsal view of a low energy, proximally located metacarpal fracture *(arrow)*.

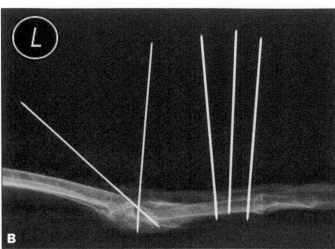

Figure 6-38B. Intra-operative caudal-cranial view. The proximal pins were crossed to obtain better purchase on the bone.

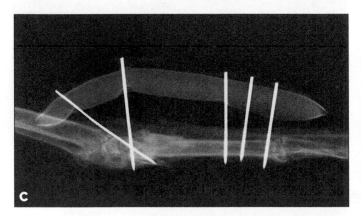

Figure 6-38C. 11 days post-operatively, caudal-cranial view.

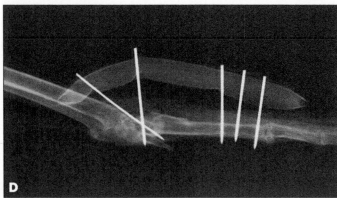

Figure 6-38D. 38 days post-operatively, caudal-cranial view – healing complete, fixation removed.

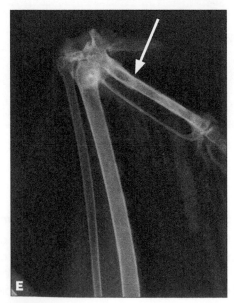

Figure 6-38E. Ventro-dorsal view of the healed fracture *(arrow)*.

Case 17.

Management of a Distal Major Metacarpal Fracture in a Juvenile Bald Eagle *(Haliaeetus leucocephalus)* (Figures 6-39A-F): The initial attempt at management was made with a curved edge splint **(Figure 6-39B1, 2)** because of the soft bones present in this young patient. The splint failed to hold the fragments in alignment. After 4 days, the curved edge splint was replaced with an IM pin normograded from the distal end of the major metacarpal bone.

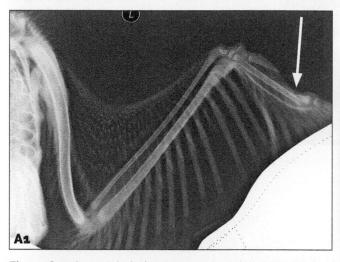
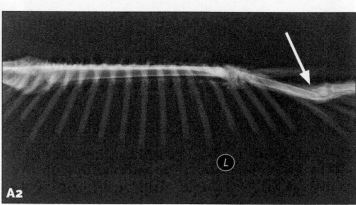

Figure 6-39A1, 2. Admission. Ventro-dorsal and caudal-cranial views. Fracture is indicated by *arrows*. Note the incompletely formed joints in this 10-week-old eaglet.

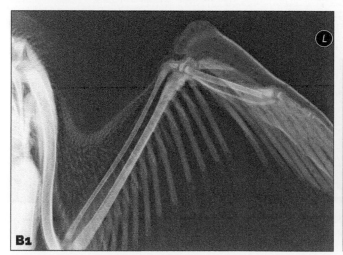
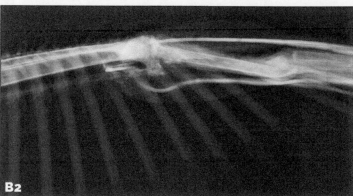

Figure 6-39B1, 2. Day 4 after application of a moldable, thermally activated splint: Ventro-dorsal and caudal-cranial views. Alignment of the fragments is poor. Further efforts at alignment and fixation were needed to adequately manage this case.

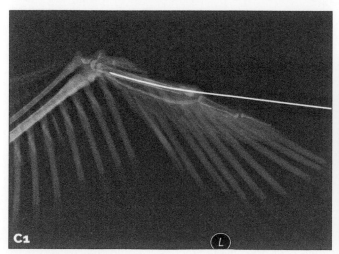
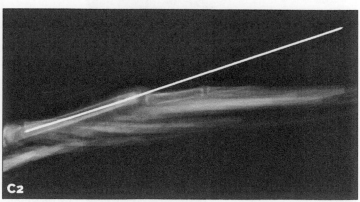

Figure 6-39C1, 2. Intra-operative ventro-dorsal and caudal-cranial views during placement of an intramedullary pin. Note introduction of IM pin at distal end of the major metacarpal.

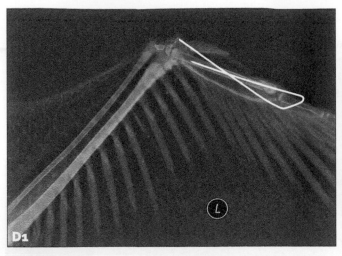

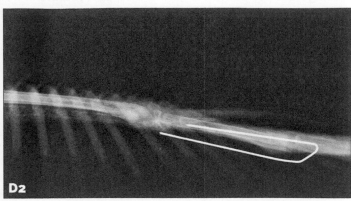

Figure 6-39D1, 2. Post-operative ventro-dorsal and caudal-cranial views. The pin is bent so that it can be captured by the over-wrapped coaptive bandage to prevent pull-out.

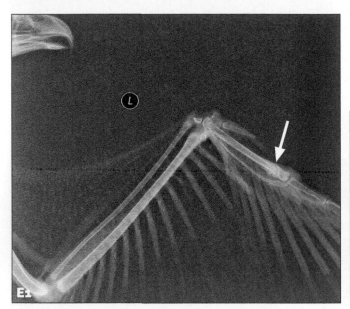

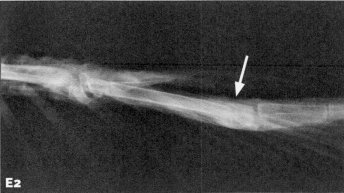

Figure 6-39E1, 2. 8 days post-operatively. Ventro-dorsal and caudal-cranial views. Callus is well-formed and bone fragments were partially healed; fixation was removed, and the wing restrained in a simple body wrap for another week. Site of the former fracture is indicated by *arrow*.

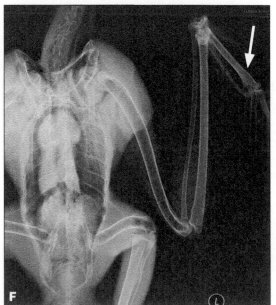

Figure 6-39F. 25 days post-operatively. Fracture is completely healed *(arrow)* and bone remodeling is complete, as is maturation of the remainder of the skeleton.

Case 18.

Management of a Metacarpal Fragment with a Short, Proximal Fragment in a Barred Owl (*Strix varia*) (Figures 6-40A-H): This injury was managed using a Type I external skeletal fixator in which a jig was employed during placement to facilitate alignment of the bone fragments.

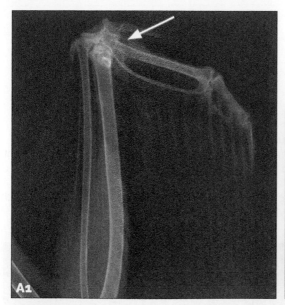
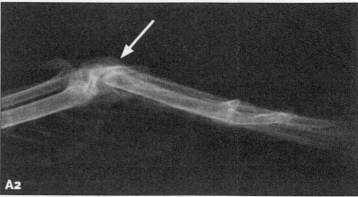

Figure 6-40A1, 2. Admission. Ventro-dorsal and caudal-cranial views. This injury resembles the one in Figure 6-38 of the Red-tailed Hawk with an asymmetric metacarpal fracture except that the proximal fragment is much shorter. The fracture location is indicated with *arrows*. A similar approach was taken for fixation. Two 0.035-in (0.7-mm) diameter interface pins were placed in a crossing over configuration into the proximal fragment to gain purchase on the small amount of bone present and prevent rotation of that fragment as would occur if only a single pin were applied. A temporary jig made from a 1/8-inch (3.175- mm) stainless steel bar and Kirschner clamps, and several intra-operative radiographs, were used to ensure alignment of the fragments.

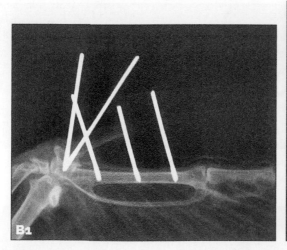
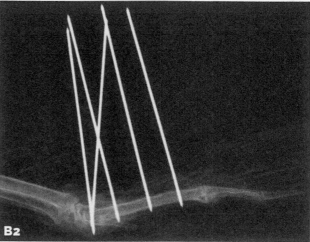

Figure 6-40B1, 2. Intra-operative radiograph for checking pin placement. Ventro-dorsal and caudal-cranial views.

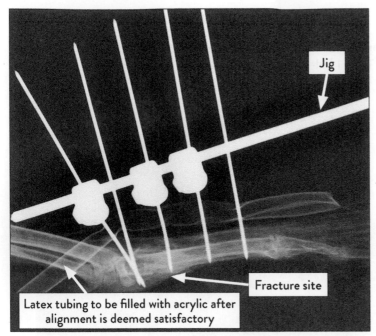

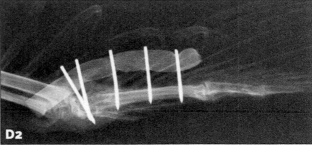

Figure 6-40C. Intra-operative caudal-cranial view: A temporary jig was used to allow alignment of fragments and hold pins in place while the acrylic bar was formed. Note the shadow of the latex tubing that was put in place before the jig was applied. The jig was removed after the acrylic in the tube had cured.

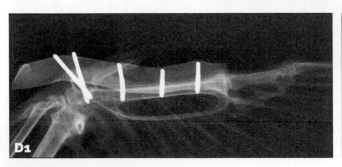

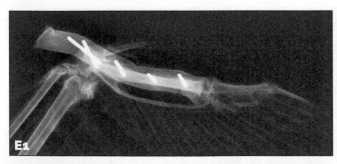

Figure 6-40D1, 2. Immediately post-operatively. Ventro-dorsal and caudal-cranial views. Alignment is good in both planes. The acrylic bar is close to the bone making for a stronger construct by creating a short working distance between the bone and fixator bar.

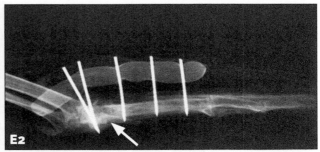

Figure 6-40E1, 2. Day 13 post-operatively. Ventro-dorsal and caudal-cranial views. Alignment was good in both planes; fixation showed no signs of loosening and there was callus formation evident at the fracture site *(arrow)*.

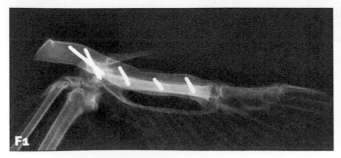

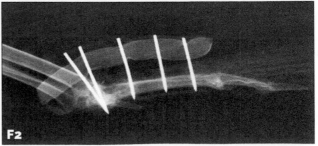

Figure 6-40F1, 2. Day 32 postop. Ventro-dorsal and caudal-cranial views. Healing was progressing, callus formation was not excessive suggesting good stability; there was good bone viability at the fracture site.

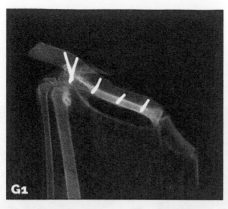

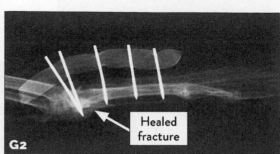

Figure 6-40G1, 2. Day 42 post-operatively. Ventro-dorsal and caudal-cranial views. Healing was complete and bone remodeling was evident. Hardware was removed at this point.

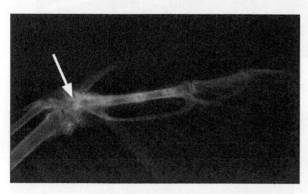

Figure 6-40H. Day 100 post-operatively. Ventro-dorsal view. Pre-release radiograph. *Arrow* indicates original fracture.

Case 19.

Conversion of a Type 1 Fixator with a Jig to a Hybrid Tie-in-Fixator in a Great Horned Owl *(Bubo virginianus)* **(Figures 6 41A-D):** A Type I Fixator with a jig was converted intra-operatively to a hybrid tie-in fixator when it became apparent that proper bone alignment was not being achieved. The midshaft location of the fracture was conducive to IM pin placement.

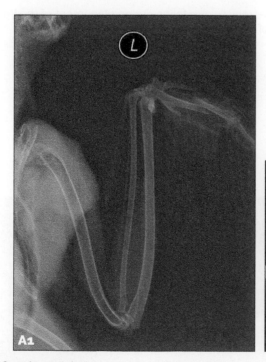

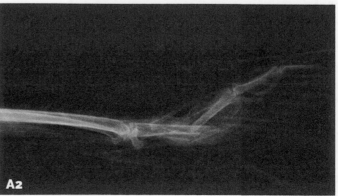

Figure 6-41A1, 2. Admission. Ventro-dorsal and caudal-cranial views. This case presented with a midshaft, transverse closed fracture of the major metacarpal bone with severe angular deviation of the distal fragment.

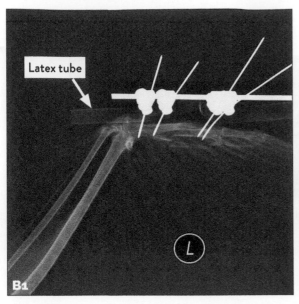
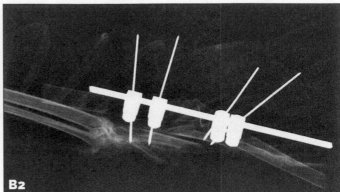

Figure 6-41B1, 2. Intra-operative radiographs. Ventro-dorsal and caudal-cranial views. The initial attempt to achieve bone alignment with the aid of a jig yielded unsatisfactory results, so another attempt was made converting to a hybrid fixator.

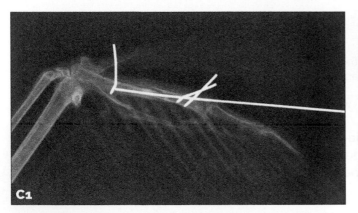
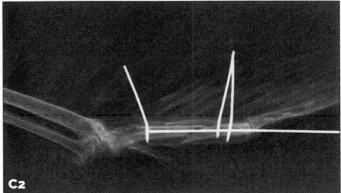

Figure 6-41C1, 2. Intra-operative radiographs. Ventro-dorsal and caudal-cranial views taken during placement of the IM pin for the hybrid fixator. Note normograde insertion of IM pin from distal end of the major metacarpal bone.

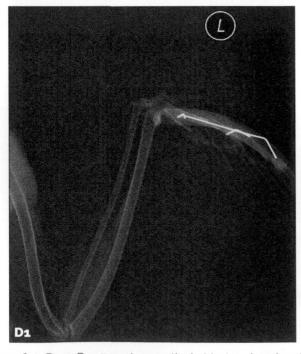
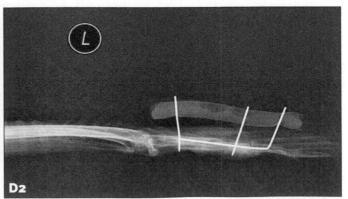

Figure 6-41D1, 2. Day 7 post-operatively. Ventro-dorsal and caudal-cranial views. These images demonstrate the complete tie-in fixator applied to the metacarpus.

Case 20.

Use of a Type 1 Transarticular Fixator to Stabilize a Major Distal Metacarpal Fracture in an American Kestrel *(Falco sparverius)* **(Figures 6-42A-E).**

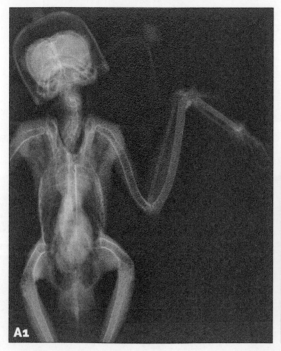

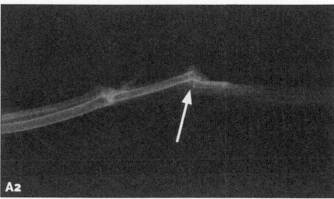

Figure 6-42A1, 2. Admission. Ventro-dorsal and caudal-cranial views. Distally located major metacarpal luxation/fracture *(arrow)*. There is no bone fragment in the distal major metacarpal to gain purchase with an ESF pin. Coaptation with a thermoplastic splint was attempted but alignment of the bones was not achieved. The splint was replaced by a transarticular fixator. This consisted of three 0.035-inch (0.7-mm) diameter Interface pins placed in the proximal fragment and two more tapping into the more distal phalange.

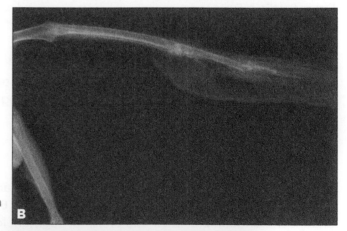

Figure 6-42B. Caudal-cranial view. The first attempt at stabilization with a thermoplastic splint did not yield satisfactory alignment.

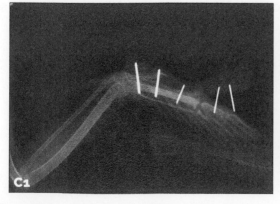

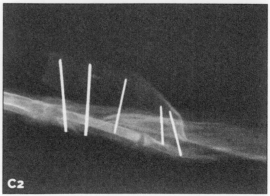

Figure 6-42C1, 2. Post-operative radiographs. Ventro-dorsal and caudal-cranial views. A Type 1 fixator was applied as a transarticular device with two pins anchored in the phalanges—note alignment of fragments in both planes.

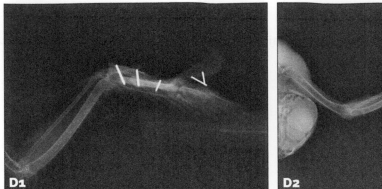
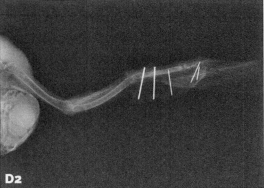

Figure 6-42D1, 2. Day 6 post-operative radiograph. Ventro-dorsal and caudal-cranial views. Alignment has been maintained and the fixator is firmly attached.

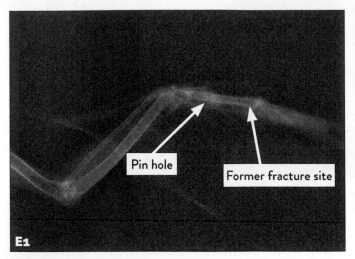
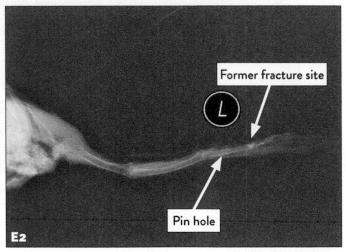

Figure 6-42E1, 2. Day 34 post-operatively. Ventro-dorsal and caudal-cranial views. Healing is complete and the wing elements are functional. The fracture is all but nondetectable – not to be confused with the immediately adjacent metacarpal-phalangeal joint.

Metacarpal Fractures Managed with Coaptation

Metacarpal fractures afford more latitude for choice between coaptation and surgical fixation. The cases in this section illustrate situations in which coaptation was regarded as a better choice than a surgical management approach.

Case 21.

Management of a Proximal Comminuted Major Metacarpal Fracture with Coaptation (Curved- Edge Splint) in a Bald Eagle *(Haliaeetus leucocephalus)* (Figures 6-43A-C): This method of fixation was chosen because of the comminution present in the proximal fragment for which installation of external skeletal fixator pins was contraindicated. The fracture healed in 6 weeks in a functional state; however, malalignment can be seen in the caudal-cranial view.

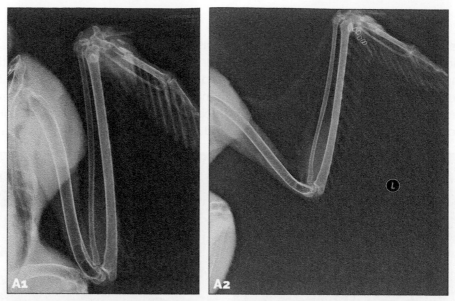

Figure 6-43A1, 2. Admission radiograph (ventro-dorsal) and at 12 days post-splinting. Alignment has been well-maintained and callus formation is evident. Note staples used for closure of an open wound. Physical therapy was begun at this point per standard protocol and continued twice weekly for the duration of recovery.

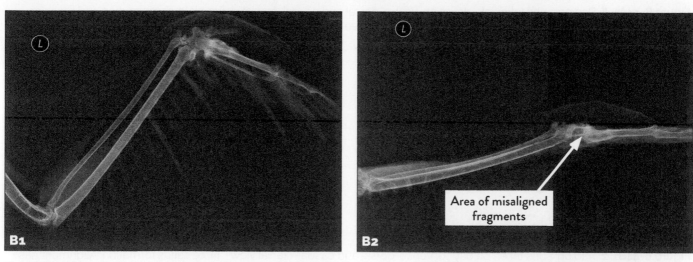

Area of misaligned fragments

Figure 6-43B1, 2. Radiographs taken at 42 days post splint application. Ventro-dorsal and caudal-cranial views. Fracture is healed, but there is malalignment evident in the caudal-cranial view; however, the wing was fully functional.

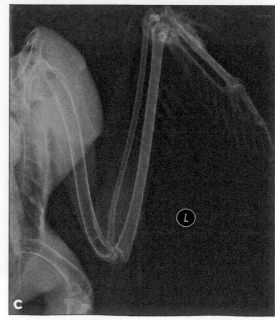

Figure 6-43C. Radiograph taken at 105 days - ventro-dorsal view. Following the regrowth of molted feathers and completion of a physical conditioning routine, this eagle was released.

Case 22.

Bald Eagle *(Haliaeetus leucocephalus)* **(Figures 6-44A-C):** This case resembles the previous case and was managed non-surgically using a curved-edge splint. The outer 7 primary feathers were cut slightly distal to the skin line to deleverage the distractive forces otherwise applied to the metacarpus by these long heavy feathers. Alignment marks were made on the feather shafts with a permanent marker prior to removal. Feathers were saved until the bone healed after which they were reattached by imping. In addition to the splint, the wing was taped to the body for the first two weeks and no physical therapy was conducted until partial healing of the fracture was evident.

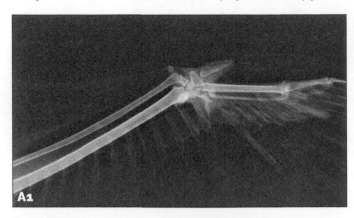
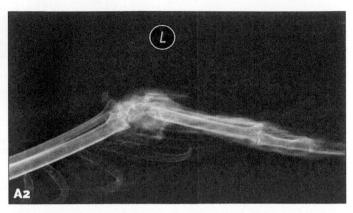

Figure 6-44A1, 2. Radiographs taken at admission: Ventro-dorsal and caudal-cranial views. Note comminution and the very short proximal fragment. The articular surfaces appear to be free of damage as viewed on the ventro-dorsal projection.

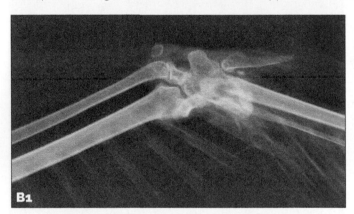
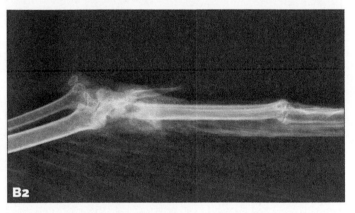

Figure 6-44B1, 2. Radiographs taken on day 16: Ventro-dorsal and caudal-cranial views. Note callus formation. Alignment has been maintained in both planes. Physical therapy (passive range of motion) was started at this point.

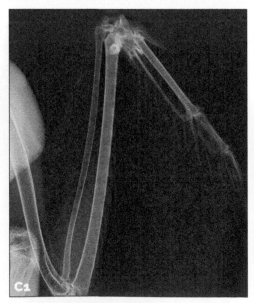
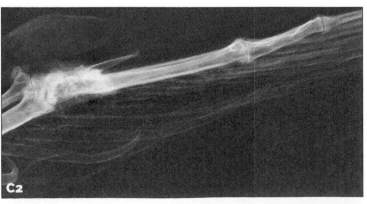

Figure 6-44C1, 2. Radiograph on day 187: Ventro-dorsal and caudal-cranial views just prior to release. Note remodeling of callus and good alignment in both planes.

Case 23.

Management of a Midshaft Major Metacarpal Fracture with Coaptation in a Sharp-shinned Hawk *(Accipiter striatus)*: This mode of stabilization was chosen owing to the small size of the bones (total body weight was 120 g) and the significant degree of edema and swelling of the soft tissues which required an extended period of time to resolve. The fracture healed adequately with good function of the wing despite the mal-alignment evident in the posterior-anterior view **(Figures 6-45A-C)**.

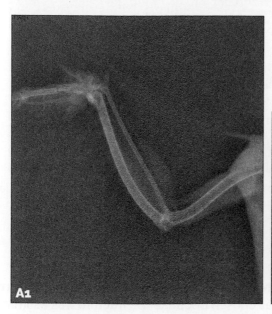

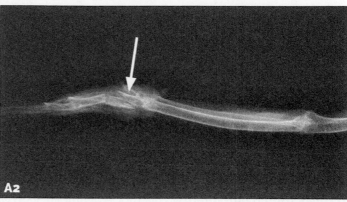

Figure 6-45A1, 2. Radiographs taken on admission: Ventro-dorsal and caudal-cranial views. Note swelling of soft tissue evident in the posterior-anterior projection *(arrow)*. DMSO was applied to the affected area for the first 3 days; light bandaging was applied, and the wing was held taped firmly to the body.

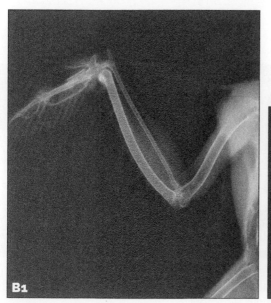

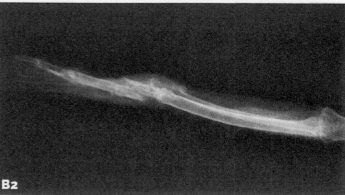

Figure 6-45B1, 2. Radiographs taken on day 25: Ventro-dorsal and caudal-cranial views. Misalignment of the fragments can be noted in the caudal-cranial view.

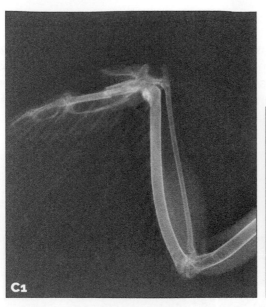
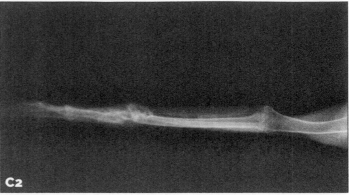

Figure 6-45C1, 2. Day 38: Ventro-dorsal and caudal-cranial views. The fracture was healed with slight malalignment evident in posterior-anterior; mechanics were good, however, and the patient was released with full flight ability. Note resolution in soft tissue swelling around the metacarpal joint as seen in the caudal-cranial view.

Case 24.

Management of Midshaft, Simple Fractures of the Major and Minor Metacarpals with Coaptation in a Broad-winged Hawk *(Buteo platypterus).* This mode of stabilization was chosen because the fracture was estimated to be 7-10 days old with considerable callus formation (arrow) and attendant stability **(Figures 6-46A-D)**.

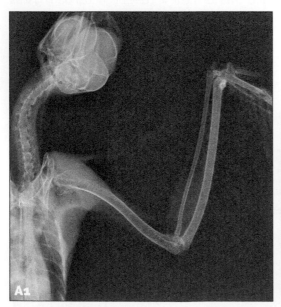
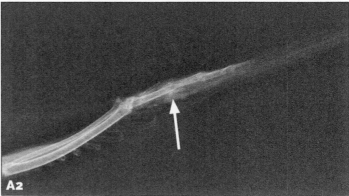

Figure 6-46A1, 2. Admission radiographs: Ventro-dorsal and caudal-cranial views. Note the callus at the fracture site and the density of the surrounding soft tissue *(arrow)* – both contributing to stability at the site. Slight bending of the soft callus during application of the coaptive bandage brought the metacarpal fragments into alignment.

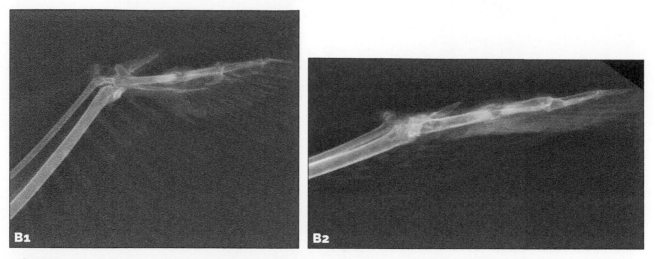

Figure 6-46B1, 2. Radiographs taken on Day 16: Ventro-dorsal and caudal-cranial views. The periosteal callus was forming well and beginning to mineralize; alignment has been maintained in both planes. Interfragmentary bone loss was evident.

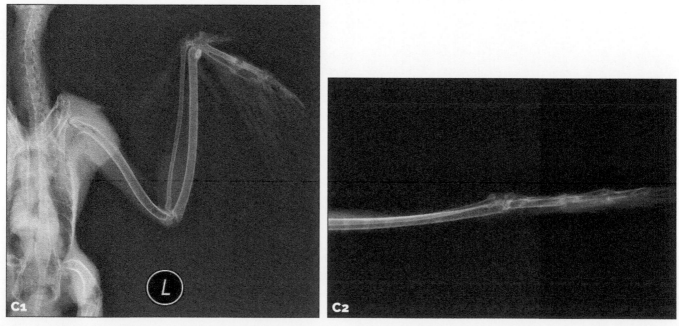

Figure 6-46C1, 2. Radiographs taken on day 28: Ventro-dorsal and caudal-cranial views. The external callus has remodeled and is holding fragments in alignment. There was a lack of endosteal callus bridging the fracture. Coaptation was maintained for 4 more weeks. Physical therapy was provided twice weekly during healing.

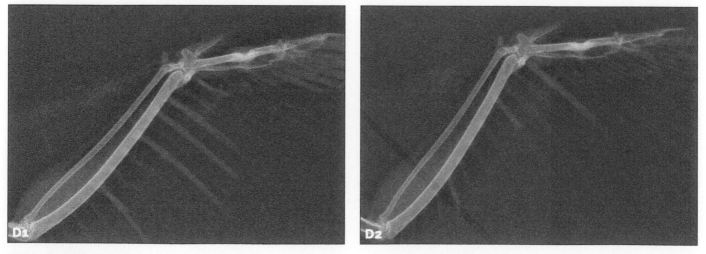

Figure 6-46D1, 2. Ventro-dorsal radiographs taken on days 51 and 76. Bridging endosteal callus has formed and the healing process was complete.

Anatomy of the Pelvic Girdle and Leg

PELVIC GIRDLE, THIGH, LEG AND PES

Lateral Skeleton

Three bones form the pelvic girdle—the ilium, the ischium, and the pubis. These bones are partially fused to each other, as well as to the synsacrum. The synsacrum represents a fusion of a number of sacral, lumbar, and caudal vertebrae. Most of the bony pelvis is derived from the ilium cranially and the ischium caudally. The acetabulum lies between the two and contains a central acetabular foramen *[foramen acetabula]*. Caudal to the acetabulum is an ilioischiatic foramen *[foramen ilioischiadicum]*, with an obturator foramen [foramen obturatum] ventrally. The two slender pubic bones attach to the ischia cranially, but curve caudally and ventrally.

The femur of birds varies in its curvature of the condyles distally, based on function. Dislocation of the knee and tendons is reduced by deep grooves and ridges over the joint surface. These factors aid in locomotion and dexterity (Fischer 1946).

There are several prominent features at both the proximal and distal ends of the femur. At the proximal end of the femur is a prominent trochanter *[trochanter femoris]* for insertion of the iliotrochantericus muscles. There is an intercondylar sulcus *[sulcus intercondylaris]* between the lateral and medial condyles. It is continuous proximally with the patellar sulcus for the patella to slide.

Notable features may also be observed for the tibiotarsus and fibula. On the proximal end of the tibiotarsus and fibula is an articular surface for the femoral condyles. Additionally, there are the cranial and lateral cnemial crests for the origins of some of the extensor muscles of the hock and digits. At the distal end of the bone on the cranial side is an extensor canal for the extensor digitorum longus. The medial and lateral condyles at the distal end of the bone articulate with the tarsometatarsus.

It is thought that during embryogenesis some of the proximal tarsal bones fuse with the tibia; hence, the term tibiotarsus. The tarsometatarsus is thought to include some of the distal tarsal bones with three metatarsal bones. Metatarsals II, III, and IV are fused in the adult (Getty 1975) with metatarsal I remaining separate.

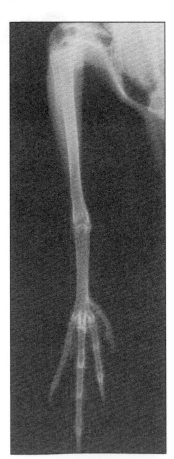

The proximal tarsometatarsus has a medial and a lateral surface for articulation with the tibiotarsus. At its distal end are three trochlea for articulation with digits II, III, and IV. There is an interosseous canal *[canalis interosseous tendineus]* for the tendon of the extensor of digit IV between the trochlea for digits III and IV. On the medial side of the tarsometatarsus is a fossa [fossa metatarsi I] for the first metatarsal.

Digits II, III, and IV usually have three, four, and five phalanges (or phalanxes), respectively. Digit I, the hallux, usually has two phalanges. Digit IV may be directed cranially or caudally, depending on the species. The last phalanx of each digit is claw shaped.

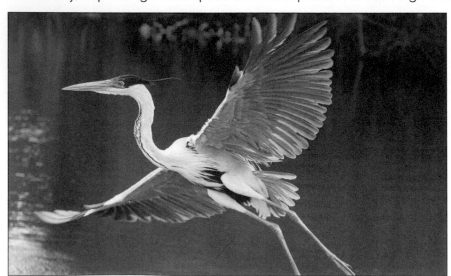

Lateral Skeleton of the Leg

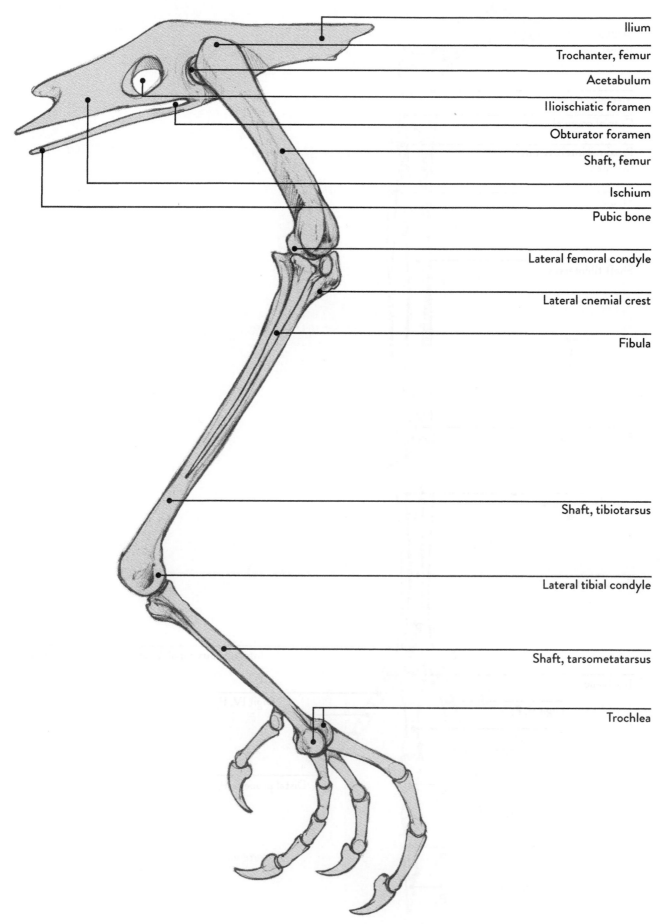

Ilium

Trochanter, femur

Acetabulum

Ilioischiatic foramen

Obturator foramen

Shaft, femur

Ischium

Pubic bone

Lateral femoral condyle

Lateral cnemial crest

Fibula

Shaft, tibiotarsus

Lateral tibial condyle

Shaft, tarsometatarsus

Trochlea

Cranial Pelvic Limb Skeleton

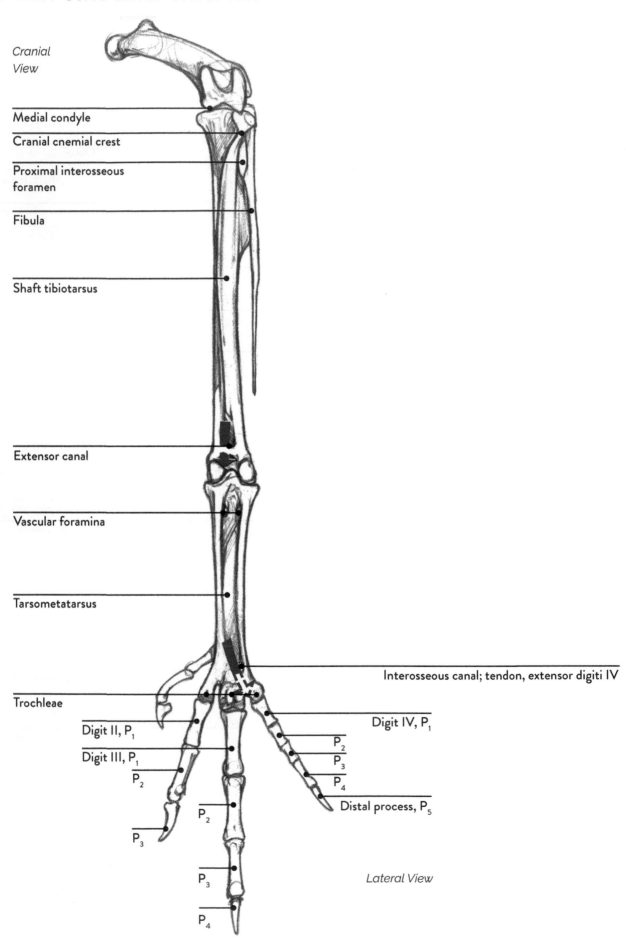

Cranial View

Medial condyle

Cranial cnemial crest

Proximal interosseous foramen

Fibula

Shaft tibiotarsus

Extensor canal

Vascular foramina

Tarsometatarsus

Trochleae

Digit II, P$_1$

Digit III, P$_1$

P$_2$

P$_3$

P$_2$

P$_3$

P$_4$

Interosseous canal; tendon, extensor digiti IV

Digit IV, P$_1$

P$_2$

P$_3$

P$_4$

Distal process, P$_5$

Lateral View

Medial View of The Skeleton of the Leg

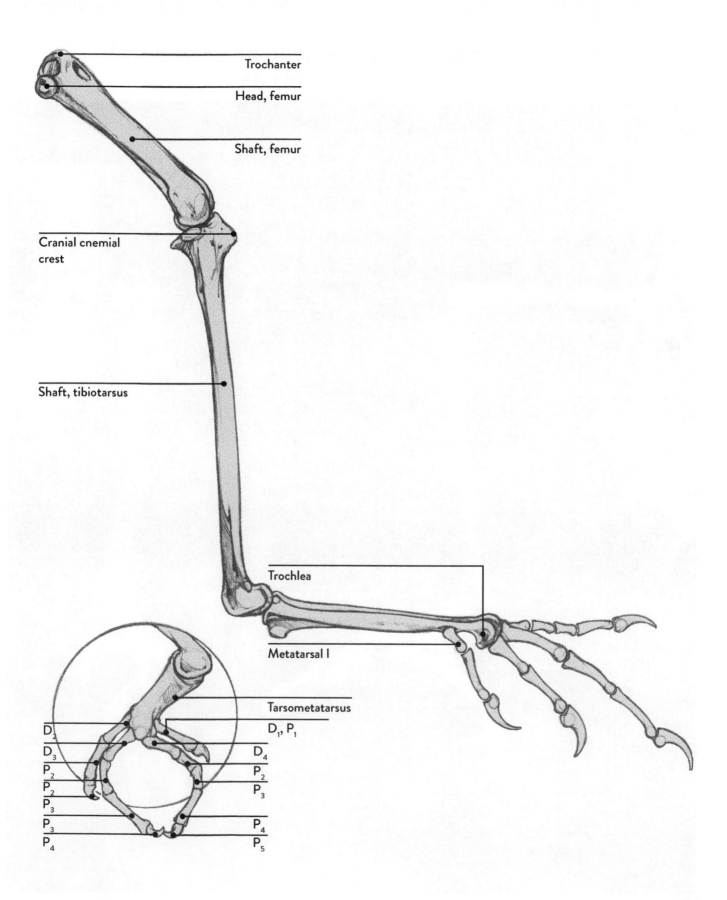

Trochanter

Head, femur

Shaft, femur

Cranial cnemial crest

Shaft, tibiotarsus

Trochlea

Metatarsal I

Tarsometatarsus

D_1, P_1

D_2

D_3

D_4

P_2

P_2

P_2

P_3

P_3

P_3

P_4

P_4

P_5

Leg: CT Images

Computed tomography images of the leg are presented for the orange-winged Amazon (*Amazona amazonica*), umbrella cockatoo *(Cacatua alba)*, military macaw *(Ara militaris)*, budgerigar *(Melopsittacus undulatus)*, pigeon *(Columba livia)*, domestic chicken *(Gallus gallus domesticus)*, red-tailed hawk *(Buteo jamaicensis)*, great horned owl *(Bubo virginianus)*, and golden eagle *(Aquila chrysaetos)*.

Orange-winged Amazon (*Amazona amazonica*)
Caudal and Medial Leg

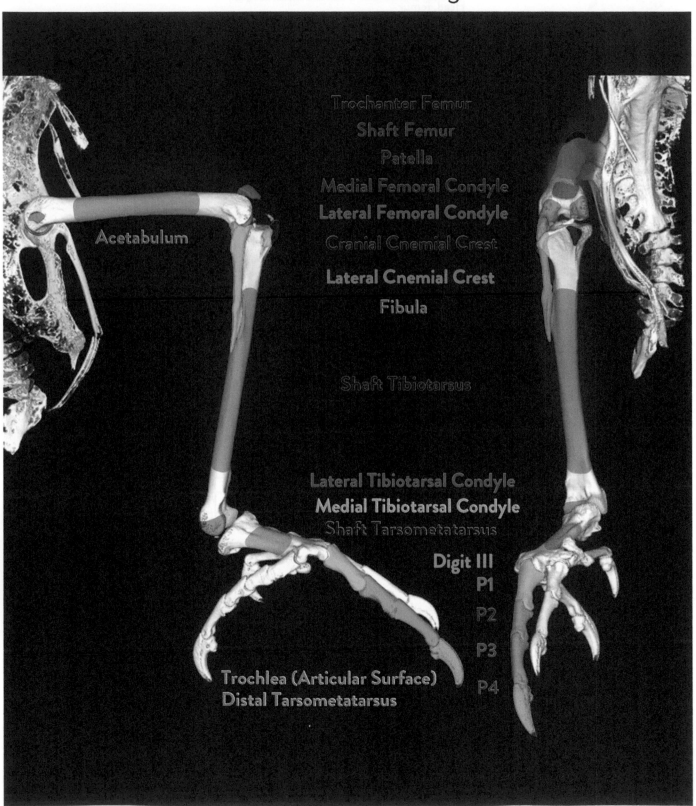

Trochanter Femur
Shaft Femur
Patella
Medial Femoral Condyle
Lateral Femoral Condyle
Cranial Cnemial Crest
Lateral Cnemial Crest
Fibula

Acetabulum

Shaft Tibiotarsus

Lateral Tibiotarsal Condyle
Medial Tibiotarsal Condyle
Shaft Tarsometatarsus

Digit III
P1
P2
P3
P4

Trochlea (Articular Surface)
Distal Tarsometatarsus

Orange-winged Amazon (*Amazona amazonica*)
Caudal and Medial Leg

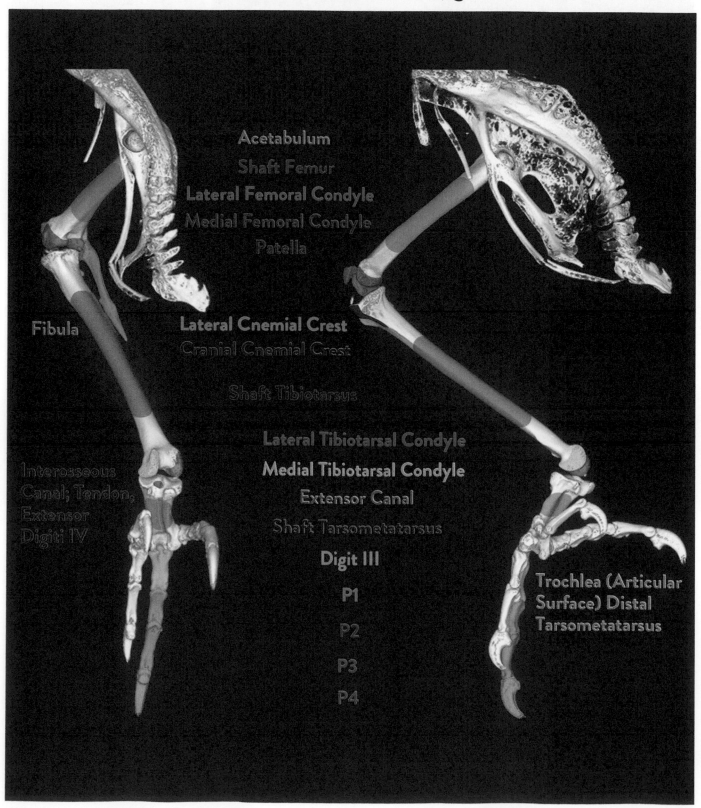

Acetabulum

Shaft Femur

Lateral Femoral Condyle

Medial Femoral Condyle

Patella

Fibula

Lateral Cnemial Crest

Cranial Cnemial Crest

Shaft Tibiotarsus

Lateral Tibiotarsal Condyle

Medial Tibiotarsal Condyle

Extensor Canal

Shaft Tarsometatarsus

Interosseous Canal; Tendon, Extensor Digiti IV

Digit III

P1

P2

P3

P4

Trochlea (Articular Surface) Distal Tarsometatarsus

Umbrella Cockatoo (*Cacatua alba*)
Lateral and Cranial Leg

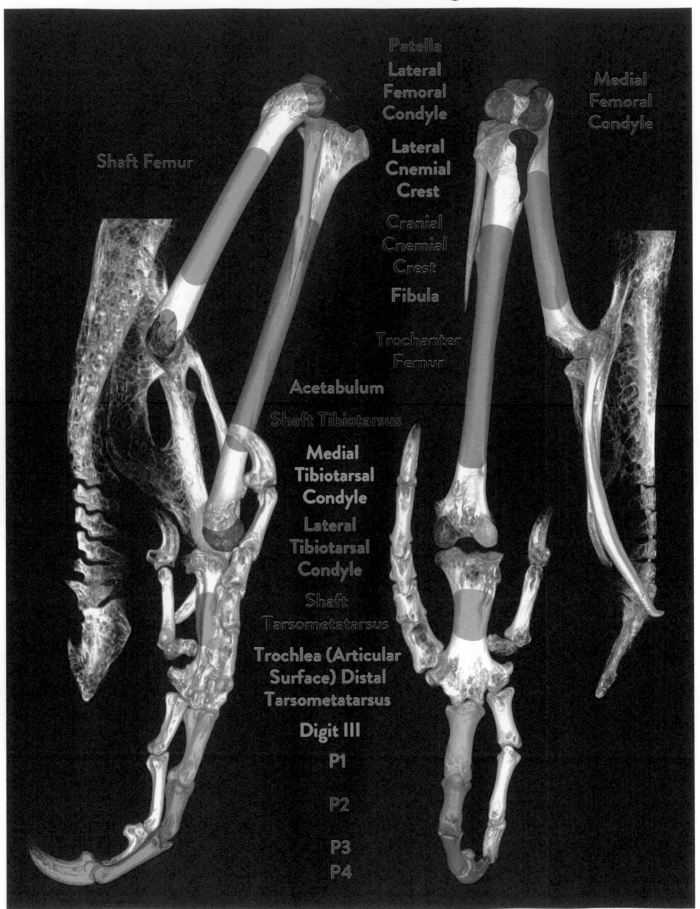

Patella

Lateral Femoral Condyle

Lateral Cnemial Crest

Cranial Cnemial Crest

Fibula

Trochanter Femur

Shaft Femur

Medial Femoral Condyle

Acetabulum

Shaft Tibiotarsus

Medial Tibiotarsal Condyle

Lateral Tibiotarsal Condyle

Shaft Tarsometatarsus

Trochlea (Articular Surface) Distal Tarsometatarsus

Digit III

P1

P2

P3

P4

Umbrella Cockatoo (*Cacatua alba*)
Caudal and Medial Leg

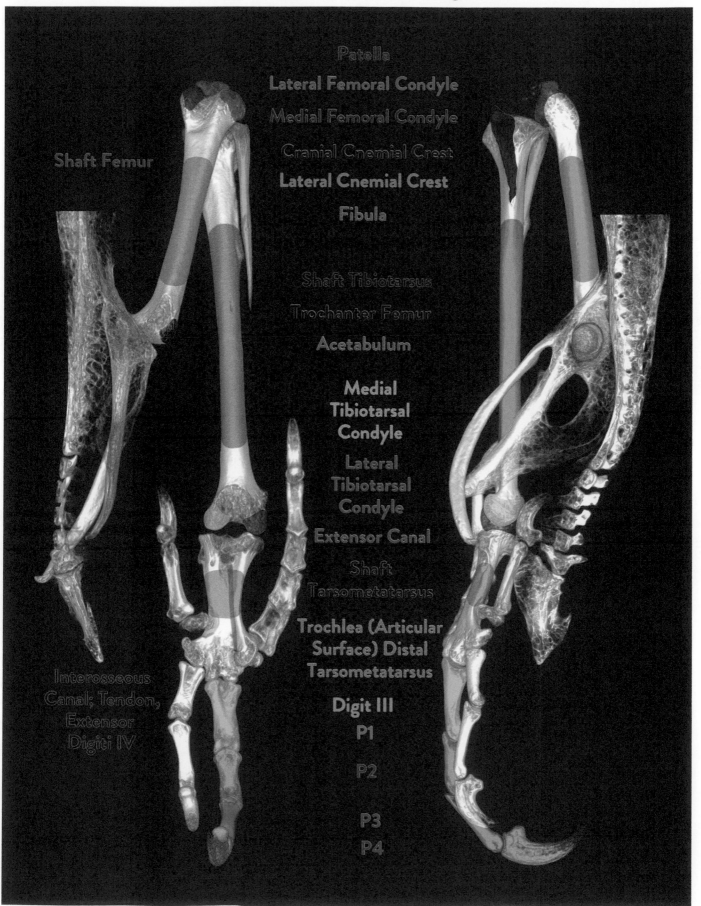

Patella
Lateral Femoral Condyle
Medial Femoral Condyle
Cranial Cnemial Crest
Lateral Cnemial Crest
Fibula

Shaft Tibiotarsus
Trochanter Femur
Acetabulum

Medial
Tibiotarsal
Condyle
Lateral
Tibiotarsal
Condyle
Extensor Canal
Shaft
Tarsometatarsus

Trochlea (Articular
Surface) Distal
Tarsometatarsus

Digit III
P1

P2

P3
P4

Shaft Femur

Interosseous
Canal; Tendon,
Extensor
Digiti IV

Military Macaw (*Ara militaris*)
Lateral and Cranial Hip

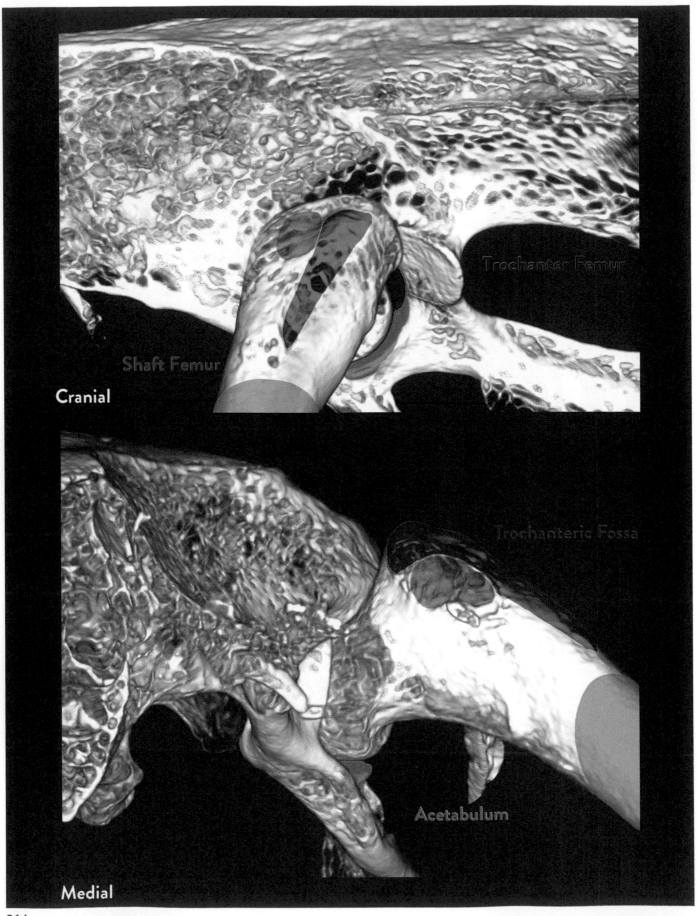

264

Military Macaw (*Ara militaris*)
Caudal and Caudal Medial Hip

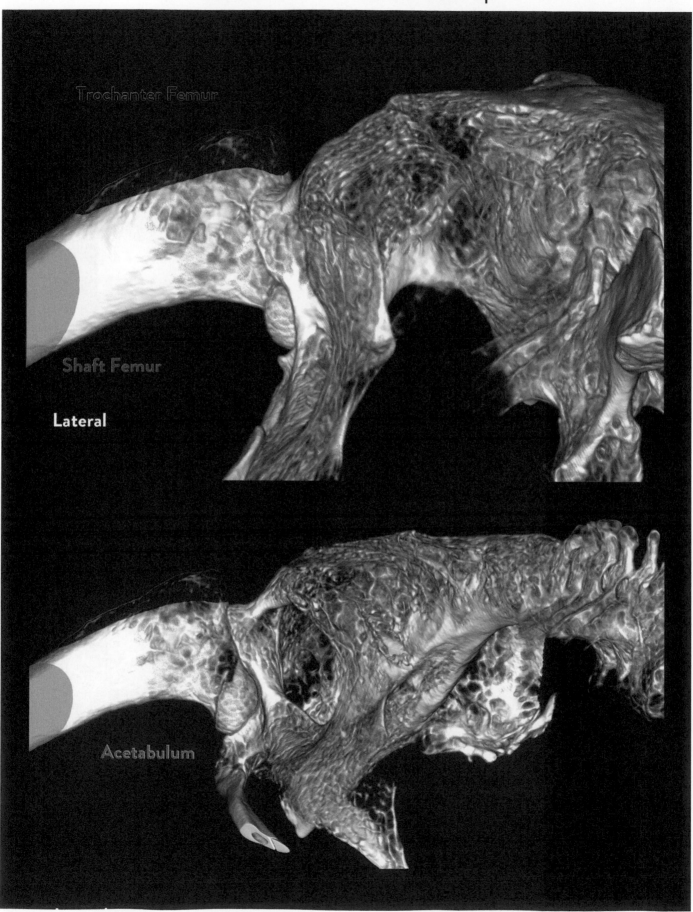

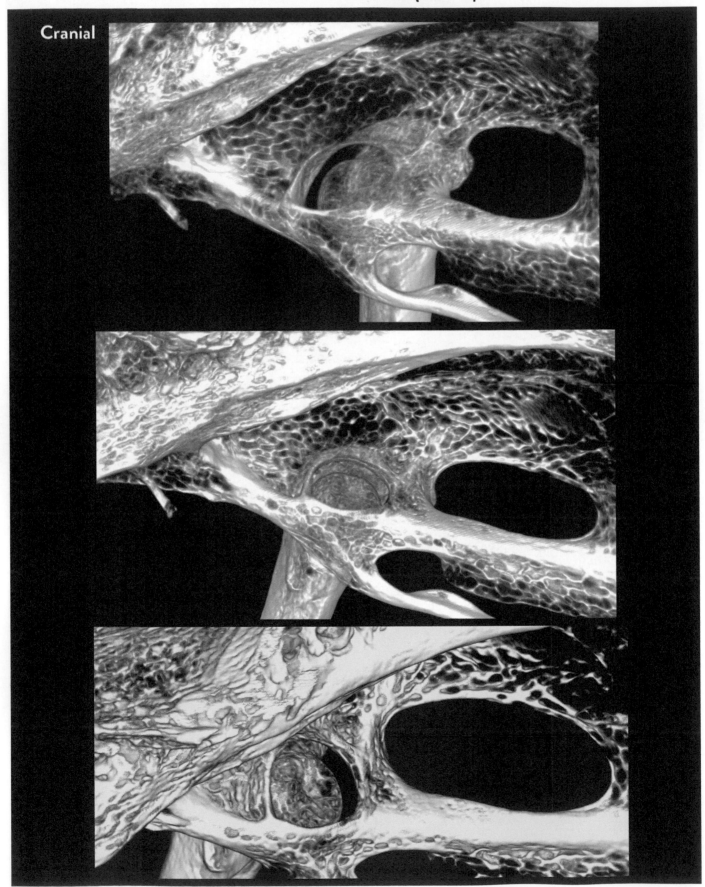

Cranial

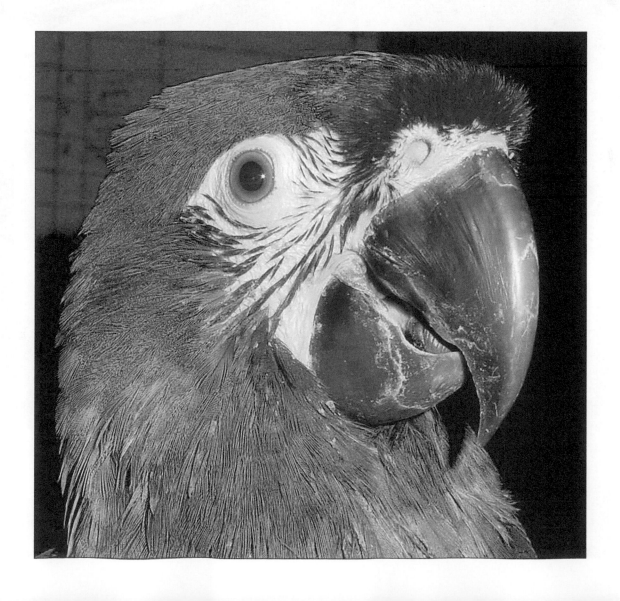

Military Macaw (*Ara militaris*)
Dorsal and Medial Hip

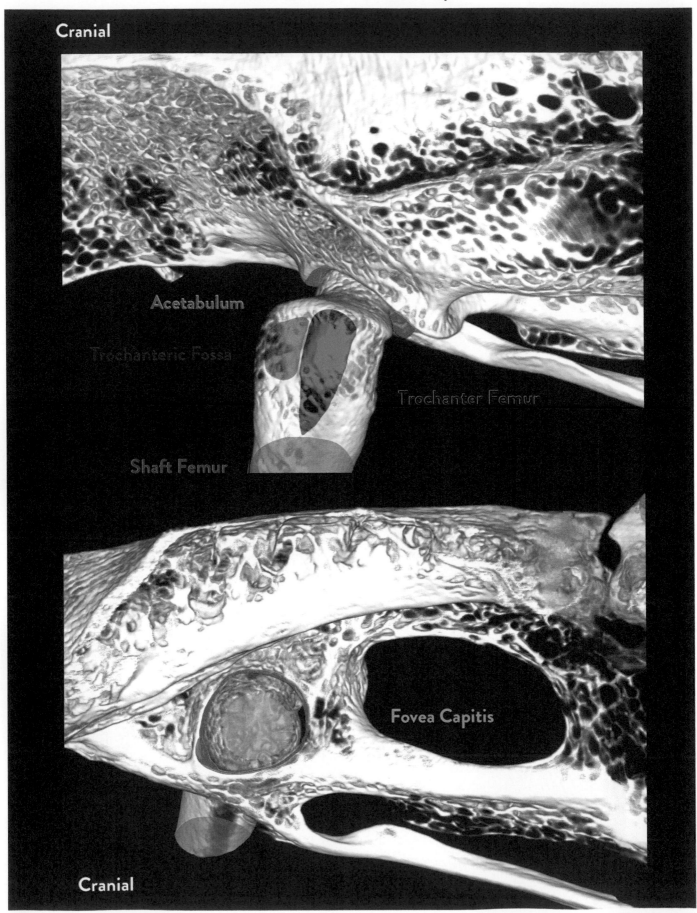

Cranial

Acetabulum

Trochanteric Fossa

Trochanter Femur

Shaft Femur

Fovea Capitis

Cranial

Military Macaw (*Ara militaris*)
Ventral and Ventral Lateral Hip

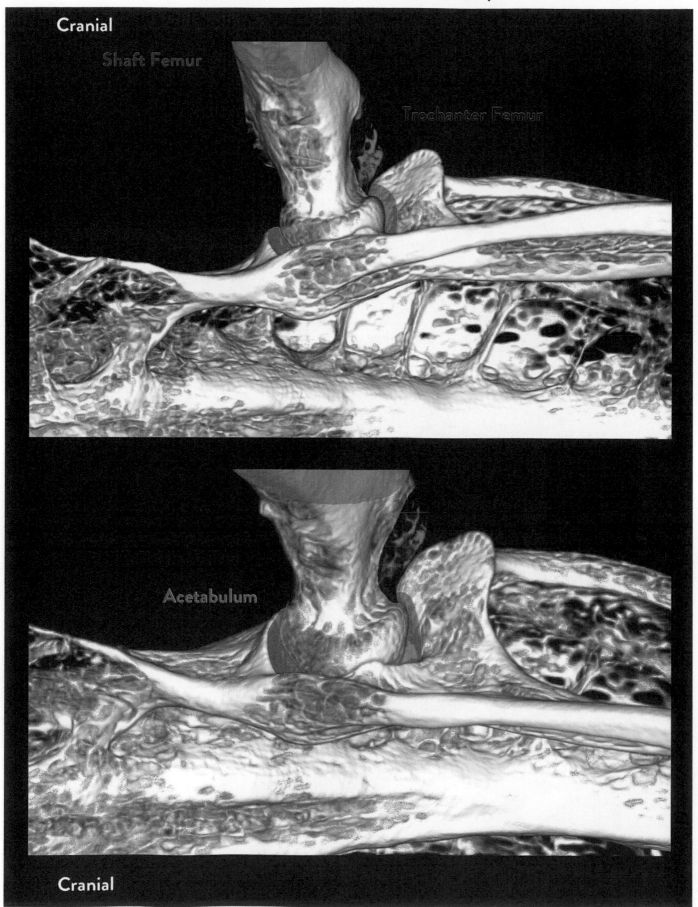

Military Macaw (*Ara militaris*)
Lateral Cranial Oblique, Lateral and Lateral Caudal Oblique Stifle

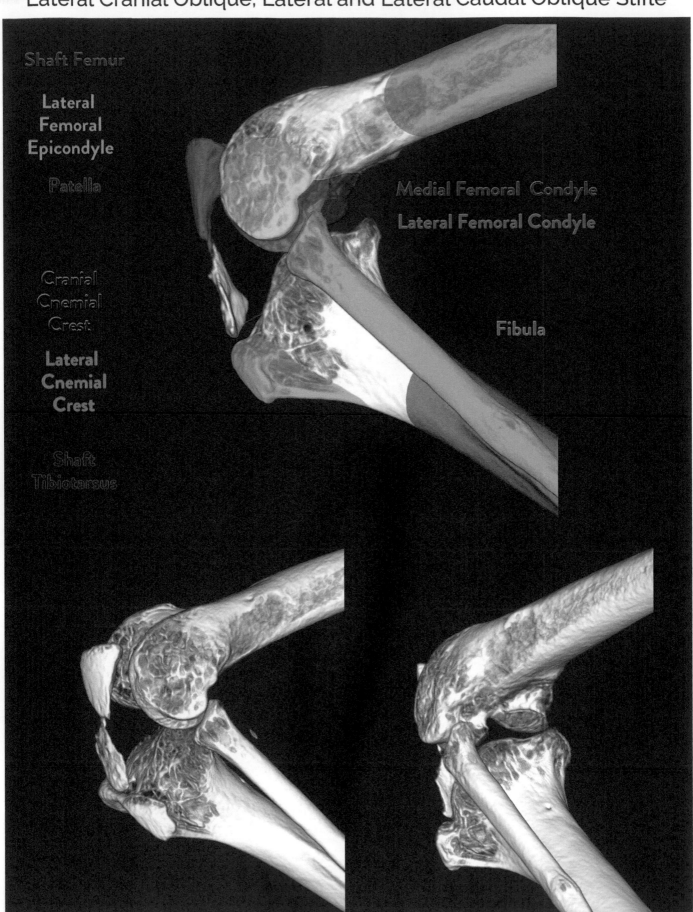

Shaft Femur

Lateral Femoral Epicondyle

Patella

Medial Femoral Condyle

Lateral Femoral Condyle

Cranial Cnemial Crest

Lateral Cnemial Crest

Fibula

Shaft Tibiotarsus

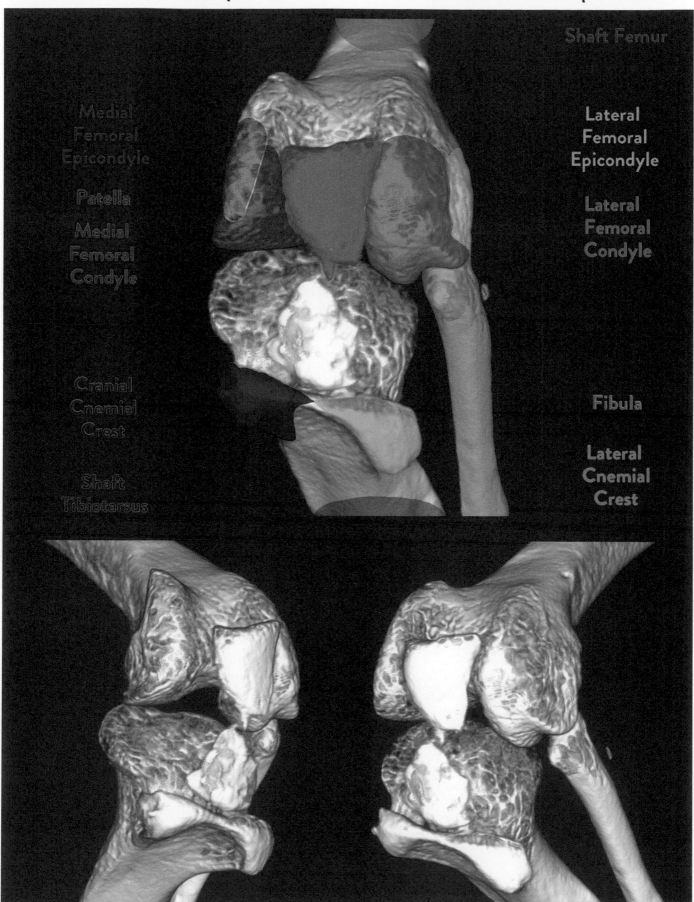

Shaft Femur

Medial Femoral Epicondyle

Patella

Medial Femoral Condyle

Cranial Cnemial Crest

Shaft Tibiotarsus

Lateral Femoral Epicondyle

Lateral Femoral Condyle

Fibula

Lateral Cnemial Crest

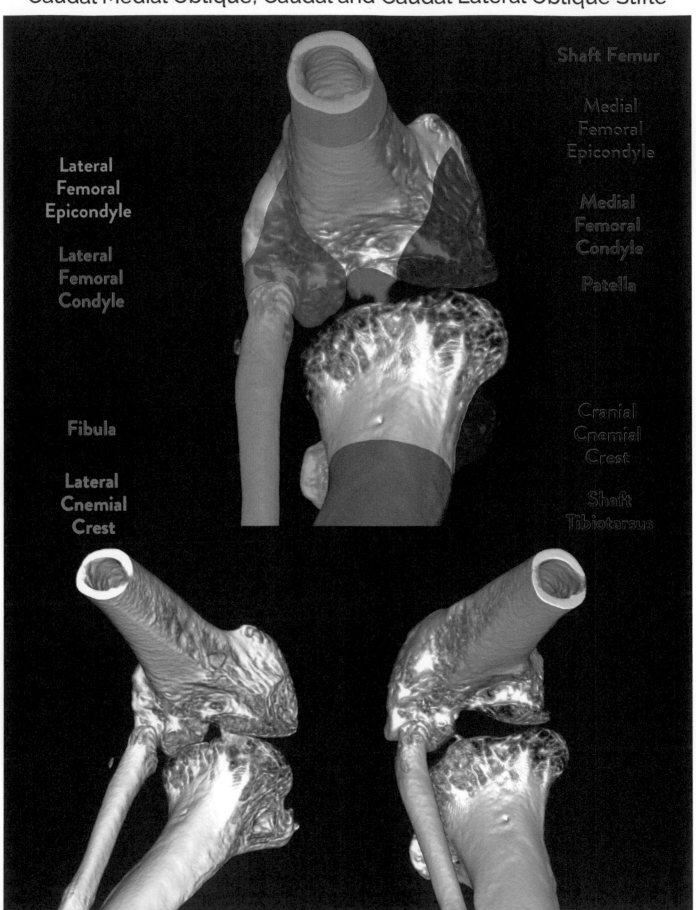

Shaft Femur

Medial Femoral Epicondyle

Medial Femoral Condyle

Patella

Lateral Femoral Epicondyle

Lateral Femoral Condyle

Fibula

Lateral Cnemial Crest

Cranial Cnemial Crest

Shaft Tibiotarsus

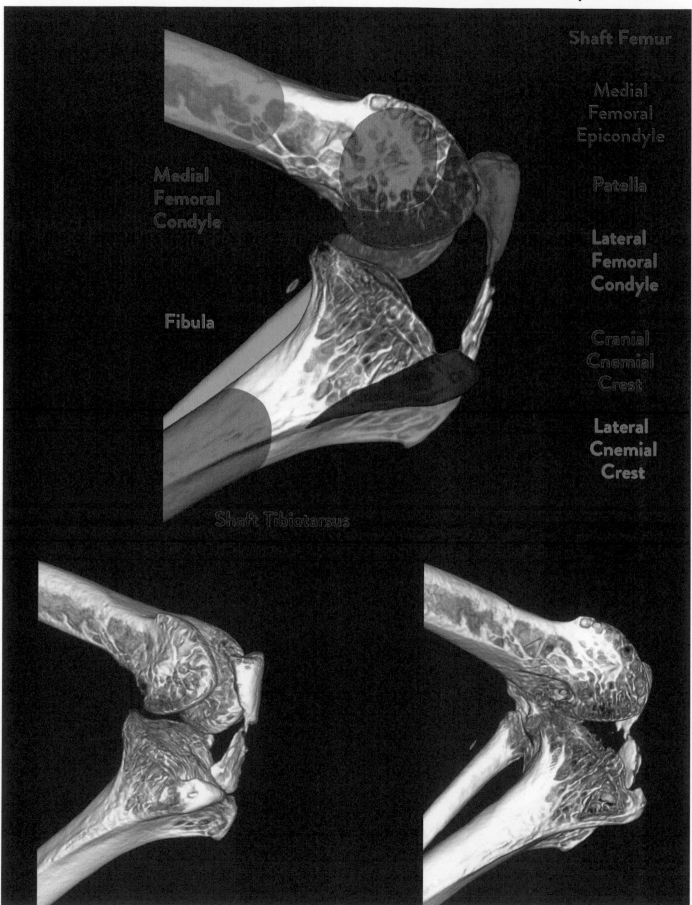

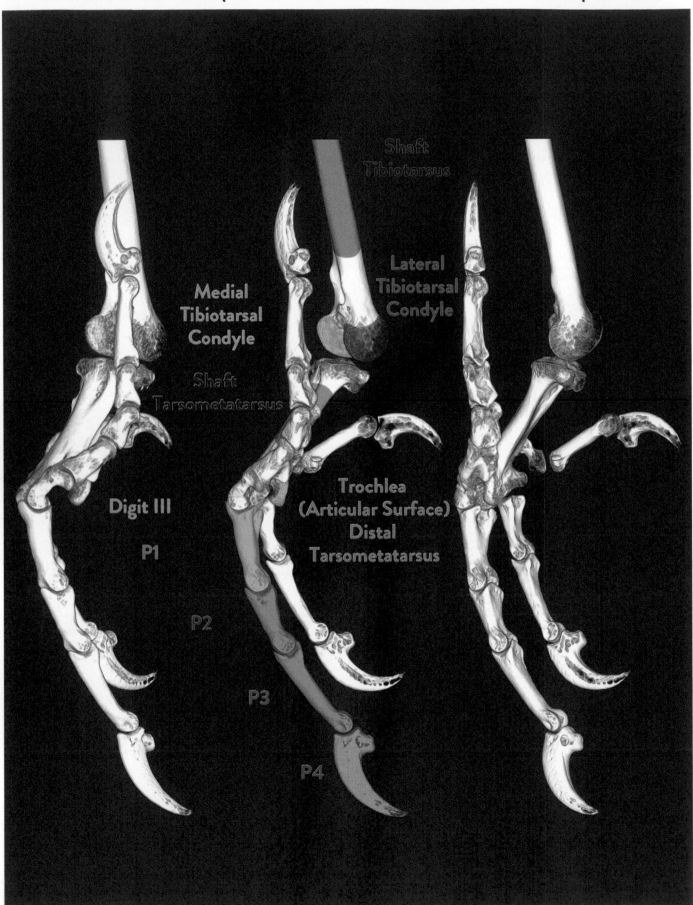

Military Macaw (*Ara militaris*)
Dorsal Medial Oblique, Dorsal and Dorsal Lateral Oblique Foot

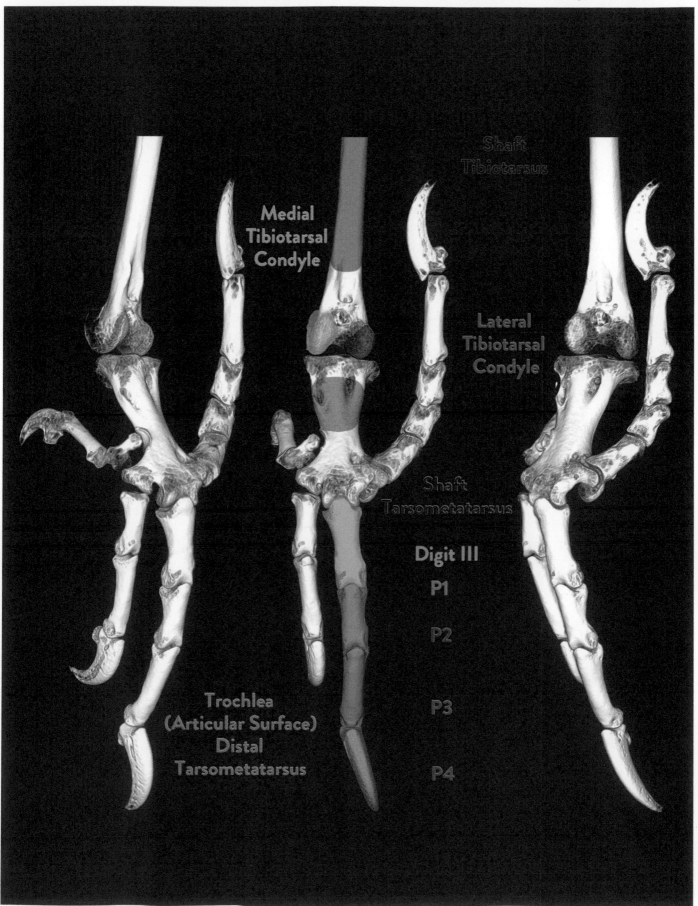

Medial Tibiotarsal Condyle

Shaft Tibiotarsus

Lateral Tibiotarsal Condyle

Shaft Tarsometatarsus

Digit III

P1

P2

P3

P4

Trochlea (Articular Surface) Distal Tarsometatarsus

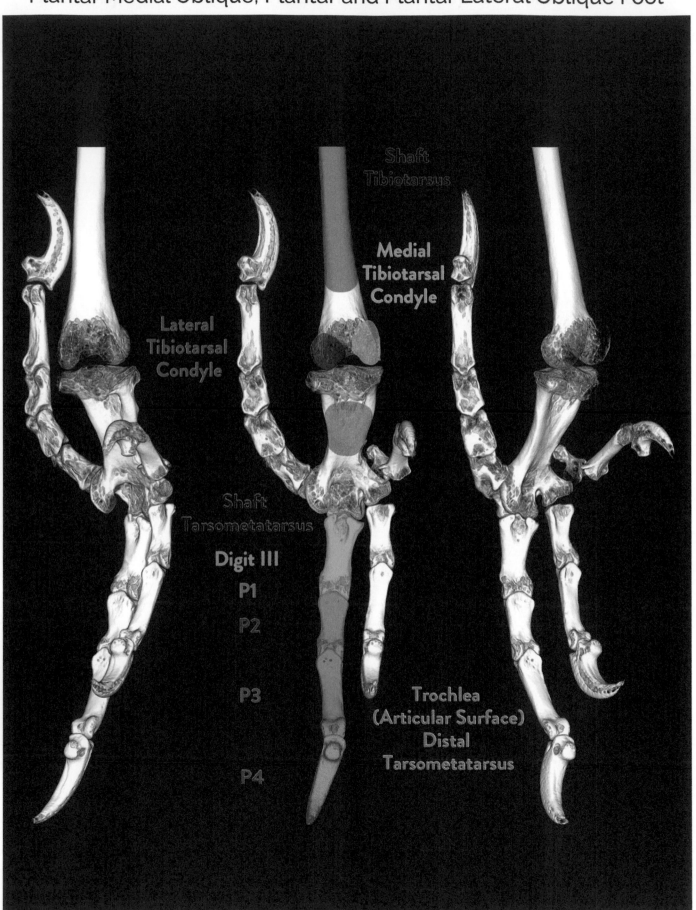

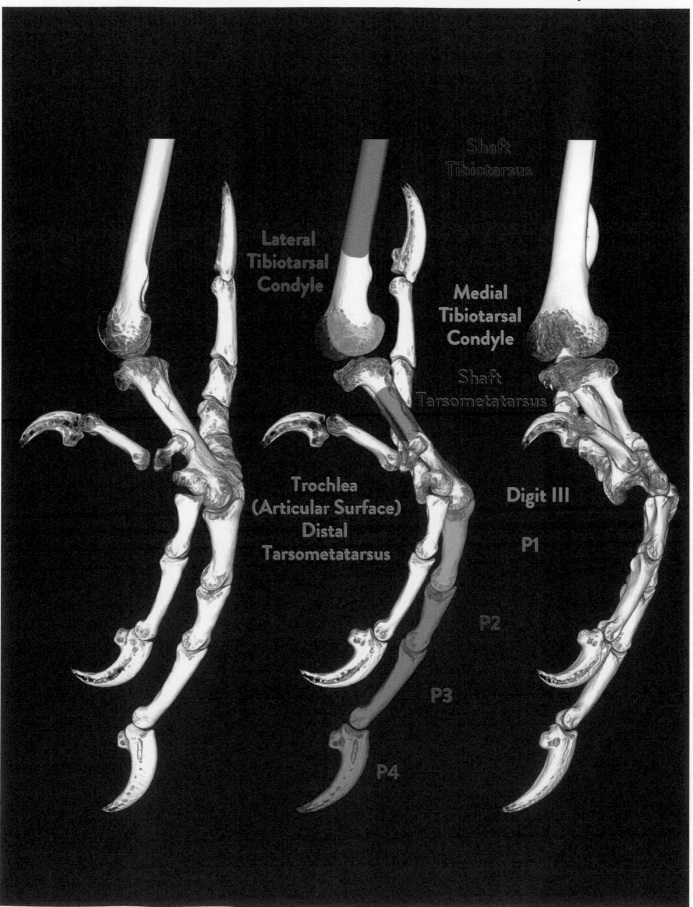

Budgerigar (*Melopsittacus undulatus*)
Lateral and Cranial View of the Leg

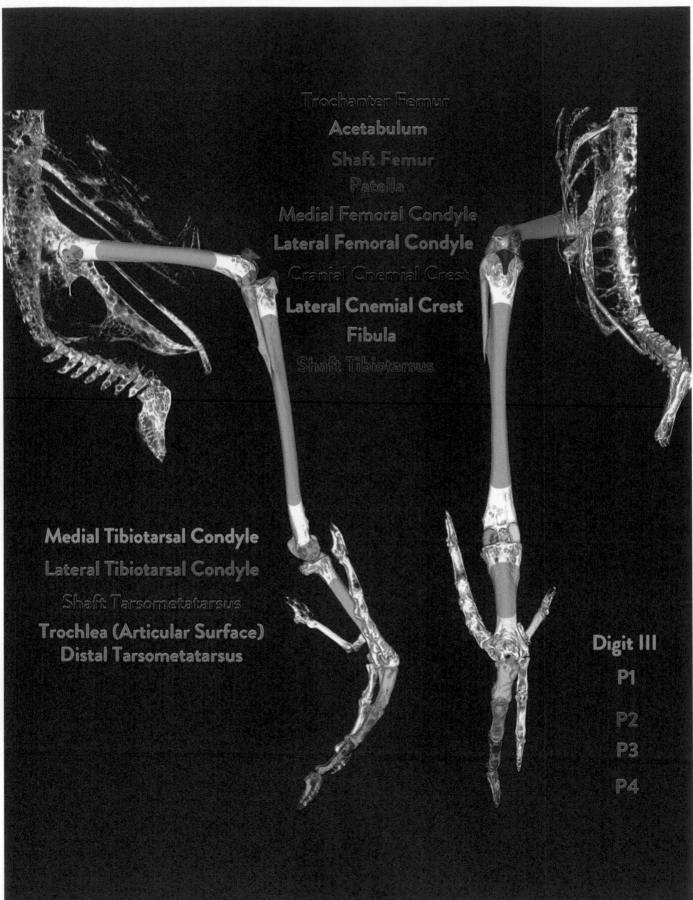

Trochanter Femur

Acetabulum

Shaft Femur

Patella

Medial Femoral Condyle

Lateral Femoral Condyle

Cranial Cnemial Crest

Lateral Cnemial Crest

Fibula

Shaft Tibiotarsus

Medial Tibiotarsal Condyle

Lateral Tibiotarsal Condyle

Shaft Tarsometatarsus

Trochlea (Articular Surface)
Distal Tarsometatarsus

Digit III

P1

P2

P3

P4

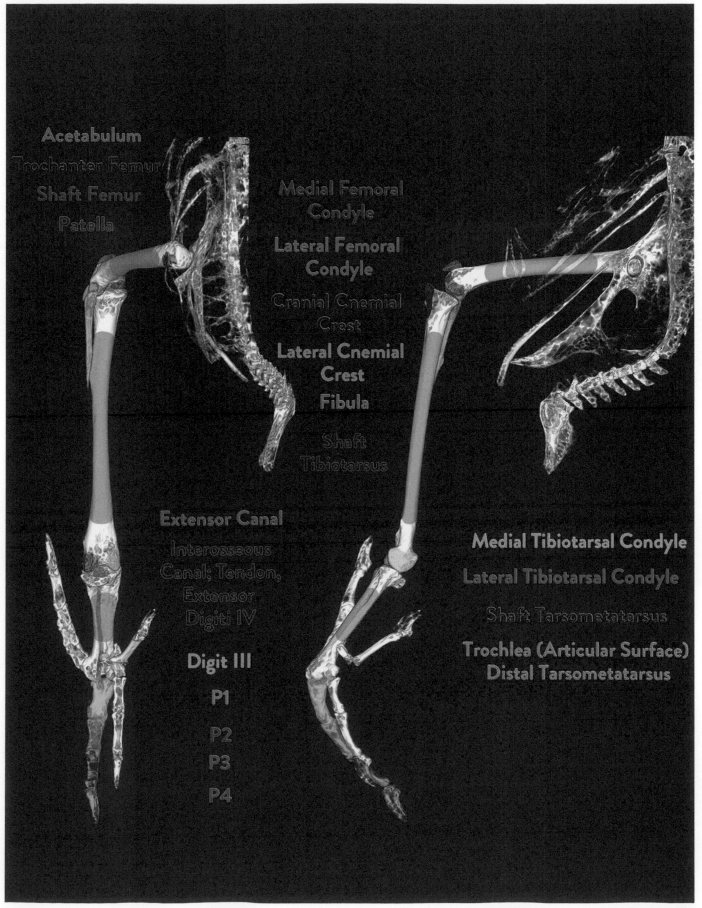

Acetabulum
Trochanter Femur
Shaft Femur
Patella

Medial Femoral Condyle
Lateral Femoral Condyle
Cranial Cnemial Crest
Lateral Cnemial Crest
Fibula
Shaft Tibiotarsus

Extensor Canal
Interosseous Canal; Tendon, Extensor Digiti IV

Digit III
P1
P2
P3
P4

Medial Tibiotarsal Condyle
Lateral Tibiotarsal Condyle
Shaft Tarsometatarsus
Trochlea (Articular Surface)
Distal Tarsometatarsus

Pigeon (*Columba livia*)
Lateral and Cranial Leg

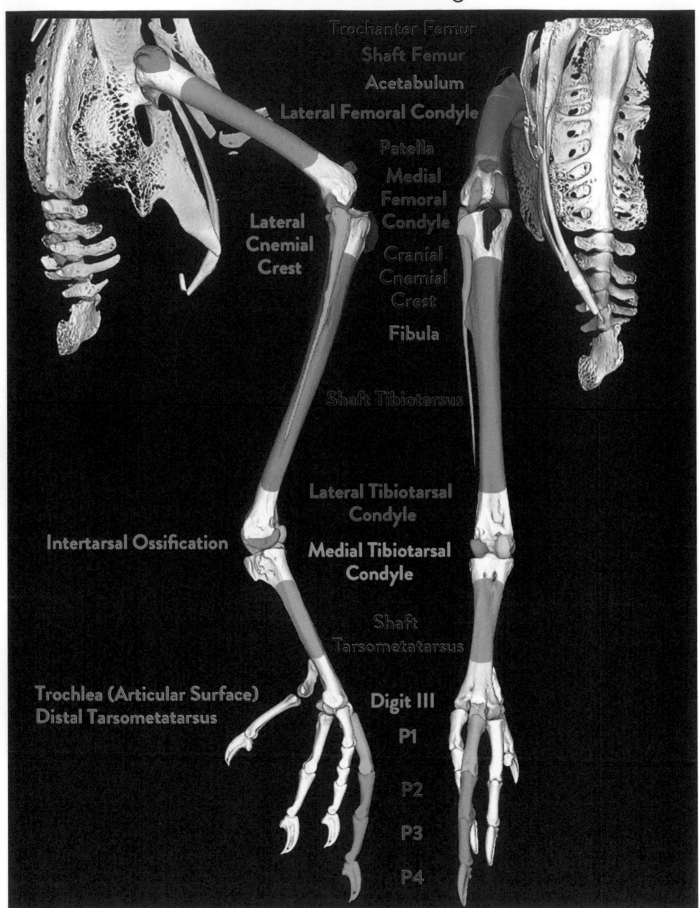

Trochanter Femur

Shaft Femur

Acetabulum

Lateral Femoral Condyle

Patella

Medial Femoral Condyle

Cranial Cnemial Crest

Fibula

Lateral Cnemial Crest

Shaft Tibiotarsus

Lateral Tibiotarsal Condyle

Medial Tibiotarsal Condyle

Intertarsal Ossification

Shaft Tarsometatarsus

Trochlea (Articular Surface) Distal Tarsometatarsus

Digit III

P1

P2

P3

P4

Pigeon (*Columba livia*)
Caudal and Medial Leg

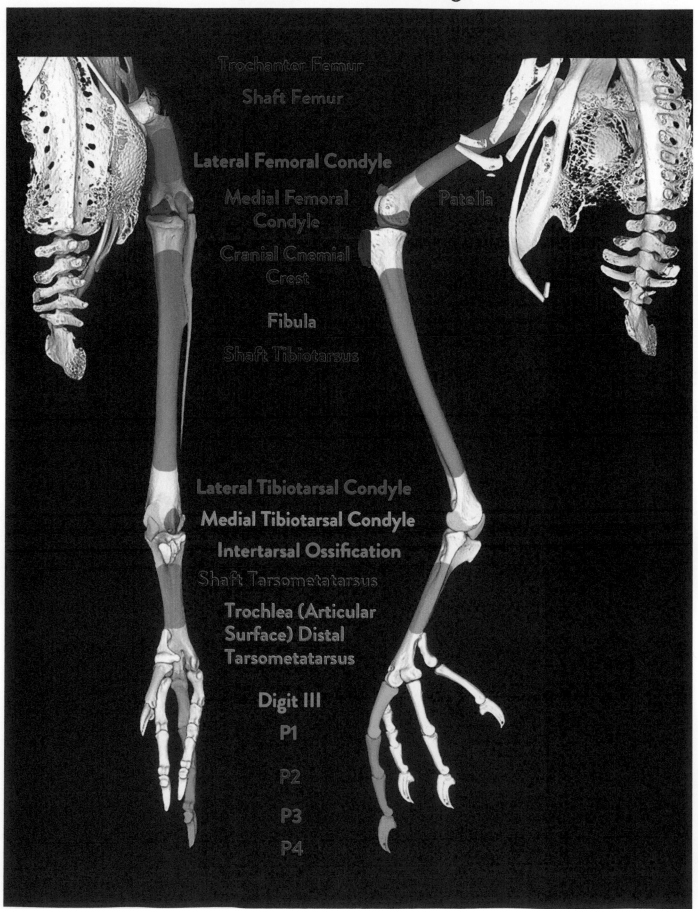

Trochanter Femur

Shaft Femur

Lateral Femoral Condyle

Medial Femoral Condyle

Patella

Cranial Cnemial Crest

Fibula

Shaft Tibiotarsus

Lateral Tibiotarsal Condyle

Medial Tibiotarsal Condyle

Intertarsal Ossification

Shaft Tarsometatarsus

Trochlea (Articular Surface) Distal Tarsometatarsus

Digit III

P1

P2

P3

P4

Domestic Chicken (*Gallus gallus domesticus*)
Lateral and Cranial Leg

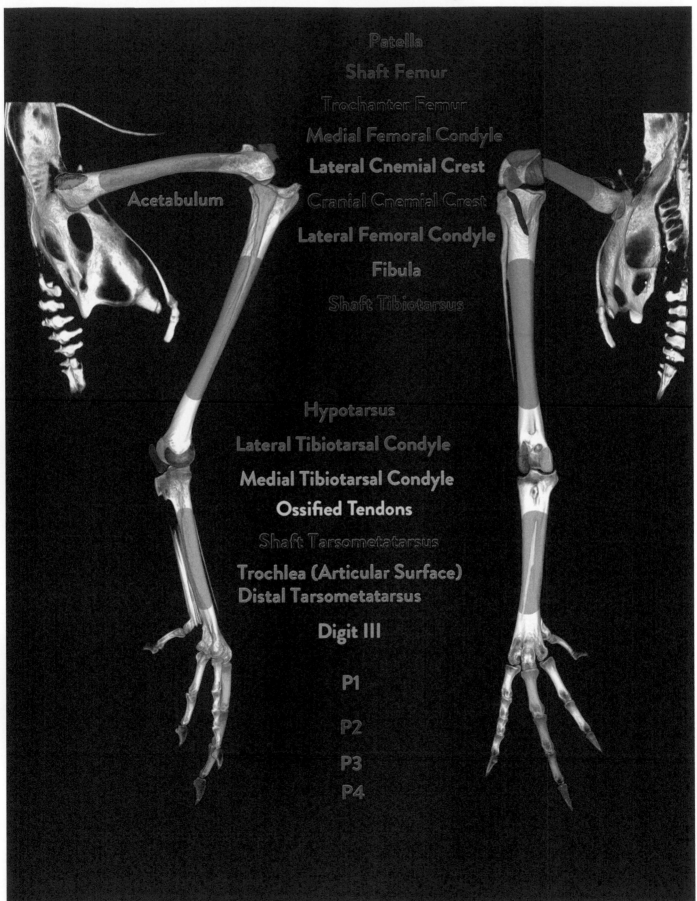

Patella

Shaft Femur

Trochanter Femur

Medial Femoral Condyle

Lateral Cnemial Crest

Cranial Cnemial Crest

Lateral Femoral Condyle

Fibula

Shaft Tibiotarsus

Acetabulum

Hypotarsus

Lateral Tibiotarsal Condyle

Medial Tibiotarsal Condyle

Ossified Tendons

Shaft Tarsometatarsus

Trochlea (Articular Surface)
Distal Tarsometatarsus

Digit III

P1

P2

P3

P4

Domestic Chicken (*Gallus gallus domesticus*)
Caudal and Medial Leg

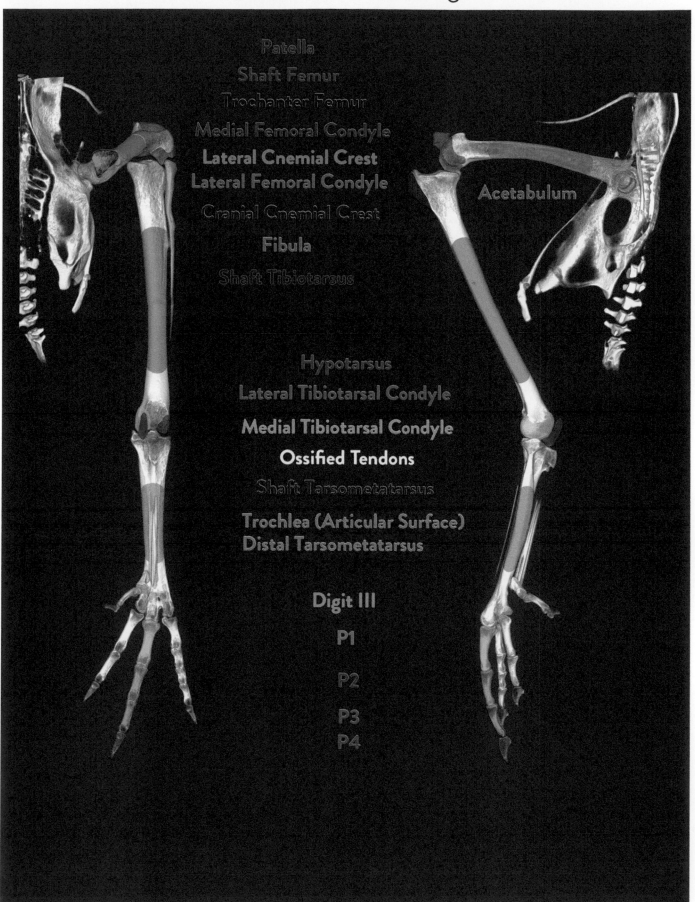

Patella
Shaft Femur
Trochanter Femur
Medial Femoral Condyle
Lateral Cnemial Crest
Lateral Femoral Condyle
Cranial Cnemial Crest
Fibula
Shaft Tibiotarsus

Acetabulum

Hypotarsus
Lateral Tibiotarsal Condyle
Medial Tibiotarsal Condyle
Ossified Tendons
Shaft Tarsometatarsus
Trochlea (Articular Surface)
Distal Tarsometatarsus

Digit III

P1

P2

P3
P4

Red-tailed Hawk (*Buteo jamaicensis*)
Lateral and Cranial Leg

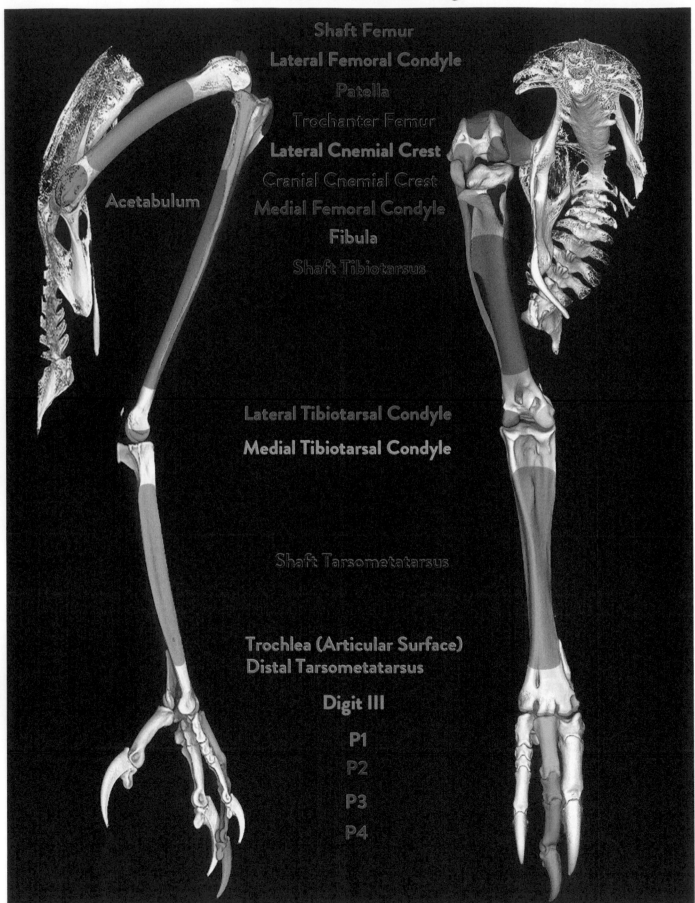

Shaft Femur

Lateral Femoral Condyle

Patella

Trochanter Femur

Lateral Cnemial Crest

Cranial Cnemial Crest

Medial Femoral Condyle

Fibula

Shaft Tibiotarsus

Acetabulum

Lateral Tibiotarsal Condyle

Medial Tibiotarsal Condyle

Shaft Tarsometatarsus

Trochlea (Articular Surface)
Distal Tarsometatarsus

Digit III

P1

P2

P3

P4

Red-tailed Hawk (*Buteo jamaicensis*)
Caudal and Medial Leg

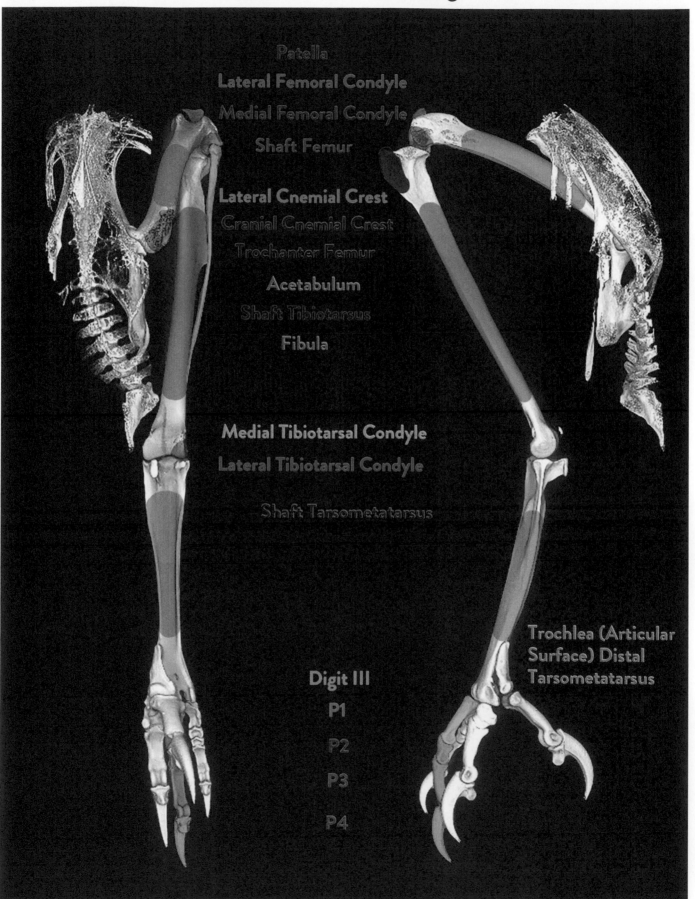

Patella
Lateral Femoral Condyle
Medial Femoral Condyle
Shaft Femur

Lateral Cnemial Crest
Cranial Cnemial Crest
Trochanter Femur
Acetabulum
Shaft Tibiotarsus
Fibula

Medial Tibiotarsal Condyle
Lateral Tibiotarsal Condyle

Shaft Tarsometatarsus

Digit III
P1
P2
P3
P4

Trochlea (Articular Surface) Distal Tarsometatarsus

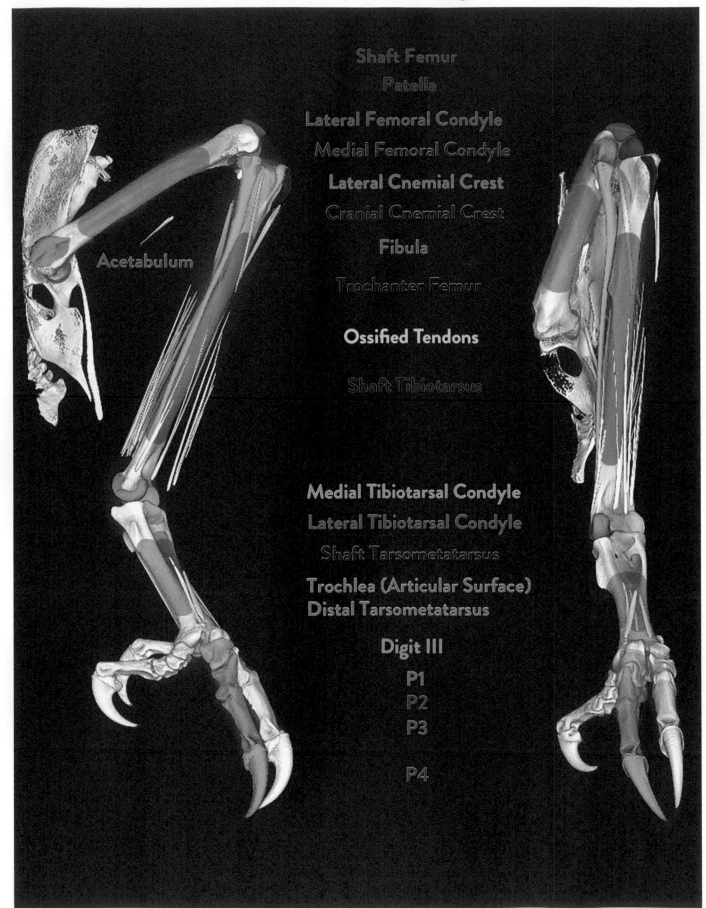

Shaft Femur
Patella
Lateral Femoral Condyle
Medial Femoral Condyle
Lateral Cnemial Crest
Cranial Cnemial Crest
Fibula
Trochanter Femur

Ossified Tendons

Shaft Tibiotarsus

Acetabulum

Medial Tibiotarsal Condyle
Lateral Tibiotarsal Condyle
Shaft Tarsometatarsus
Trochlea (Articular Surface)
Distal Tarsometatarsus

Digit III
P1
P2
P3

P4

Great Horned Owl (*Bubo virginianus*)
Caudal and Medial Leg

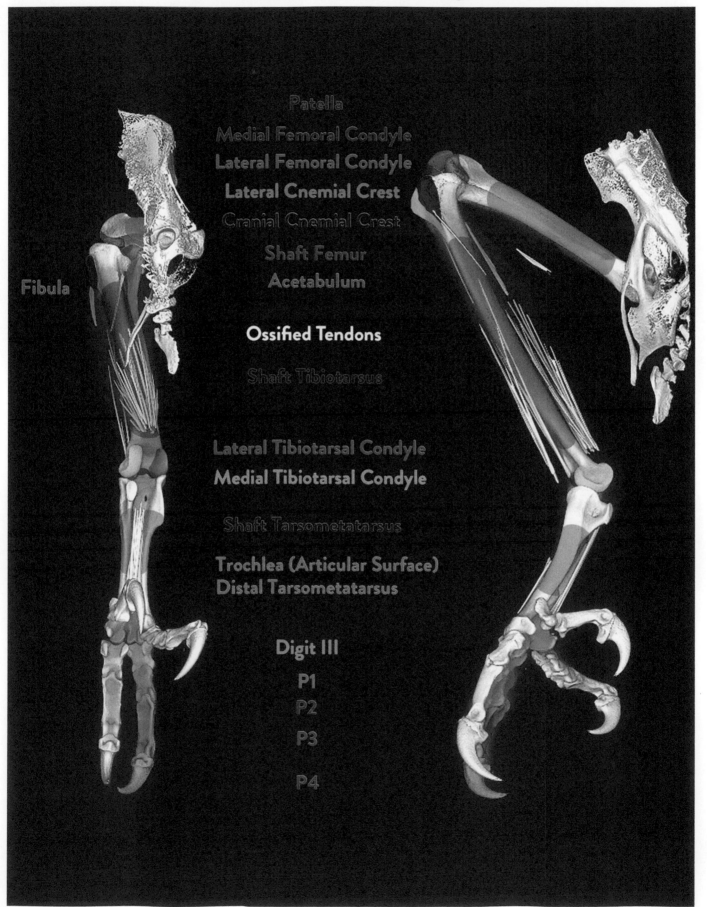

Patella
Medial Femoral Condyle
Lateral Femoral Condyle
Lateral Cnemial Crest
Cranial Cnemial Crest
Shaft Femur
Acetabulum

Fibula

Ossified Tendons

Shaft Tibiotarsus

Lateral Tibiotarsal Condyle
Medial Tibiotarsal Condyle

Shaft Tarsometatarsus

Trochlea (Articular Surface)
Distal Tarsometatarsus

Digit III

P1

P2

P3

P4

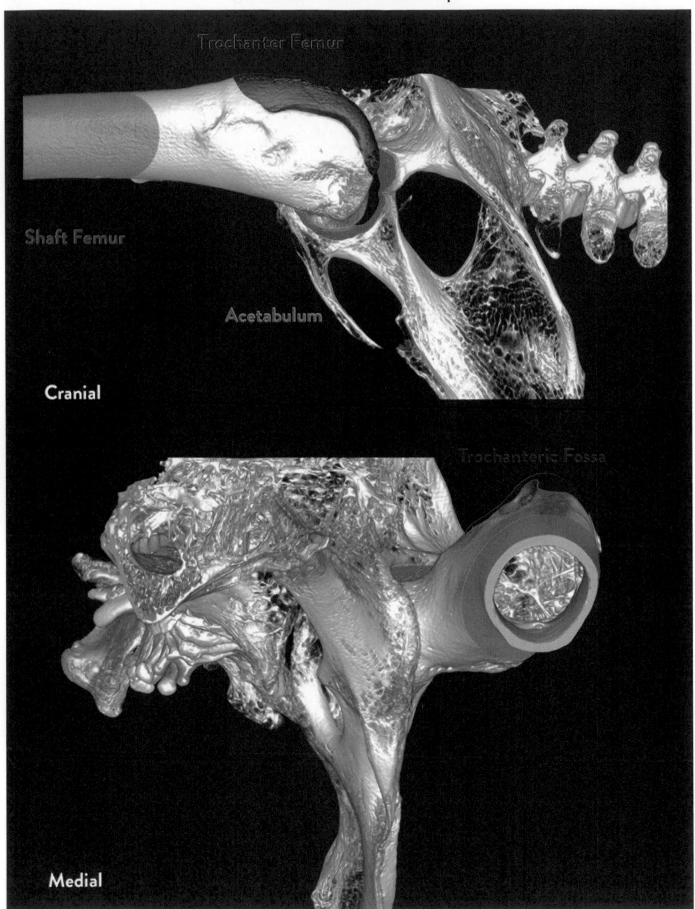

Trochanter Femur

Shaft Femur

Acetabulum

Cranial

Trochanteric Fossa

Medial

Golden Eagle (*Aquila chrysaetos*)
Caudal and Caudal Medial Hip

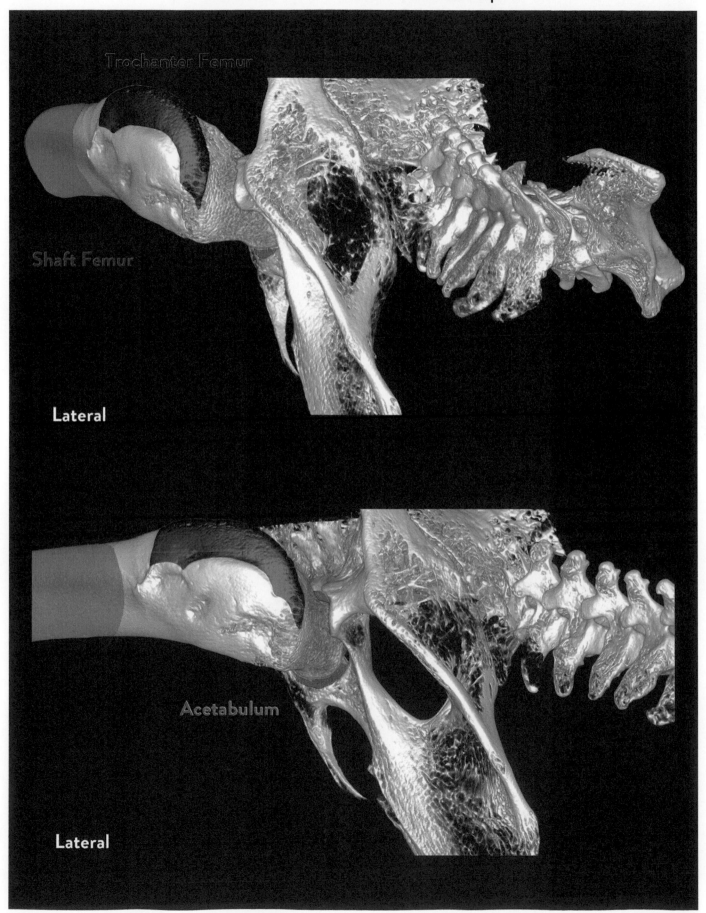

Trochanter Femur

Shaft Femur

Lateral

Acetabulum

Lateral

Golden Eagle (*Aquila chrysaetos*)
Medial Cranial Oblique, Medial Dorsal Oblique and Medial Caudal Oblique Hip

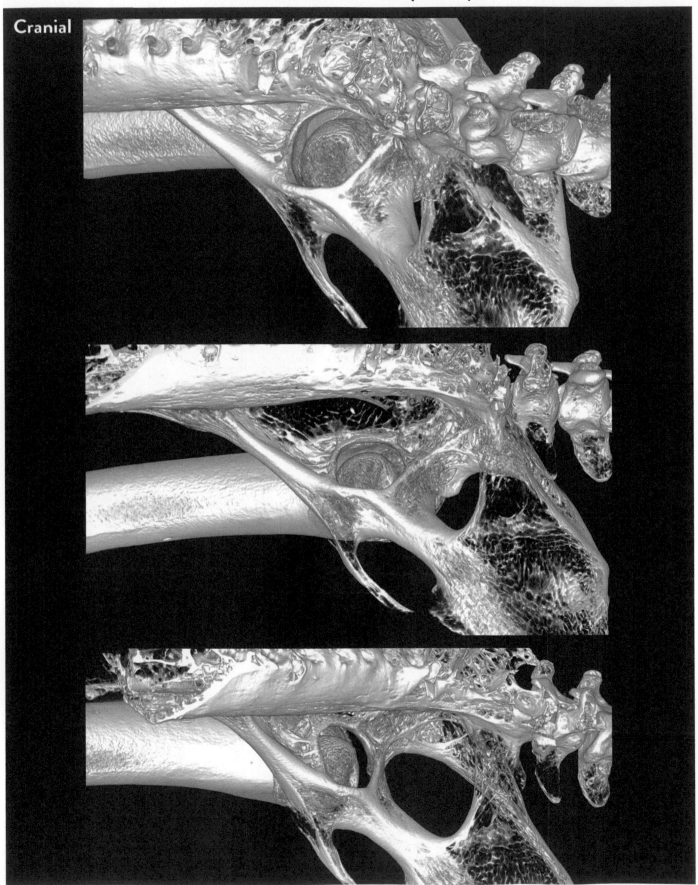

Cranial

Golden Eagle (*Aquila chrysaetos*)
Dorsal and Medial Hip

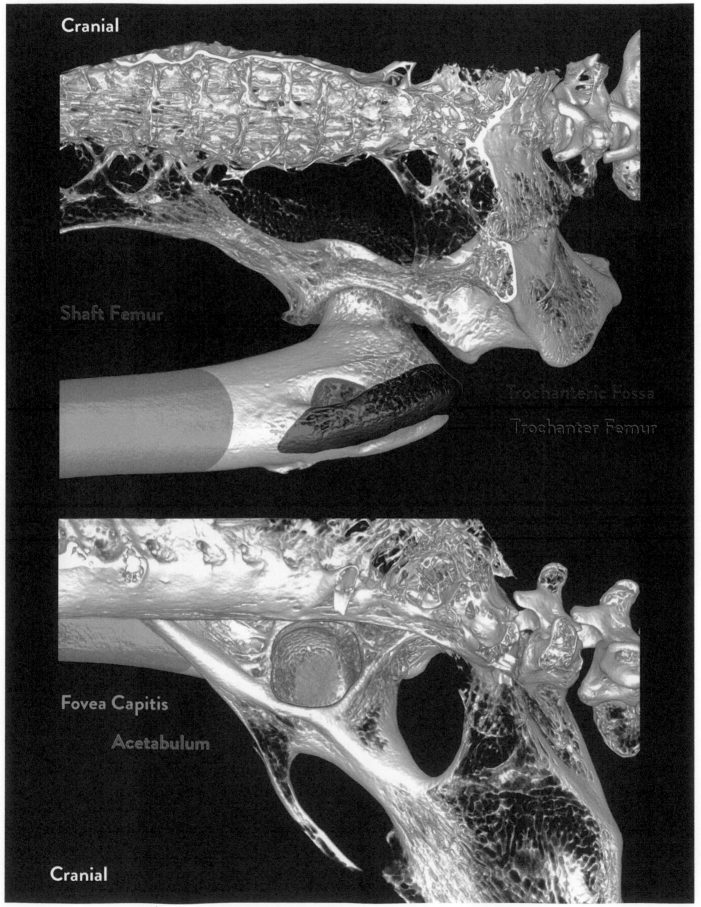

Cranial

Shaft Femur

Trochanteric Fossa

Trochanter Femur

Fovea Capitis

Acetabulum

Cranial

Golden Eagle (*Aquila chrysaetos*)
Ventral and Ventral Lateral Hip

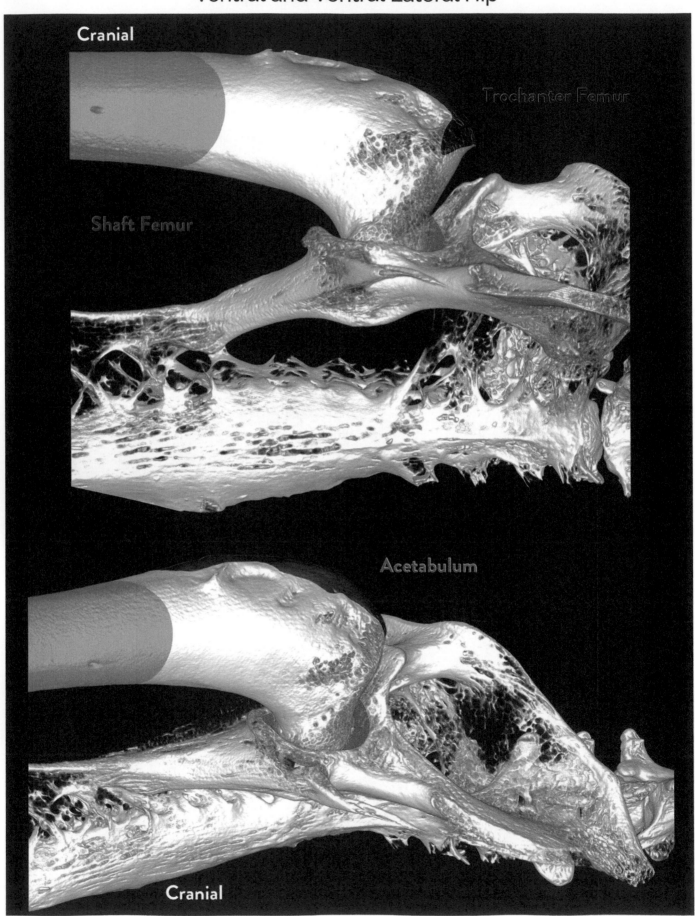

Cranial

Trochanter Femur

Shaft Femur

Acetabulum

Cranial

292

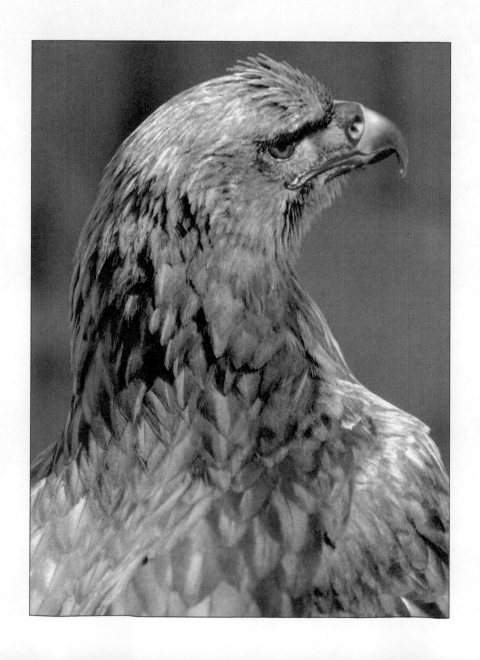

Golden Eagle (*Aquila chrysaetos*)
Lateral Cranial Oblique, Lateral and Lateral Caudal Oblique Views of Stifle

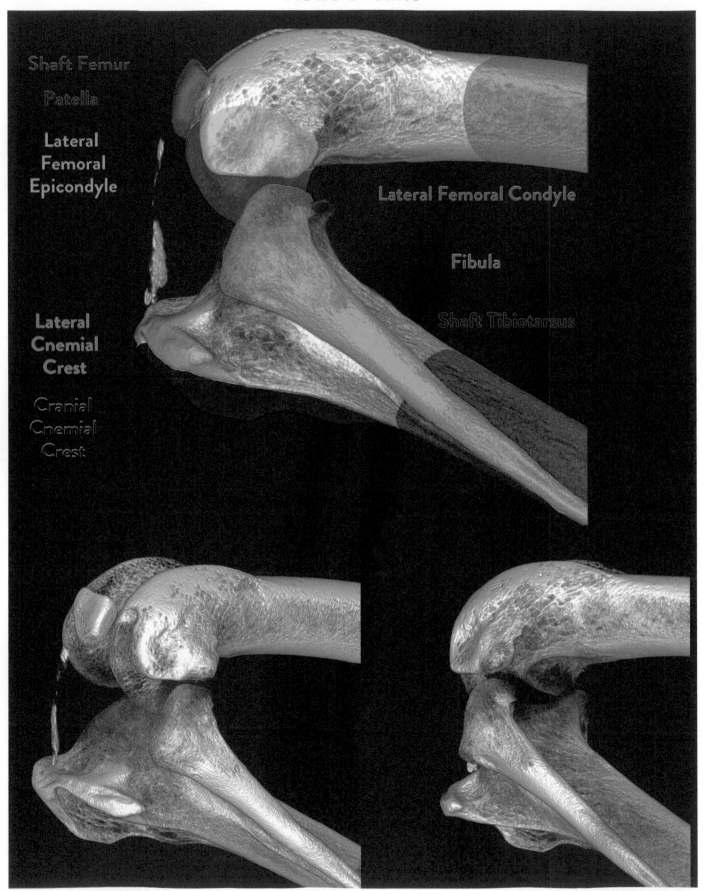

Shaft Femur

Patella

Lateral Femoral Epicondyle

Lateral Cnemial Crest

Cranial Cnemial Crest

Lateral Femoral Condyle

Fibula

Shaft Tibiotarsus

Golden Eagle (*Aquila chrysaetos*)
Cranial Medial Oblique, Cranial and Cranial Lateral Oblique Views of Stifle

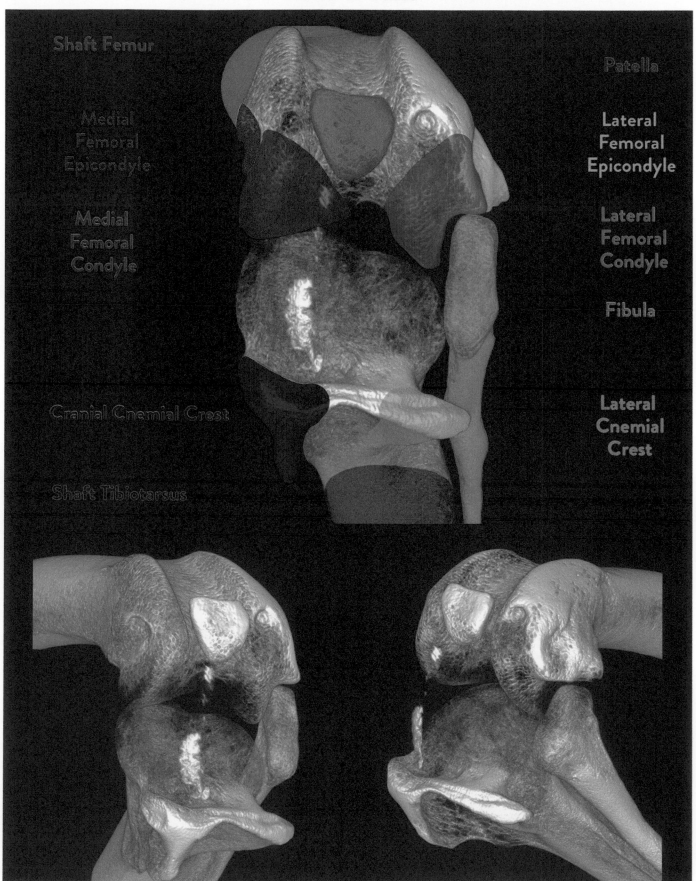

Shaft Femur

Patella

Medial Femoral Epicondyle

Lateral Femoral Epicondyle

Medial Femoral Condyle

Lateral Femoral Condyle

Fibula

Cranial Cnemial Crest

Lateral Cnemial Crest

Shaft Tibiotarsus

Golden Eagle (*Aquila chrysaetos*)
Caudal Medial Oblique, Caudal and Caudal Lateral Oblique Views of Stifle

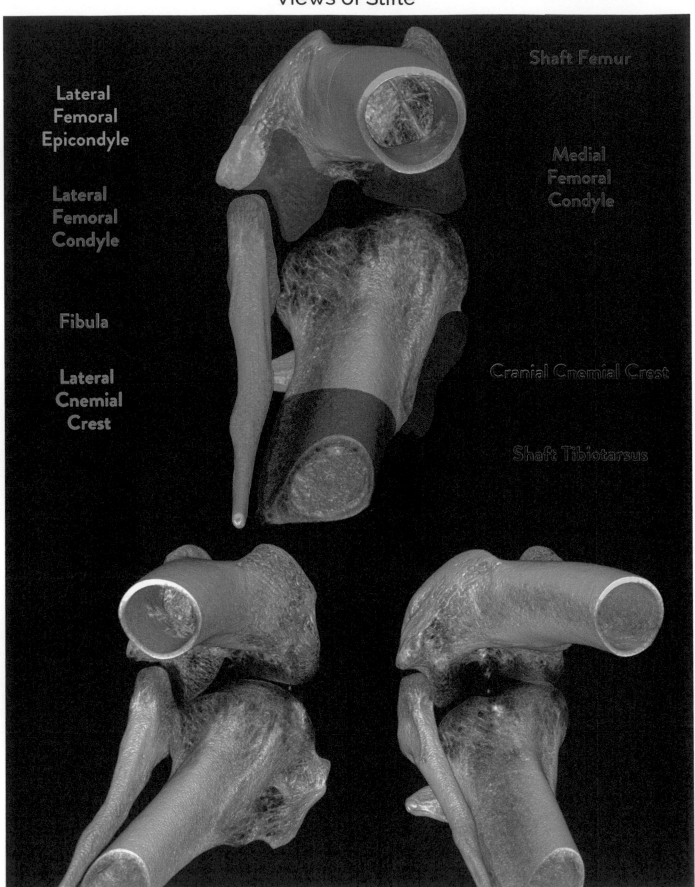

Lateral Femoral Epicondyle

Lateral Femoral Condyle

Fibula

Lateral Cnemial Crest

Shaft Femur

Medial Femoral Condyle

Cranial Cnemial Crest

Shaft Tibiotarsus

Golden Eagle (*Aquila chrysaetos*)
Medial Cranial Oblique, Medial and Medial Caudal Oblique Views of Stifle

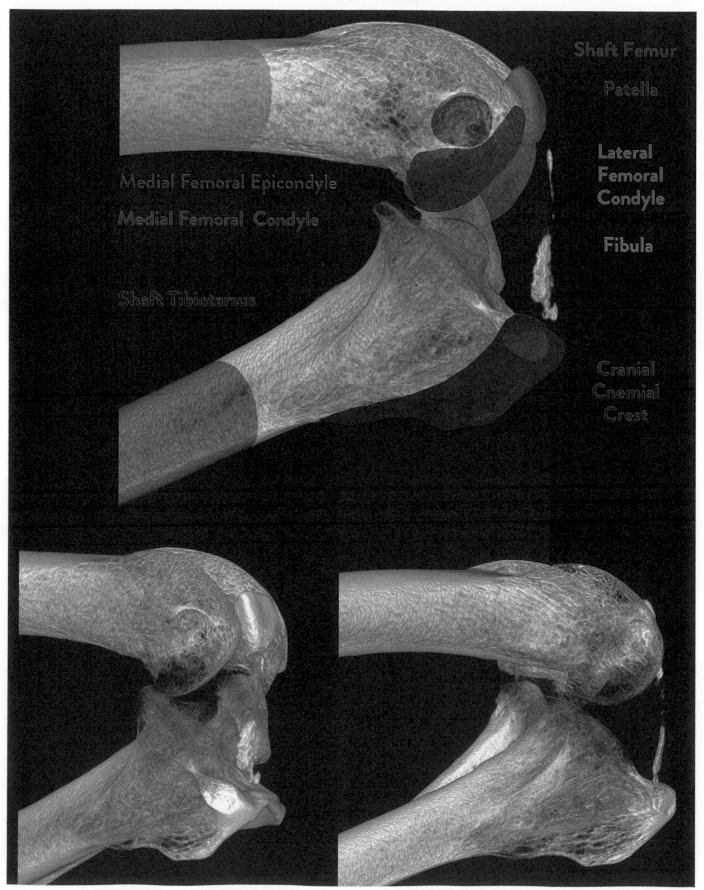

Medial Femoral Epicondyle

Medial Femoral Condyle

Shaft Tibiotarsus

Shaft Femur

Patella

Lateral Femoral Condyle

Fibula

Cranial Cnemial Crest

Golden Eagle (*Aquila chrysaetos*)
Lateral Dorsal Oblique, Lateral and Lateral Plantar Oblique Views of Foot

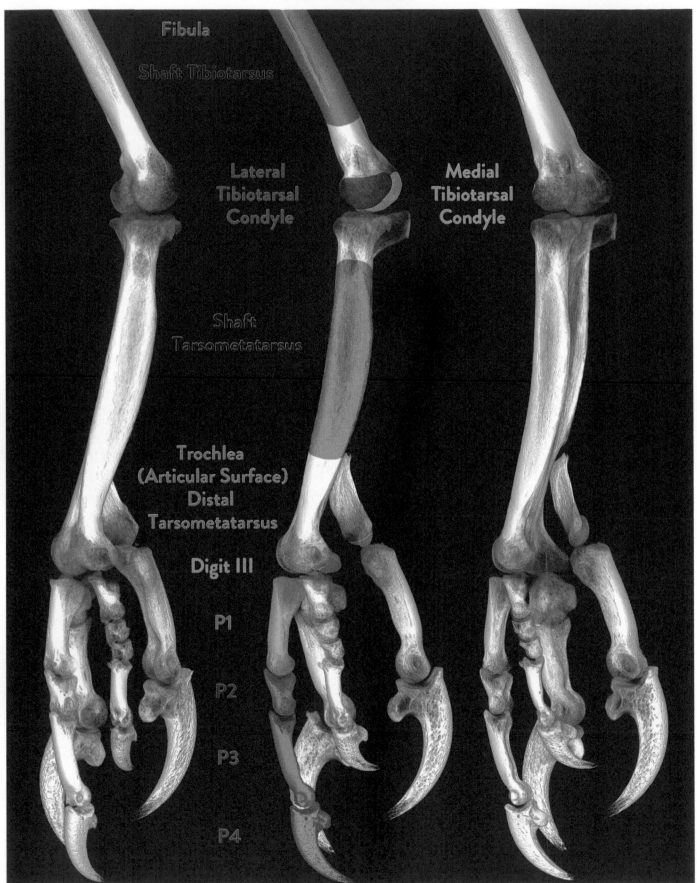

Fibula

Shaft Tibiotarsus

Lateral Tibiotarsal Condyle

Medial Tibiotarsal Condyle

Shaft Tarsometatarsus

Trochlea (Articular Surface) Distal Tarsometatarsus

Digit III

P1

P2

P3

P4

Golden Eagle (*Aquila chrysaetos*)
Dorsal Medial Oblique, Dorsal and Dorsal Lateral Oblique Views of Foot

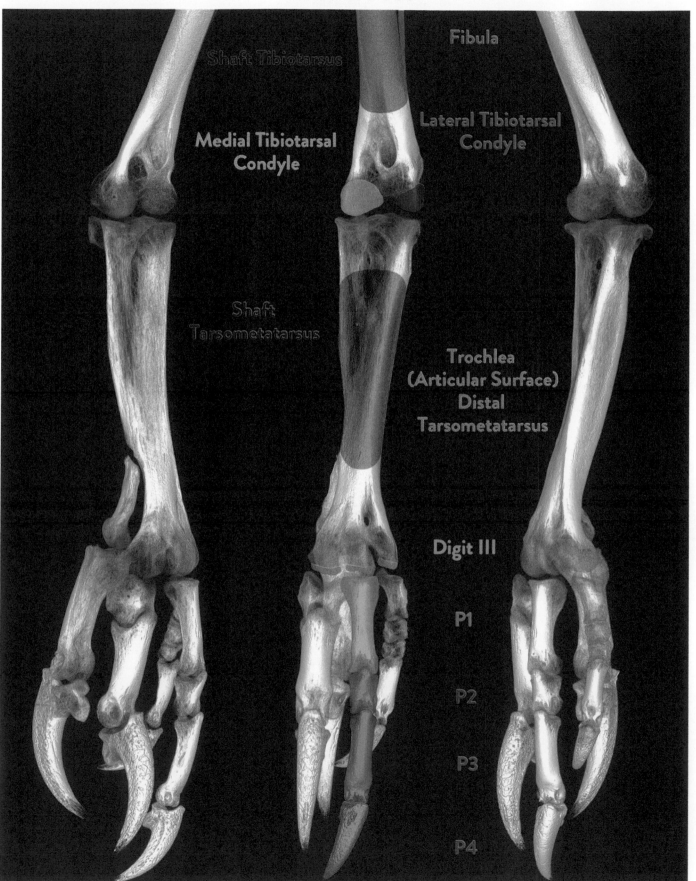

Golden Eagle (*Aquila chrysaetos*)
Plantar Medial Oblique, Plantar and Plantar Lateral Oblique Views of Foot

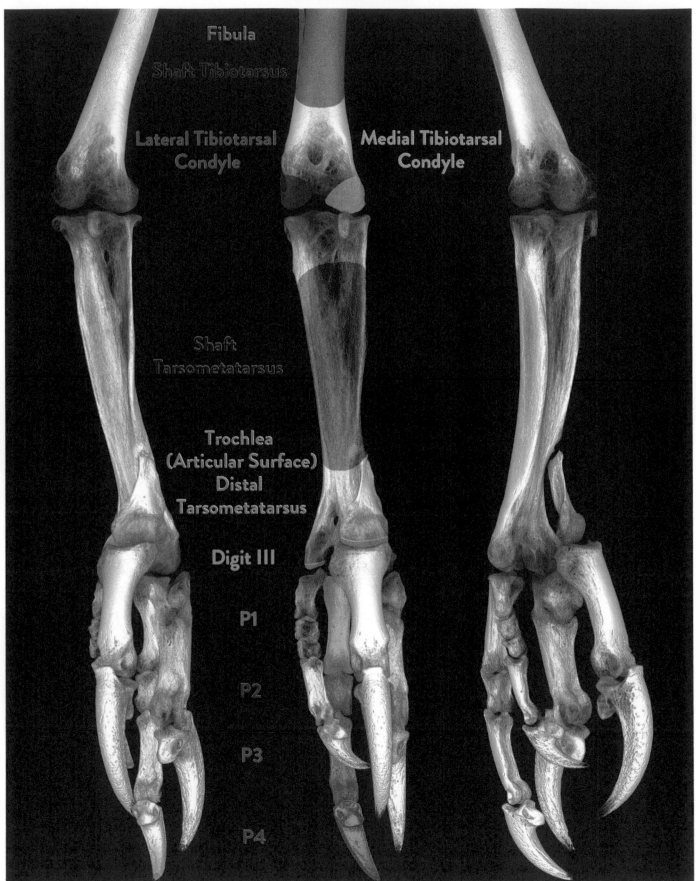

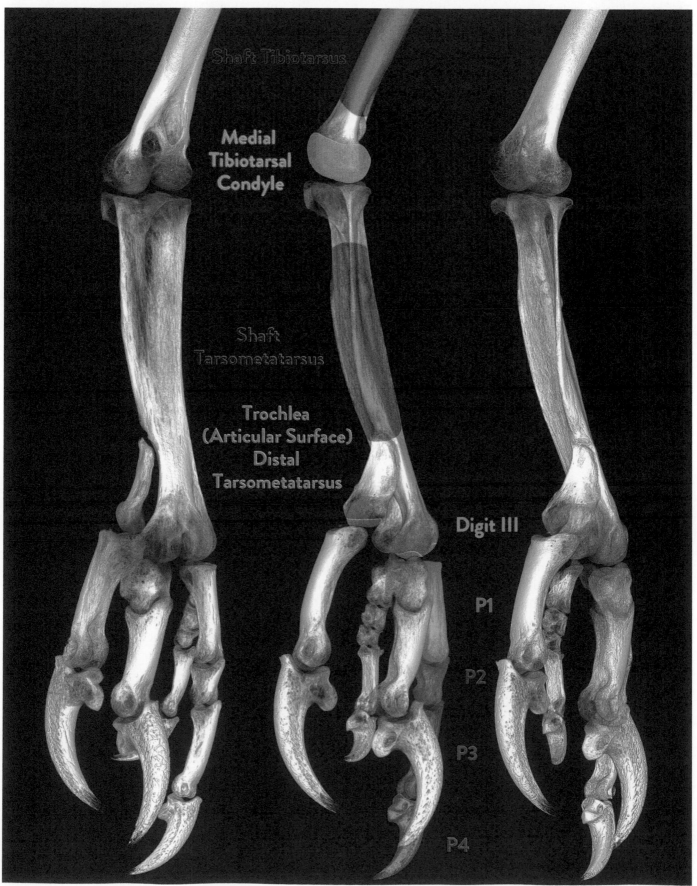

Shaft Tibiotarsus

Medial Tibiotarsal Condyle

Shaft Tarsometatarsus

Trochlea (Articular Surface) Distal Tarsometatarsus

Digit III

P1

P2

P3

P4

Superficial Layer of the Lateral leg—Cathartidae and Galliformes

Itiotibialis cranialis [sartorius]

This strap-like muscle is comparable to the sartorius of mammals, although it is not a direct homologue. It originates on the craniodorsal surface of the ilium and inserts on the craniomedial patella. Some fibers may insert on the cranial cnemial crest of the tibia. The iliotibialis cranialis extends the stifle while flexing the hip (Fischer 1946, Getty 1975). It is innervated by the femoral nerve.

Iliotibialis lateralis

In cathartids, galliformes and charadriiforms, this muscle is large, with a central aponeurotic zone. It partially covers the iliofibularis muscle (International Committee on Avian Anatomical Nomenclature 1983). It arises from the crest of the ilium to insert on the lateral cnemial crest and by a fascial attachment to the iliotibialis cranialis or sartorius muscle as a part of the patellar tendon (Fischer 1946). This muscle is commonly fused to the underlying femorotibialis externus and medius muscles. It may be further subdivided anatomically into three heads (Getty 1975); however, in this text, it will be described as a single muscle. Depending on the muscular origin in relation to the hip, this muscle can flex or extend the hip and may turn the leg slightly laterally. It is innervated by the femoral nerve.

Fibularis longus [peroneus longus]

The fibularis or peroneus longus muscle is the most cranial muscle of the crus or the tibiotarsus. However, there is considerable variation among species. It may be absent in some (owls and ospreys), small (pigeons and parakeets) or large (fowl and vultures) species (Fischer 1946, Getty 1975). In hawks, it is found deep to the tibialis cranialis. The muscle arises from the lateral side of the tibiotarsus along the cnemial crests. There are two insertions—one on the tibial cartilage [cartilago tibialis], and a second on the tendon of the flexor perforatus digiti III muscle. The two points of insertion reflect two different actions. Its insertion on the tibial cartilage allows the muscle to extend and abduct the intertarsal joint or hock. It also helps to flex digit III (Fischer 1946). It is innervated by the fibular or peroneal nerve.

Gastrocnemius

The muscle can be divided into two or three muscle groups but can have four heads. If there are three heads, two heads usually arise from the femur and one arises from the tibiotarsus (Getty 1975). The drawing on the next page (Middle layer of the lateral leg--Cathartidae and Galliformes) illustrates two muscular heads with the intermediate head (pars intermedia) fused to the medial head (pars medialis). While there are numerous heads with varying origins, the insertion is often a common tendon on the plantar surface of the tarsometatarsus and to the flexor tendons by attachments between. The gastrocnemius muscle is innervated by the medial and lateral tibial nerves. The muscle is a strong extensor of the hock and flexor of the digits due to its numerous aponeurotic attachments to the digital flexors (Fischer 1946). It is innervated by the medial and lateral tibial nerves.

Flexor perforans et perforatus digiti III

The tendon of this muscle (flexor p. et p. digiti III) moves from a lateral position on the tibiotarsus to one beneath the gastrocnemius tendon at the tarsus. It gives off a branch to the tendon of the flexor perforatus digiti III, before continuing down the tarsometatarsus, where it passes over the trochlea of the third digit deep to the tendon of the perforatus. It passes through the split tendon of insertion of the flexor perforatus digiti III at the first phalanx before inserting on the ventral surface of the third phalanx of digit III. At its insertion, it is perforated by the deep flexor tendon, which inserts onto the base of the claw. The flexor perforans et perforatus digiti III perforates and is perforated by two separate flexors. It extends the hock, but mainly flexes the distal end of the third digit. It is innervated by the lateral tibial nerve.

Superficial Layer of the Lateral leg—Cathartidae and Galliformes

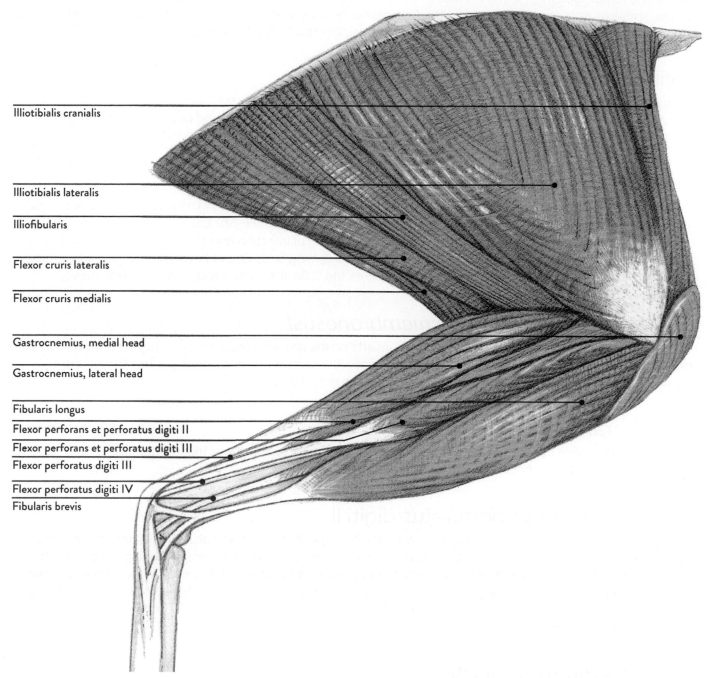

Illiotibialis cranialis

Illiotibialis lateralis

Illiofibularis

Flexor cruris lateralis

Flexor cruris medialis

Gastrocnemius, medial head

Gastrocnemius, lateral head

Fibularis longus
Flexor perforans et perforatus digiti II
Flexor perforans et perforatus digiti III
Flexor perforatus digiti III
Flexor perforatus digiti IV
Fibularis brevis

Middle Layer of the Lateral Leg--Cathartidae and Galliformes

Quadriceps Femoris Group

The femorotibialis externus muscle along with the femorotibialis medius and internus muscles represents the quadriceps complex of mammals. The externus and medius muscles are often partially fused to the overlying iliotibialis lateralis muscle, particularly over its aponeurotic portion.

The femorotibialis externus muscle takes origin from the lateral surface of the ilium and the femoral head, proximally. It inserts on the cnemial crests of the tibiotarsus. This muscle is innervated by the femoral nerve and acts to extend the stifle.

The femorotibialis medius is continuous with the femorotibiailis internus muscle. The medius muscle takes origin from the cranial surface of most of the femur while the internus takes origin from the medial surface of most of the femur (Getty 1975). The medius muscle directly inserts onto the cnemial crest as part of the patellar tendon. These muscles are innervated by the femoral nerve. They work in concert with the femorotibialis externus to extend the stifle. The medial head acts to medially rotate the tibiotarsus.

Iliofibularis

This triangular muscle is similar to the biceps femoris of mammals and is distinguished by its retinaculum, which surrounds its tendon of insertion caudolaterally on the fibula. The fibular nerve and popliteal vein also course through this tendinous loop. It is innervated by the ischiatic nerve.

Flexor cruris lateralis *[semitendinosus]*

This muscle, along with the medialis muscle, represents the hamstring muscles in mammals. The major portion of this muscle inserts onto the medial head of the gastrocnemius and the flexor cruris lateralis muscles. There may be an accessory head that originates from the main tendon of insertion and courses perpendicular to the principal fibers. The muscle is absent in hawks and owls; swimming birds do not have an accessory head (Getty 1975). The flexor cruris lateralis extends the hip and flexes the stifle. It is innervated by the ischiatic nerve.

Flexor cruris medialis *[semimembranosus]*

This flat muscle originates at the ventral ilium and inserts on the proximal medial tibiotarsus in common with the flexor cruris lateralis muscle. Like the flexor cruris lateralis, the medialis extends the hip while flexing the stifle. It also adducts the limb (Fischer 1946). It is innervated by the ischiatic nerve.

Tibialis cranialis

This muscle is covered by the fibularis longus muscle. It is an important flexor of the intertarsal joint (*see* page 305). It is innervated by the fibular or peroneal nerve.

Flexor perforans et perforatus digiti II

Flexor perforans et perforatus digiti II lies caudal to the flexor perforans et perforatus digiti III muscle. Its tendon courses along with flexor p. et p. digiti III to the hock, where it goes through a separate cartilaginous canal. It continues medially to perforate through the tendon of insertion of flexor perforatus digiti II. Flexor p. et p. digiti II continues down digit II to split at its insertion onto the base of its distal phalanx. At this point, it is perforated by the deep flexor tendon. The muscle flexes digit II while extending the intertarsal joint (Fischer 1946). The intermediate digital flexors are innervated by the lateral tibial nerve (Getty 1975).

Flexor perforatus digiti IV

This perforatus muscle originates caudal to the flexor perforans et perforatus digiti II. The tendon crosses over the distal end of the tibiotarsus and hock to gain a lateral position on the metatarsus. When it passes over the trochlea for digit IV, it divides into three parts. The inner tendon inserts on the medial, proximal end of phalanx 1, while the lateral one inserts on the distal lateral end of phalanx 1. The central tendon is perforated at its insertion site on phalanx 2 by the deep digital flexor tendon (Fischer 1946). This superficial digital flexor is innervated by the lateral tibial nerve (Getty 1975).

Middle Layer of the Lateral Leg--Cathartidae and Galliformes

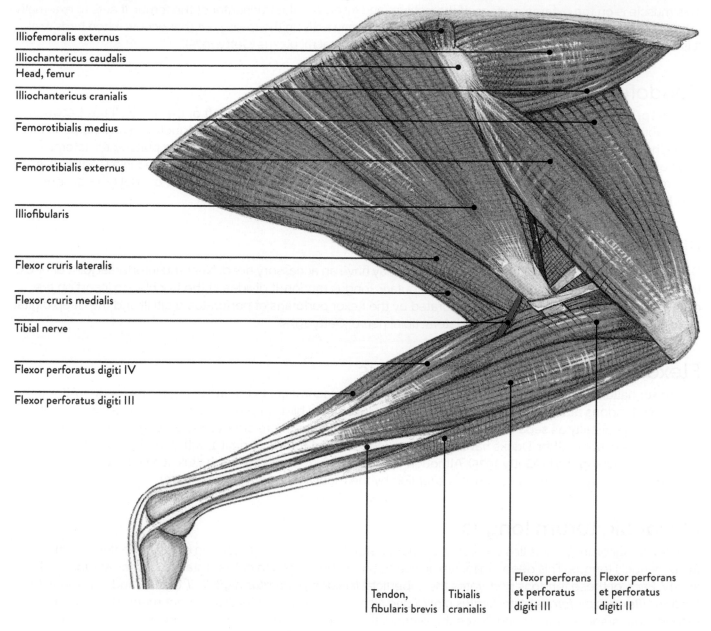

Illiofemoralis externus

Illiochantericus caudalis

Head, femur

Illiochantericus cranialis

Femorotibialis medius

Femorotibialis externus

Illiofibularis

Flexor cruris lateralis

Flexor cruris medialis

Tibial nerve

Flexor perforatus digiti IV

Flexor perforatus digiti III

Tendon, fibularis brevis

Tibialis cranialis

Flexor perforans et perforatus digiti III

Flexor perforans et perforatus digiti II

Deep Layer of the Lateral Leg--Cathartidae and Galliformes

Iliotrochantericus cranialis and caudalis *[gluteus profundus and medius]*

The iliotrochantericus cranialis (*gluteus profundus*) is a thin muscle that courses along the lateral ilium ventral to the iliotrochantericus caudalis. The muscle inserts on the lateral femur along the trochanter and its distal continuation, the iliotrochanteric impression. Both muscles serve to rotate the tibiotarsus and flex the hip (Fischer 1946). These 2 flexors are innervated by the cranial gluteal nerve which is a branch of the femoral nerve (Getty 1975).

Iliofemoralis externus *[piriformis]*

The iliofemoralis externus is comparable to the piriformis of mammals. It is a small triangular muscle that lies over the dorsolateral hip joint. Due to its small size, it probably has limited abilities for abduction. There is considerable variation between species and may be absent. This muscle when present is innervated by the femoral nerve (Getty 1975).

Ischiofemoralis *[obturator externus]*

This muscle is on the external surface of the ischium and inserts on the trochanter of the femur. It acts to externally rotate the distal limb and extend the hip (Fischer 1946). It may assist in the toeing out that occurs when birds walk. It is supplied by the ischiofemoral nerve which comes off the sacral plexus (Getty 1975).

Caudofemoralis

This strap-like muscle runs from the pygostyle of the tail to the caudolateral shaft of the femur. It lies between the flexor cruris lateralis and the iliofibularis and the flexor cruris medialis and the adductors. The insertion can be fleshy or tendinous. Although it pulls the femur caudally, its major function may be to pull the tail laterally and ventrally. This muscle would cause the tail to be depressed as the legs are outstretched in a landing. It is absent in some vultures and the California condor (Fischer 1946). It is innervated by the caudal gluteal nerve which is a branch of the sacral plexus (Getty 1975).

Flexor perforatus digiti III

Depending on the species of bird, this perforatus may have an accessory head. Near the intertarsal joint or hock, the major tendon is joined by a branch of the fibularis longus tendon. It divides at the trochlea to insert on the distal end of phalanx 1 of digit III. It is perforated by the flexor perforans et perforatus digiti III and the deep digital flexor. This muscle is innervated by the lateral tibial nerve (Getty 1975).

Flexor hallucis profundis or longus

The flexor hallucis profundus or longus muscle may have attachments to the flexor digitorum longus. Although these two tendons attach in a fibrous retinaculum or vinculum in birds of prey, gallinaceous birds, and parrots, they continue distally as separate tendons. In finches and canaries, there are two separate tendons with no attachments to each other. Ducks have only a small tendon that travels to digit 1, with the major supply going to the three remaining digits (Getty 1975). Although this muscle flexes digit I or the hallux, it also helps to flex the other digits by way of its retinaculum. It is supplied by the medial tibial nerve (Getty 1975).

Flexor digitorum longus

The flexor digitorum longus lies against the caudolateral tibiotarsus with its tendon of insertion deep to the flexor hallucis longus. This deep digital flexor inserts on the base of each of the distal processes of digits II, III, and IV. Each of these tendons perforates the superficial *[flexores perforatus digiti II, III, and IV]* and intermediate tendons *[flexores perforans et perforatus digiti II and III]* before inserting at its distal attachment. The muscle extends the tarsometatarsus and flexes the second, third and fourth digits. There can be accessory fibroelastic slips to the subterminal phalanges. When there is a vinculum between the flexor digitorum longus and the flexor hallucis profundus, this allows for independent flexion of the forward toes independent of the hallux. But if there is flexion of the hallux the attachments result in flexion of the forward toes. The nerve supply is the medial tibial nerve (Getty 1975).

Blood supply and innervation

The major blood and nerve supply to the leg is found at this deep layer. The ischiatic nerve *[n. ischiadicus]* travels through the ilioischiatic foramen *[foramen ilioischiadicum]* to enter the lateral leg just caudal to the shaft of the femur. The ischiatic artery *[a. ischiadica]* accompanies the nerve. The vein *[v. ischiadica]* enters the lateral leg just proximal to insertion of the caudofemoralis and is the closest neurovascular structure to the femoral shaft.

At the distal end of the femur, the ischiatic nerve divides into the fibular nerve *[n. fibularis]* cranially and the tibial nerve *[n. tibialis]* caudally. In this region, the vascular supply changes names to the popliteal artery and vein *[a. and v. popliteal]* and the sural artery and vein *[a. and v. suralis]*.

Deep Layer of the Lateral Leg--Cathartidae and Galliformes

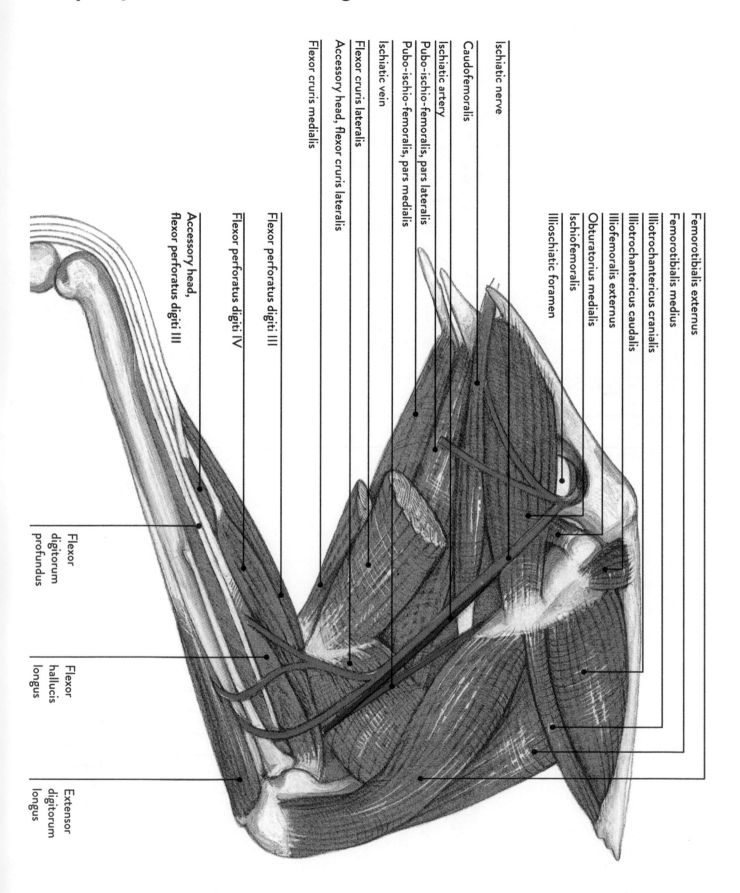

Ischiatic nerve

Caudofemoralis

Ischiatic artery

Pubo-ischio-femoralis, pars lateralis

Pubo-ischio-femoralis, pars medialis

Ischiatic vein

Flexor cruris lateralis

Accessory head, flexor cruris lateralis

Flexor cruris medialis

Femorotibialis externus

Femorotibialis medius

Iliotrochantericus cranialis

Iliotrochantericus caudalis

Iliofemoralis externus

Obturatorius medialis

Ischiofemoralis

Ilioschiatic foramen

Accessory head, flexor perforatus digiti III

Flexor perforatus digiti IV

Flexor perforatus digiti III

Flexor digitorum profundus

Flexor hallucis longus

Extensor digitorum longus

Lateral Femur of Cathartidae and Galliformes

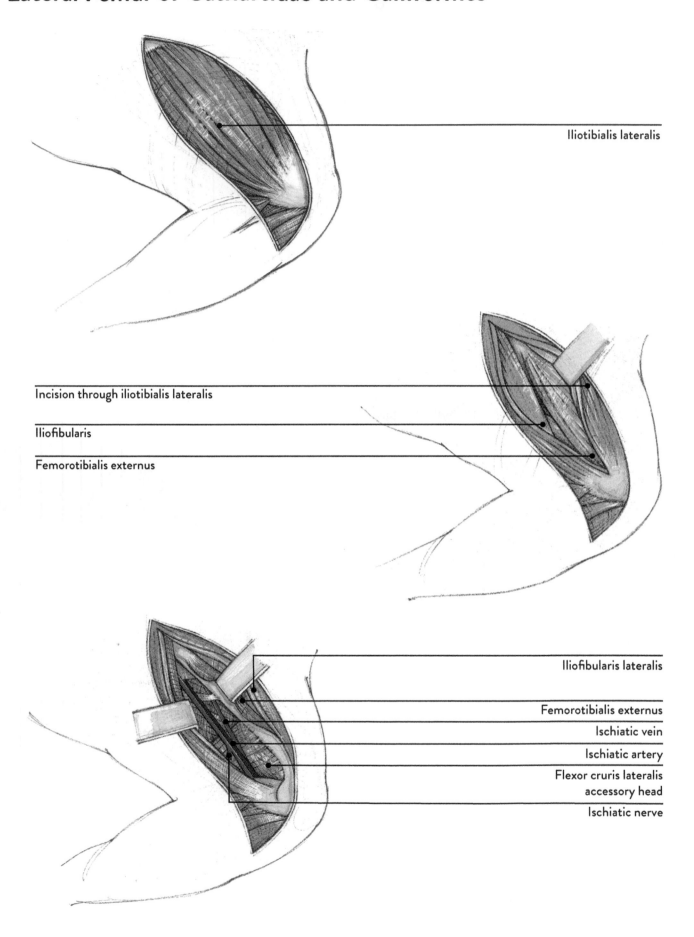

Iliotibialis lateralis

Incision through iliotibialis lateralis

Iliofibularis

Femorotibialis externus

Iliofibularis lateralis

Femorotibialis externus

Ischiatic vein

Ischiatic artery

Flexor cruris lateralis
accessory head

Ischiatic nerve

Coxofemoral Joint

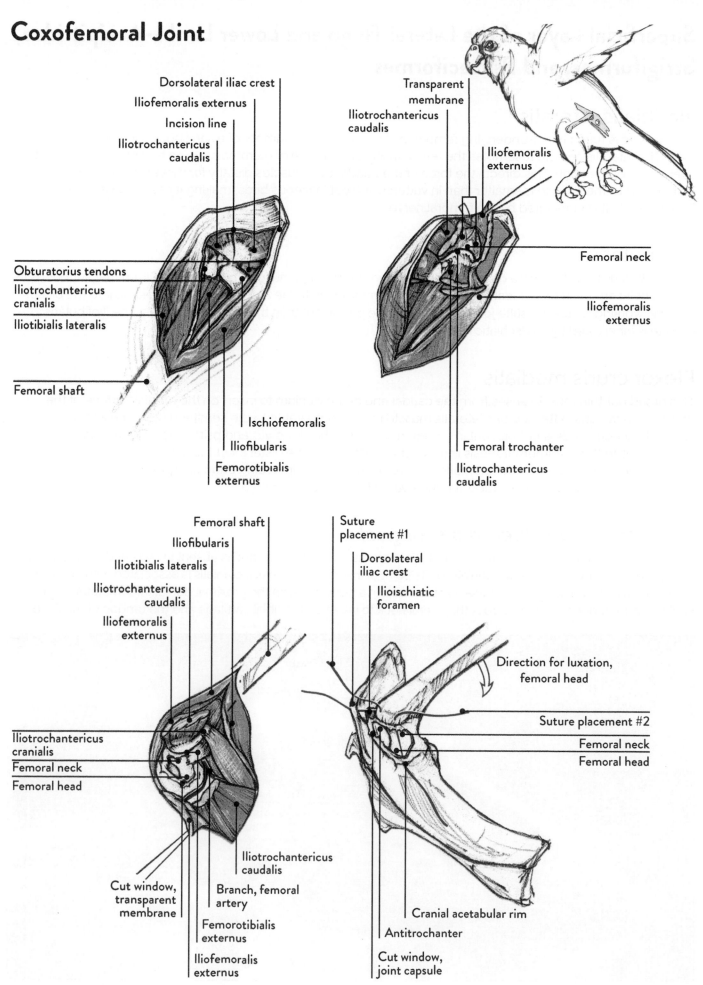

Dorsolateral iliac crest
Iliofemoralis externus
Incision line
Iliotrochantericus caudalis

Obturatorius tendons
Iliotrochantericus cranialis
Iliotibialis lateralis

Femoral shaft

Ischiofemoralis
Iliofibularis
Femorotibialis externus

Transparent membrane
Iliotrochantericus caudalis
Iliofemoralis externus

Femoral neck

Iliofemoralis externus

Femoral trochanter
Iliotrochantericus caudalis

Femoral shaft
Iliofibularis
Iliotibialis lateralis
Iliotrochantericus caudalis
Iliofemoralis externus

Iliotrochantericus cranialis
Femoral neck
Femoral head

Cut window, transparent membrane
Iliotrochantericus caudalis
Branch, femoral artery
Femorotibialis externus
Iliofemoralis externus

Suture placement #1
Dorsolateral iliac crest
Ilioischiatic foramen

Direction for luxation, femoral head

Suture placement #2
Femoral neck
Femoral head

Cranial acetabular rim
Antitrochanter
Cut window, joint capsule

Superficial Layer of the Lateral Thigh and Lower Limb--Accipitridae, Strigiformes, and Psittaciformes

Iliotibialis lateralis

This muscle is fused to the underlying femorotibialis externus in a number of avian species including hawks and owls. The lateralis muscle resembles the tensor fascia lata muscle of mammals, which tenses the fascia on the lateral side of the thigh. This directs the force of the quadriceps muscles distally for movement of the stifle joint. In these birds, the muscle is smaller than in vultures and gallinaceous birds, making it easier to visualize the femoral shaft. It is innervated by the femoral nerve.

Iliofibularis

The iliofibularis muscle can be distinguished from the surrounding muscles by the retinaculum that surrounds its tendon of insertion on the caudal fibula. In psittaciformes, Accipitridae and strigiformes it is similar to the biceps femoris, working to flex the stifle joint. It appears more prominent than the iliotibialis laterals. The iliofibularis muscle is innervated by the ischiatic nerve.

Flexor cruris medialis

This broad but thin muscle arises from the caudal end of the ischium to insert on the medial surface of the proximal tibiotarsus. A flexor cruris lateralis muscle that is comparable to the semitendinosis muscle of vultures and gallinaceous birds is not present in common species of hawks, owls, and psittacines. The medialis muscle is comparable to the semimembranosis muscle of mammals. It is the distal most muscle on the caudal portion of the femur in birds and acts as a landmark for several procedures, including endoscopy of the caudal thoracic air sac and placement of an air sac tube. It is innervated by the ischiatic nerve.

Fibularis longus *[peroneus longus]*

This muscle is found deep to the tibialis cranialis in hawks and psittacines and is absent in owls and osprey. It can be distinguished from the tibialis cranialis by its point of insertion; the tibialis cranialis is associated with an extensor retinaculum as it crosses the intertarsal joint to insert in a bony canal on the proximal dorsal tarsometatarsus. The fibularis muscle goes caudally across the lateral hock to insert on the tibial cartilage and the tendon of the flexor

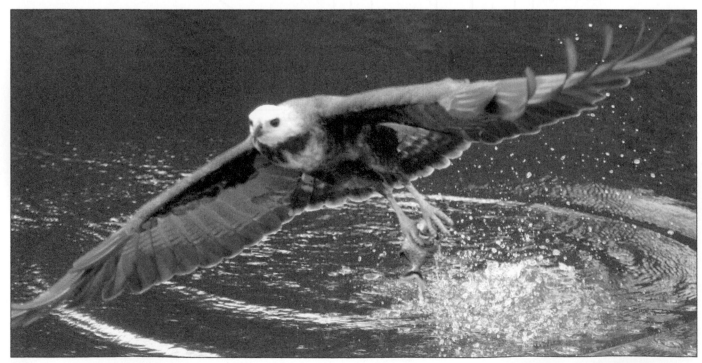

perforatus digiti III. Its insertion on the tibial cartilage acts to extend and abduct the hock. Its other insertion onto the tendon of the flexor acts to help in the flexion of the third digit. Its origin is on the lateral side of the tibiotarsus from the lateral to the cranial cnemial crests. It is innervated by the fibular nerve.

Flexor perforatus digiti IV

In psittacines this muscle has two muscle bellies that form a single tendon of insertion. The tendon of insertion usually attaches to the base of the first phalanx. It then divides into lateral, middle and medial tendons to the first, second and third interphalangeal joint capsules respectively. The deep digital flexor tendon passes through the middle and medial branch where it inserts onto the ungual phalanx in the galliforms that are anisodactylous species. This muscle is supplied by the lateral tibial nerve (Getty 1975).

Superficial Layer of the Lateral Thigh and Lower Limb--Accipitridae, Strigiformes, and Psittaciformes

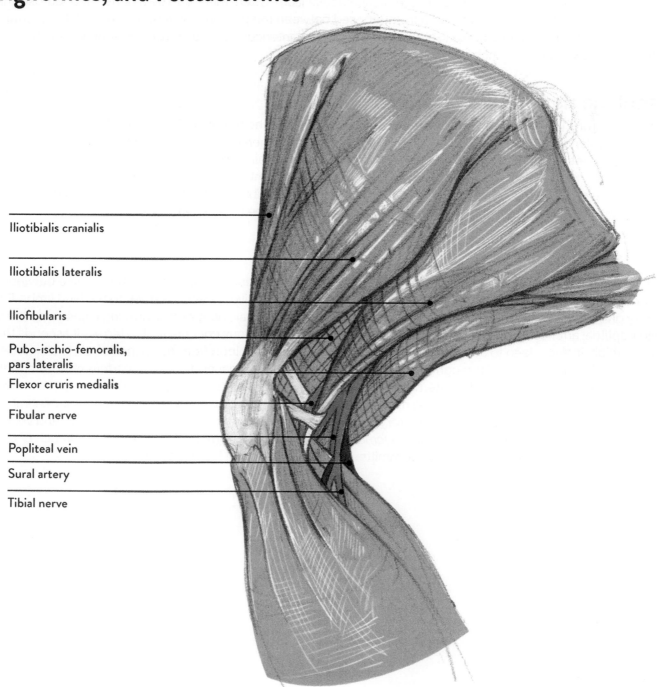

Iliotibialis cranialis

Iliotibialis lateralis

Iliofibularis

Pubo-ischio-femoralis, pars lateralis

Flexor cruris medialis

Fibular nerve

Popliteal vein

Sural artery

Tibial nerve

Deep Layer of the Lateral Femur in Accipitridae, Strigiformes, and Psittaciformes

Caudofemoralis

The caudofemoralis is a strap-like muscle that depresses and moves the tail fan laterally when the leg is advanced. This muscle is supplied by the caudal gluteal nerve which branches from the sacral plexus (Getty 1975).

Iliotrochantericus caudalis *[gluteus medius]*

The iliotrochantericus caudalis muscle takes origin from the lateral surface of the preacetabular ilium. This muscle inserts on the trochanteric ridge on the lateral surface of the femur just distal to the trochanter. The iliotrochantericus may rotate the femur medially while flexing it. It is thought to resist overextension during landing thereby acting as a shock absorber as the muscle is stretched during landing. The shape of the muscle varies in relation to the shape of the preacetabular ilium. Often, there can be a dense aponeurosis that contributes to a strong tendon of insertion. Interposed between the tendon of insertion and the lateral femur is a large bursa, the trochanteric bursa (Getty 1975). The iliotrochantericus caudalis muscle is supplied by the cranial gluteal nerve which is a branch of the femoral nerve (Getty 1975).

Ischiatic nerve *[n. ischiadicus]*

This nerve runs laterally from cranial to caudal along the shaft of the femur. At its distal end, the nerve divides into the fibular nerve [n. fibularis] or peroneal nerve and the tibial nerve *[n. tibialis]*. The fibular nerve courses through the retinaculum of the iliofibularis to innervate the muscles of the craniolateral tibiotarsus. These muscles are mainly involved in flexion of the hock or intertarsal joint and extension of the digits. In addition, the nerve has a superficial branch, which innervates the craniolateral tibiotarsus and hock. The larger tibial nerve innervates the extensors of the intertarsal joint and the flexors of the digits (Getty 1975).

Blood supply

The terminal ends of the abdominal aorta are the paired ischiatic arteries *[a. ischiadica]*. They course between the middle and caudal divisions of the kidney before exiting through the ilioischiatic foramen to the hind limbs. Each artery gives branches to the hips and the muscles of the flexor compartment before dividing distally into the sural and popliteal arteries. The ischiatic vein *[v. ischiadica]* is the major venous channel for the leg. As it ascends the lateral thigh, it dives deep to the caudofemoralis. The majority of the blood from the ischiatic vein is diverted to the femoral vein *[v. femoralis]* through a communicating vein (caudal renal portal vein *[v. portalis renalis caudalis]*). The femoral vein continues as the external iliac vein *[v. iliaca externa]* before going through a renal portal valve *[valva portalis renalis]*. Blood from the leg must traverse the renal portal system before entering the general systemic circulation. The cranial femoral artery and vein are terminal branches of the femoral artery and vein. The cranial cutaneous femoral nerve *[n. cutaneus femoralis cranialis]* arises from the femoral nerve, a branch of the lumbar plexus (Getty 1975, International Committee on Avian Anatomical Nomenclature 1979).

Deep Layer of the Lateral Femur in Accipitridae, Strigiformes, and Psittaciformes

Iliotrochantericus caudalis

Iliotrochantericus cranialis

Obturatorius medialis

Ischiofemoralis

Iliofibularis

Femorotibialis externus

Caudofemoralis

Ischiatic vein

Pubo-ischio-femoralis, pars lateralis

Ischiatic artery

Tibial nerve

Fibular nerve

Musculature of the Lateral Femur in Accipitridae, Strigiformes and Psittaciformes

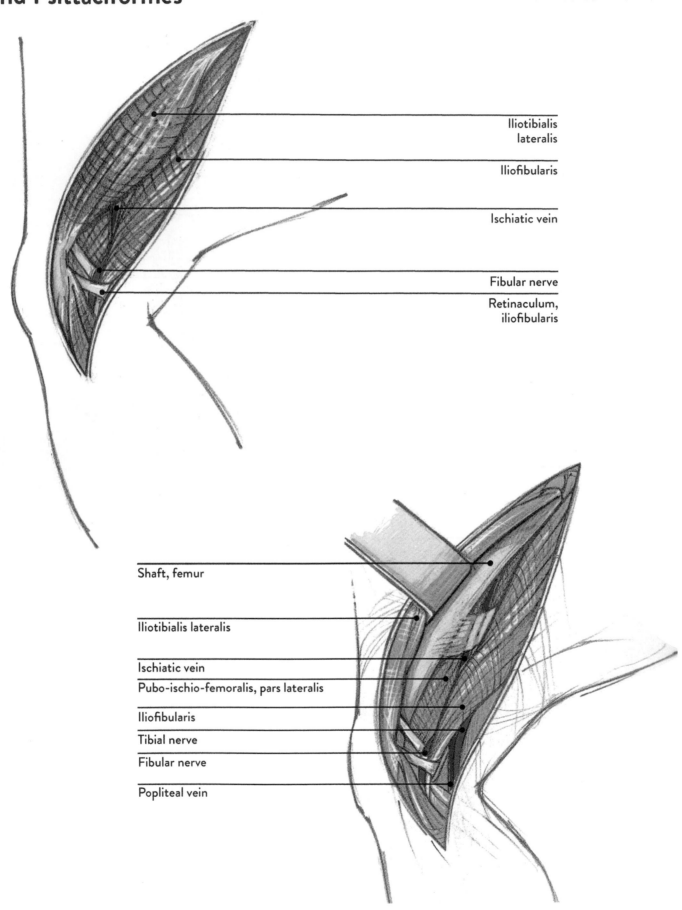

Iliotibialis lateralis

Iliofibularis

Ischiatic vein

Fibular nerve

Retinaculum, iliofibularis

Shaft, femur

Iliotibialis lateralis

Ischiatic vein

Pubo-ischio-femoralis, pars lateralis

Iliofibularis

Tibial nerve

Fibular nerve

Popliteal vein

Medial Leg: Superficial Layer of the Thigh (Femur)--Cathartidae and Galliformes

Flexor cruris medialis *[semimembranosus]*

This muscle, comparable to the semimembranosus muscle of mammals, originates mainly on the ischium. The medialis muscle is thin and flat and is closely associated with the flexor cruris lateralis. It inserts between the medial and intermediate heads of the gastrocnemius muscle onto the caudal proximal tibiotarsus. Its tendon may insert in common with the flexor cruris lateralis or semitendinosus muscle, if the latter is present. The medialis muscle is a strong flexor of the hip and abductor of the femur (Fischer 1946). It may also act to resist extension of the tibiotarsus as other extensor muscles contract. It is innervated by the ischiatic nerve.

Pubo-ischio-femoralis, pars medialis *[adductor magnus et brevis]*

This muscle may be closely adhered to the underlying pubo-ischio-femoralis, pars lateralis muscle. The pars medialis muscle is comparable to the adductor magnus et brevis muscle of mammals, based on its medial location. Both muscles insert on the caudal surface of the femur, including the medial femoral condyle and popliteal fossa. They adduct the femur and extend the hip. The pubo-ischio-femoralis, pars medialis is innervated by the obturator nerve.

Ambiens *[pectineus]*

The ambiens muscle is homologous to the pectineus of mammals and is found in birds and in reptiles. Its muscle belly originates from the ilium and narrows to a tendon that crosses the patella. From there, it inserts onto the heads of the long flexors of the digits. It may not go beyond the patella in some species, and it may be absent in others (finches, canaries, and other passerines; some species of psittacines, pigeons, and doves) (Getty 1975). Additionally, in some Psittacidae there is an ambiens while in other genera there is none. The ambiens has been described as the "perching muscle," because it helps to flex the toes for grasping when the intertarsal joint is flexed (Getty 1975). It however may have other functions including extension of the tibiotarsus and adduction of the leg. It is innervated by the femoral nerve (Getty 1975).

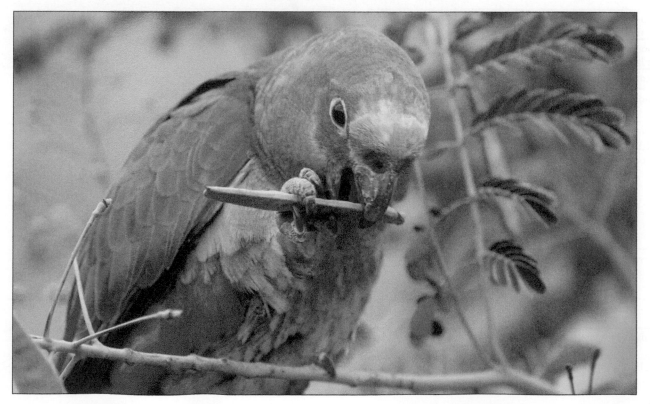

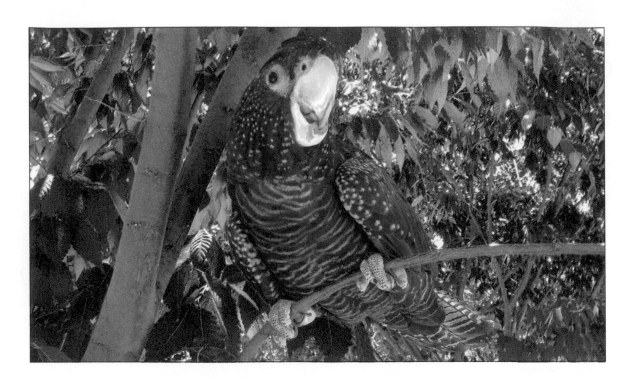

Medial Leg: Superficial Layer of the Thigh (Femur)

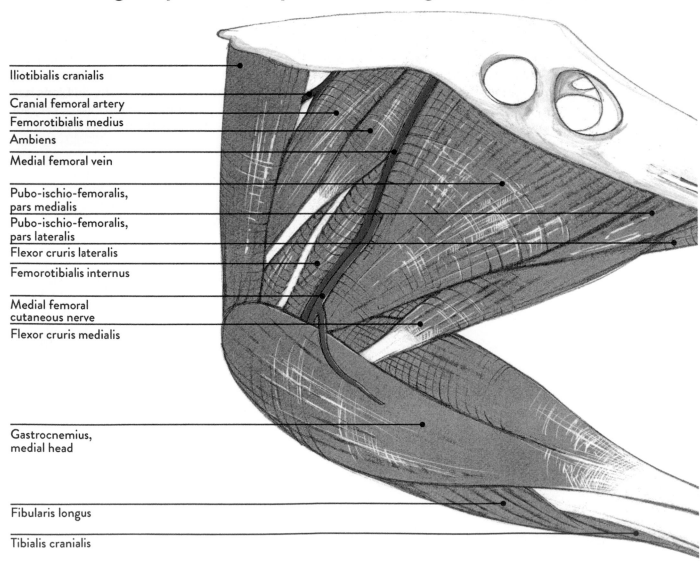

Iliotibialis cranialis

Cranial femoral artery

Femorotibialis medius

Ambiens

Medial femoral vein

Pubo-ischio-femoralis,
pars medialis

Pubo-ischio-femoralis,
pars lateralis

Flexor cruris lateralis

Femorotibialis internus

Medial femoral
cutaneous nerve

Flexor cruris medialis

Gastrocnemius,
medial head

Fibularis longus

Tibialis cranialis

Deep Muscle Layer, Medial Thigh--Cathartidae and Galliformes

Femorotibialis internus *[vastus medialis]*

This muscle is one of the three muscles in birds that composes the quadriceps femoris in mammals. It is the most medial muscle of this group, and it is caudal to the ambiens muscle and cranial to both the pubo-ischio femoralis, pars medialis muscle and the pubo-ischio-femoralis, pars lateralis muscle. It takes origin from the medial surface of the femoral shaft and inserts on the medial portion of the cnemial crest of the tibiotarsus. It contributes to a small part of the patellar tendon. These muscles together extend the stifle and the medial internal head is important for the medial rotation of the entire leg (Getty 1975).

Femorotibialis medius *[femorotibialis medius]*

This muscle, combined with the rectus femoris muscle, is considered in birds to represent one of the four heads of the quadriceps femoris. However, the rectus femoris originates on the femur, not the ilium, as in mammals. This muscle is continuous with the femorotibialis externus (also called the vastus lateralis), which is deep. This muscle takes origin from the trochanteric ridge distally over the entire surface of the femur. The medius muscle inserts on the cnemial crest of the tibiotarsus as the cranial and medial part of the patellar tendon to extend the stifle. The internus and medius muscles are innervated by the femoral nerve.

Medial Leg: Deep Muscle Layer of the Thigh (Femur)

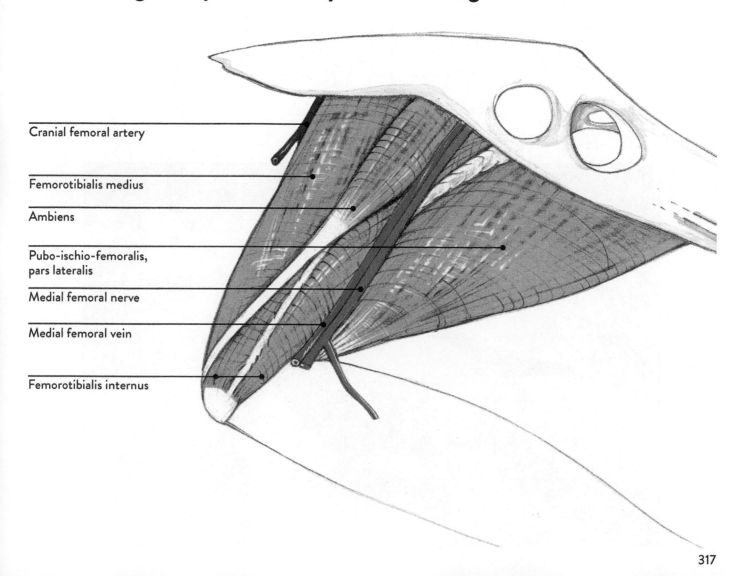

Cranial femoral artery

Femorotibialis medius

Ambiens

Pubo-ischio-femoralis, pars lateralis

Medial femoral nerve

Medial femoral vein

Femorotibialis internus

Blood supply and innervation

The medial femoral artery *[a. femoralis medialis]* can be seen running with the most medial femoral vein *[v. femoralis medialis]*, between the pubo-ischio-femoralis, pars medialis and the femorotibialis internus muscles. This artery is a branch of the femoral artery, which is the extra-abdominal continuation of the external iliac artery. It anastomoses distally with the medial tibial artery, a branch of the popliteal artery. The medial femoral vein ascends the thigh to drain into the femoral vein. The medial femoral cutaneous nerve *[n. cutaneous femoralis]* is found running with the artery and vein (Getty 1975, International Committee on Avian Anatomical Nomenclature 1979). This nerve is a branch of the femoral nerve. Deep on the medial side of the thigh distally is the tibial nerve. This nerve runs with the popliteal vessels medially. The tibial nerve divides into the medial and lateral tibial nerves. The lateral tibial nerve provides branches to the lateral head of the gastrocnemius, flexors p. et p. digiti II and III and flexor perforates digiti II, III, IV. The medial tibial nerve continues with the popliteal artery and gives off several branches. It supplies the deeper muscles including the flexor digitorum longus and the flexor hallicus longus (Getty 1975).

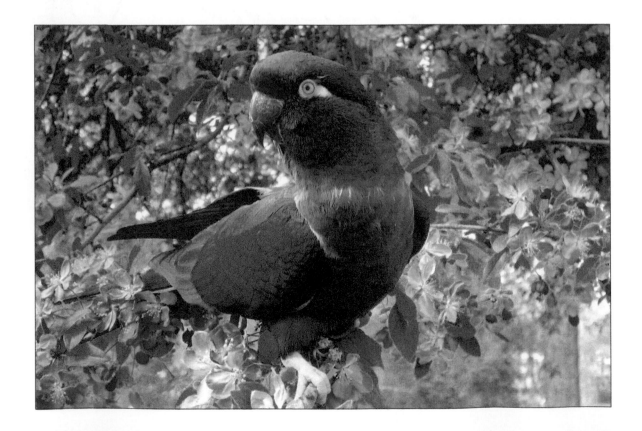

Superficial Layer of the Cranial Leg and Digits--Accipitridae, Strigiformes, and Psittaciformes

Fibularis longus *[peroneus longus]*

The fibularis longus of birds is comparable to the peroneus longus muscle of mammals. This muscle is superficial in vultures and gallinaceous birds. In Accipitridae, Strigiformes, and Psittaciformes, it is deep to the tibialis cranialis muscle as it is reduced in size. This muscle is absent in owls and osprey and some other birds. The origin can be fleshy or by an aponeurosis from the patellar tendon, the tibiotarsus including the medial and cranial cnemial crests. It can have aponeurotic connections with the tibialis cranialis muscle and some of the flexors of the leg. It inserts on the tibial cartilage and another portion becomes continuous with the tendon of insertion of the flexor perforates digiti III at the tarsometatarsus. It extends the hock by means of its connections with the tibial cartilage and through its common tendon of insertion acts to assist flexion of digit III. It is innervated by the fibular or peroneal nerve.

Tibialis cranialis

Located deep to the fibularis longus muscle in most birds except psittacines and hawks, the tibialis cranialis muscle is an important flexor of the hock and foot. It has two heads—one that takes origin on the lateral femoral condyle, and another that takes origin on the lateral cnemial crest. These muscle bellies fuse to form a single strong tendon that inserts in a groove on the dorsal cranial tarsometatarsus. The tibialis cranialis muscle flexes the intertarsal or hock joint and is also a powerful flexor of the foot. It is innervated by the fibular or peroneal nerve, as it is known in mammals.

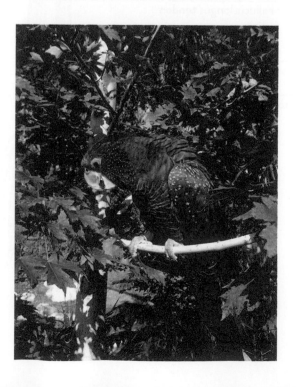

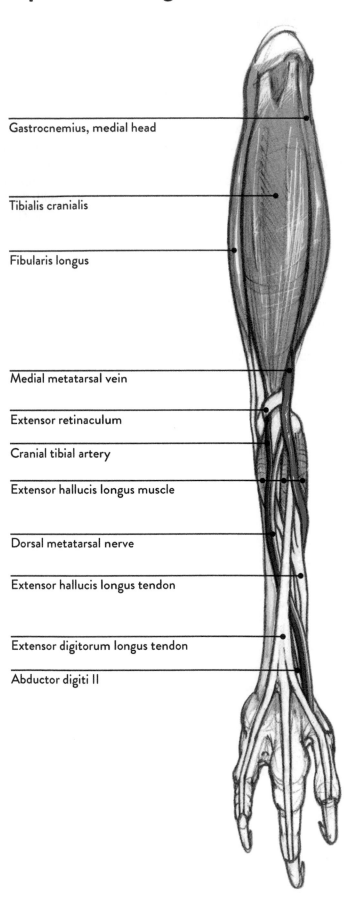

Gastrocnemius, medial head

Tibialis cranialis

Fibularis longus

Medial metatarsal vein

Extensor retinaculum

Cranial tibial artery

Extensor hallucis longus muscle

Dorsal metatarsal nerve

Extensor hallucis longus tendon

Extensor digitorum longus tendon

Abductor digiti II

Superficial Muscle Layer of the Cranial Leg and Digits--Cathartidae and Galliformes

Fibularis brevis [peroneus brevis]

The fibularis or peroneus brevis muscle is located distally on the lateral shaft of the tibiotarsus and fibula. It is mostly covered by the other muscles of the crus or leg. Its size is significant in vultures, falcons, and some psittacines, but it is absent or smaller in storks and flamingoes (Getty 1975). Its origin is mostly aponeurotic from the lateral surface of the tibiotarsus distal to the fibular crest. It also attaches to the fibula and occupies most of the space between the fibula and the tarsometatarsus. The fibularis brevis has a short tendon that inserts on the proximal lateral tarsometatarsus, more on the plantar surface. This muscle by its insertion contributes to flexion of the intertarsal or hock joint and with its plantar insertion causes some medial rotation or toeing in as the hock is flexed. It is innervated by the fibular or peroneal nerve (Getty 1975).

Extensor digitorum longus

This muscle is the extensor of digits II, III, and IV and flexor of the tarsometatarsus. It originates on the cranial tibiotarsus between the medial and lateral cnemial crests and the shaft of the tibiotarsus and passes through the bony extensor canal to emerge deep to the extensor retinaculum which can be fibrous or boney. The tendons of insertion are held in place by deep fascia. This tendon then divides into three tendons that insert on each of the distal processes, digits II, III, and IV. There are also smaller accessory attachments to the proximal portion of each of the interphalangeal joint capsules prior to the main insertion onto the claw of each of the digits. Since it originates on the dorsal tibiotarsus, it acts to flex the hock while extending digits II, III and IV. The extensor is innervated by the fibular nerve (Getty 1975).

Extensor brevis digiti III

This muscle takes origin on the distal end of the dorsal tarsometatarsus and inserts on the base of the proximal phalanx of digit III. As its name implies, it extends digit III. It is innervated by the superficial fibular nerve (Getty 1975).

Extensor hallucis longus

This muscle is the major extensor of the hallux or digit I. It originates on the dorsomedial surface of the tarsometatarsus and inserts on the distal process or ungual phalanx or claw of digit I. The tendon of insertion is held against the digit by deep fascia. The longus muscle extends the hallux or digit I and is innervated by the deep fibular nerve. Accessory heads may be found in some species (Getty 1975).

Blood supply and innervation

The tendon of the tibialis cranialis courses through a ligamentous loop. It is accompanied by the deep fibular nerve [n. fibularis profundus] and the cranial tibial artery and vein [a. and v. tibialis cranialis]. The cranial tibial artery is the major vascular supply to the lower leg and digits. However, the major venous drainage is via the caudal tibial vein. After the artery and vein cross the hock or intertarsal joint, they are designated the dorsal metatarsal artery and vein. [a. and v. metatarsales dorsales]. The dorsal metatarsal nerves [n. metatarsales dorsales] are derived from branches of both the superficial and deep fibular nerves.

Cranial Leg--Cathartidae and Galliformes

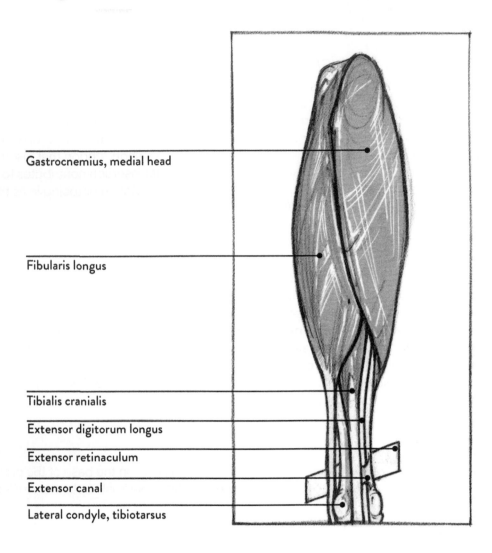

Gastrocnemius, medial head

Fibularis longus

Tibialis cranialis

Extensor digitorum longus

Extensor retinaculum

Extensor canal

Lateral condyle, tibiotarsus

Cranial Leg and Digits
MIDDLE LAYER
Most Species

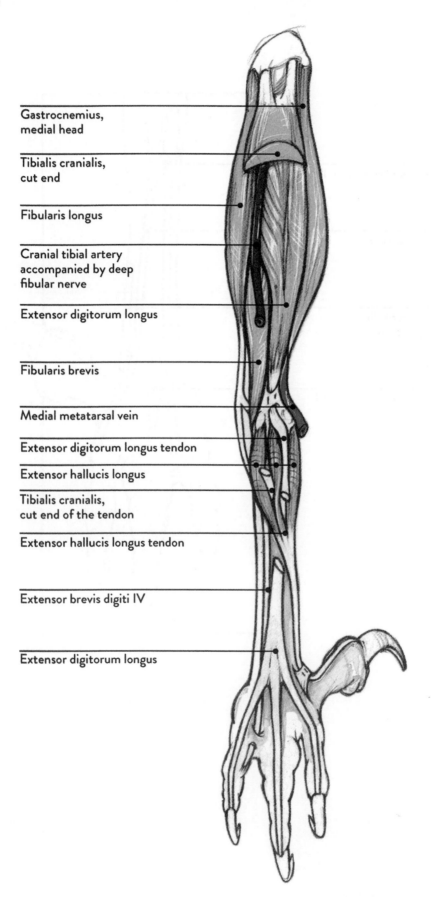

Gastrocnemius, medial head

Tibialis cranialis, cut end

Fibularis longus

Cranial tibial artery accompanied by deep fibular nerve

Extensor digitorum longus

Fibularis brevis

Medial metatarsal vein

Extensor digitorum longus tendon

Extensor hallucis longus

Tibialis cranialis, cut end of the tendon

Extensor hallucis longus tendon

Extensor brevis digiti IV

Extensor digitorum longus

Cranial Leg and Digits
DEEP LAYER
Most Species

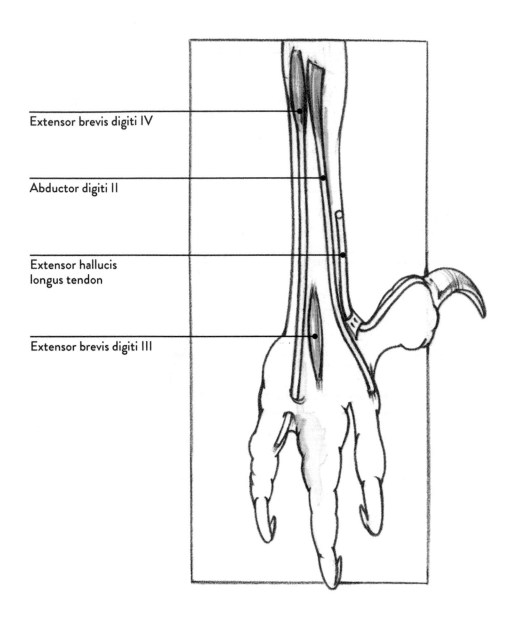

Extensor brevis digiti IV

Abductor digiti II

Extensor hallucis
longus tendon

Extensor brevis digiti III

Caudal Leg and Digits
SUPERFICAL LAYER

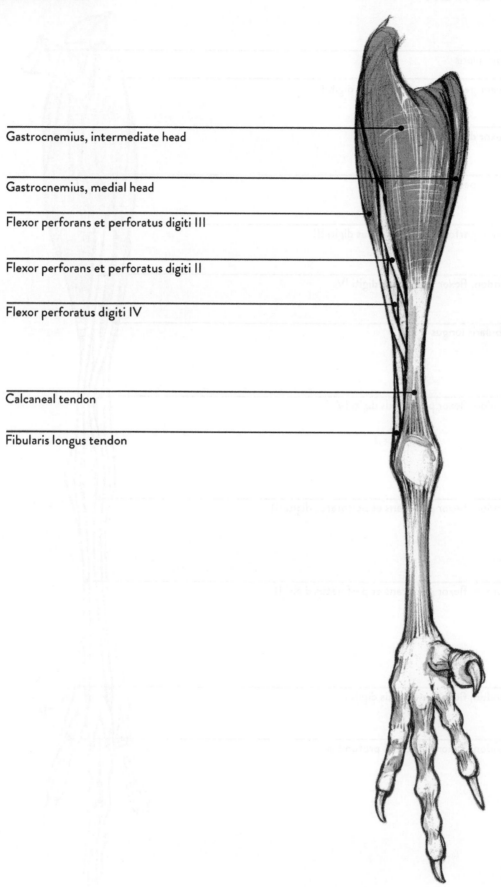

Gastrocnemius, intermediate head

Gastrocnemius, medial head

Flexor perforans et perforatus digiti III

Flexor perforans et perforatus digiti II

Flexor perforatus digiti IV

Calcaneal tendon

Fibularis longus tendon

Caudal Leg and Digits
SECOND LAYER

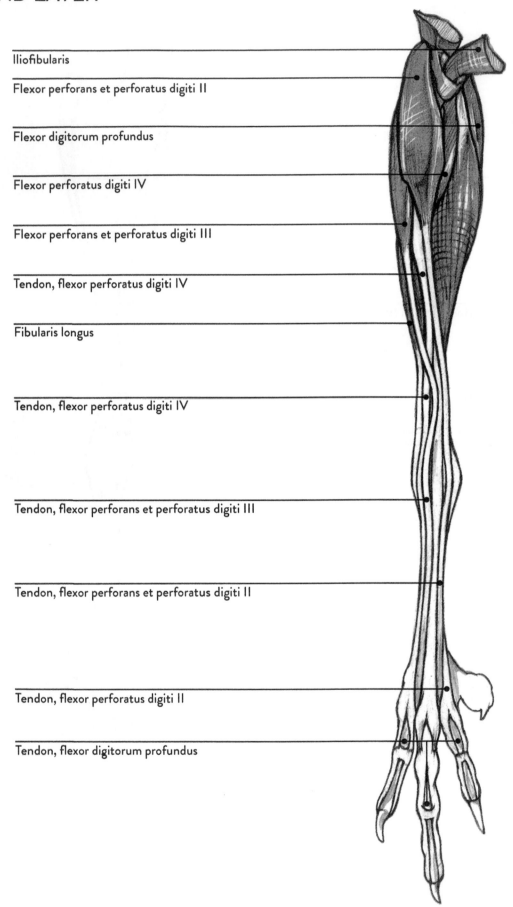

Iliofibularis

Flexor perforans et perforatus digiti II

Flexor digitorum profundus

Flexor perforatus digiti IV

Flexor perforans et perforatus digiti III

Tendon, flexor perforatus digiti IV

Fibularis longus

Tendon, flexor perforatus digiti IV

Tendon, flexor perforans et perforatus digiti III

Tendon, flexor perforans et perforatus digiti II

Tendon, flexor perforatus digiti II

Tendon, flexor digitorum profundus

Caudal Leg and Digits
THIRD LAYER

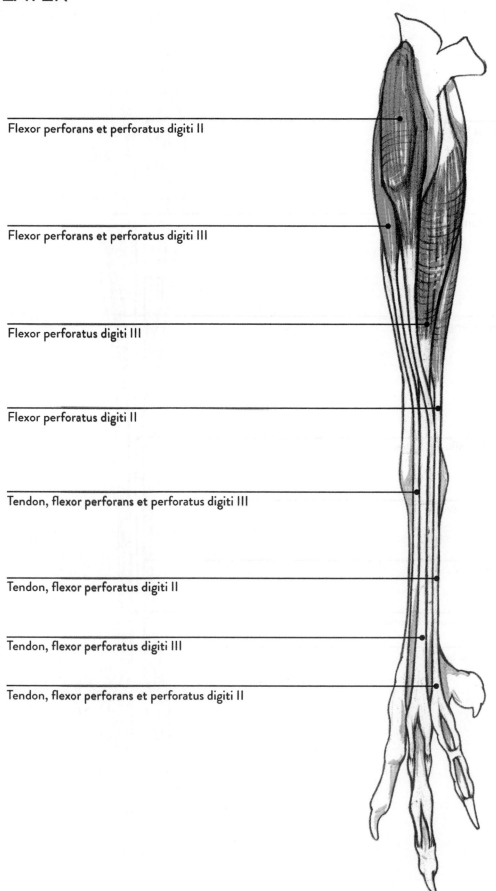

Flexor perforans et perforatus digiti II

Flexor perforans et perforatus digiti III

Flexor perforatus digiti III

Flexor perforatus digiti II

Tendon, flexor perforans et perforatus digiti III

Tendon, flexor perforatus digiti II

Tendon, flexor perforatus digiti III

Tendon, flexor perforans et perforatus digiti II

Caudal Leg and Digits
DEEP LAYER

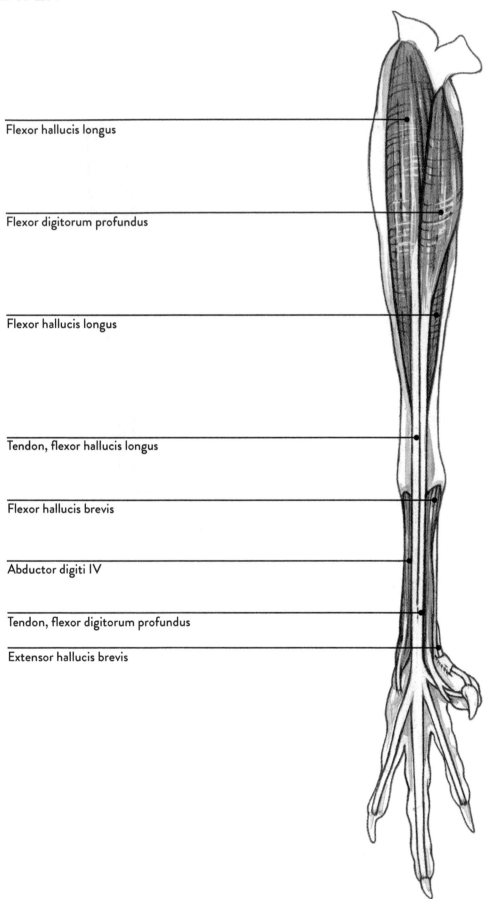

Flexor hallucis longus

Flexor digitorum profundus

Flexor hallucis longus

Tendon, flexor hallucis longus

Flexor hallucis brevis

Abductor digiti IV

Tendon, flexor digitorum profundus

Extensor hallucis brevis

Medial Tibiotarsus, Cathartidae, and Galliformes

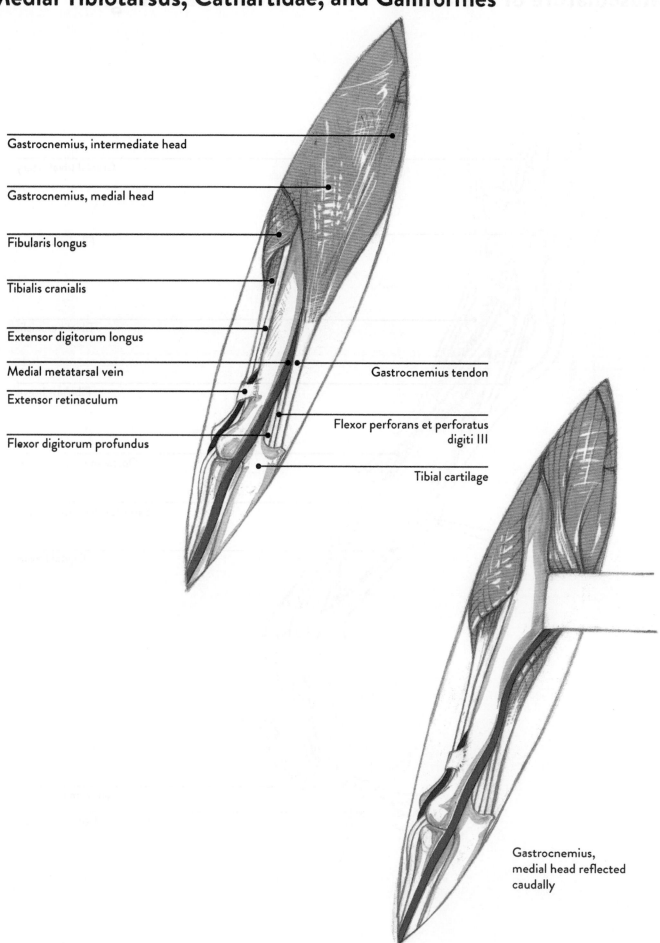

Gastrocnemius, intermediate head

Gastrocnemius, medial head

Fibularis longus

Tibialis cranialis

Extensor digitorum longus

Medial metatarsal vein

Extensor retinaculum

Flexor digitorum profundus

Gastrocnemius tendon

Flexor perforans et perforatus digiti III

Tibial cartilage

Gastrocnemius, medial head reflected caudally

Musculature of the Lateral Tarsometatarsus and Digits

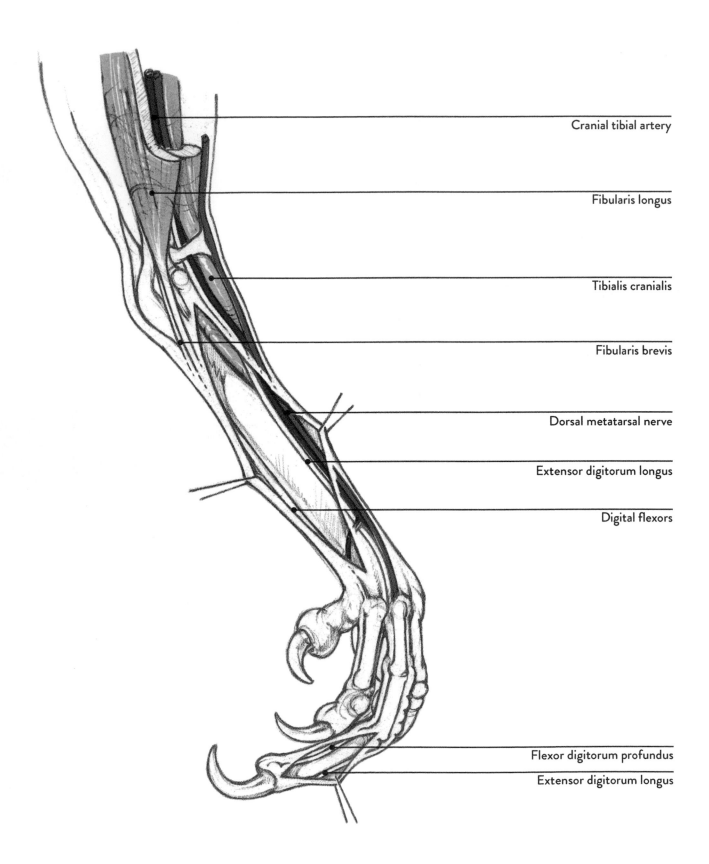

Cranial tibial artery

Fibularis longus

Tibialis cranialis

Fibularis brevis

Dorsal metatarsal nerve

Extensor digitorum longus

Digital flexors

Flexor digitorum profundus

Extensor digitorum longus

Vasculature Contrast Images of the Leg

Vasculature contrast images of the leg are presented for four species: the pigeon *(Columba livia)*, painted stork *(Mycteria leucoephala)*, African goose *(Anser anser domesticus)*, and barn owl *(Tyto alba)*. Images of the distal tibiotarsus and foot are not available on the barn owl due to extensive trauma to this bird.

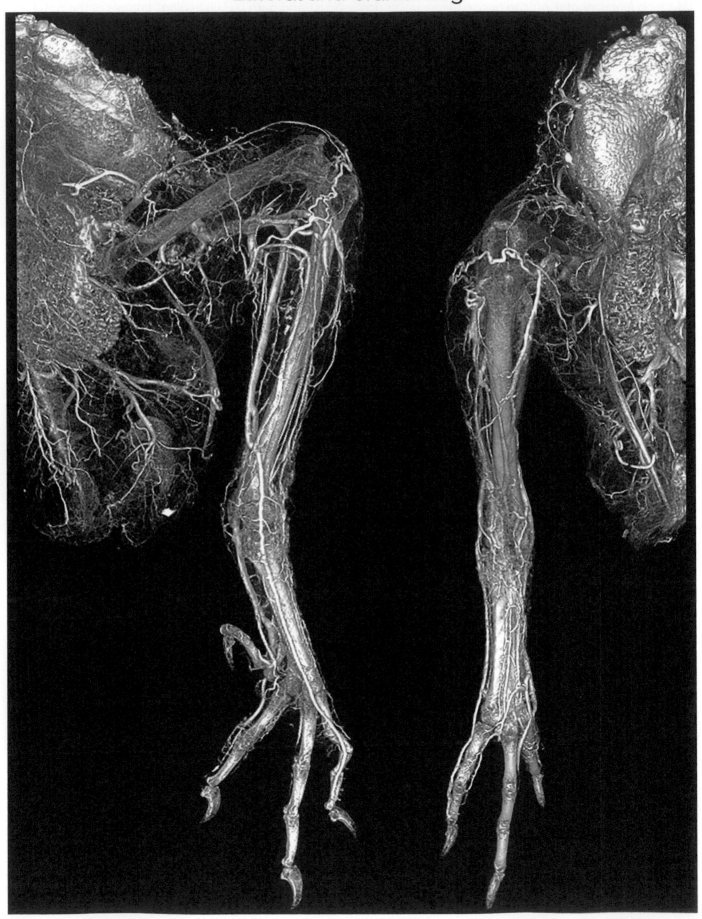

Pigeon (*Columba livia*)
Caudal and Medial Leg

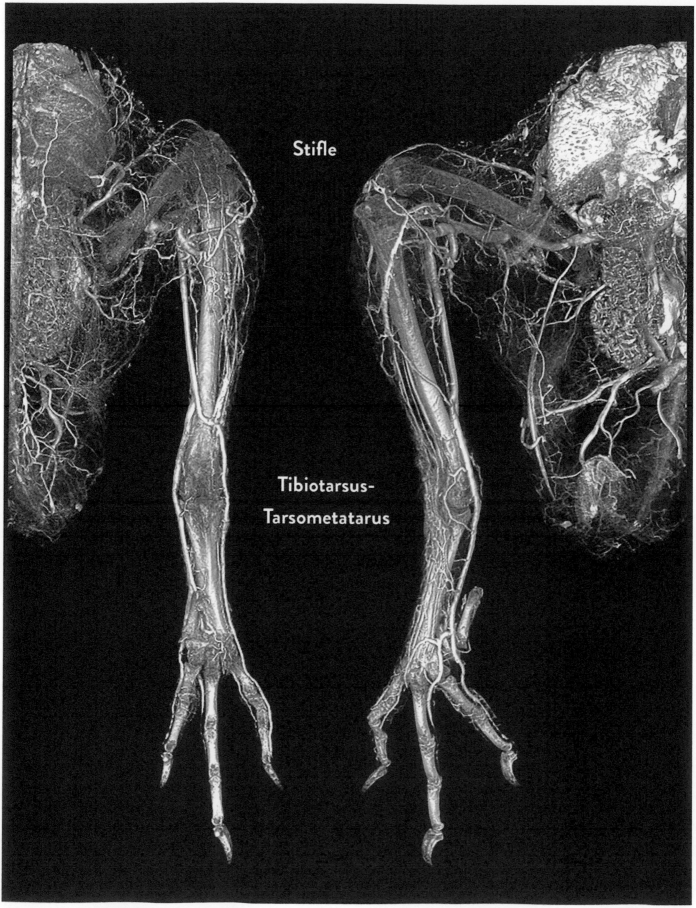

Stifle

Tibiotarsus-

Tarsometatarus

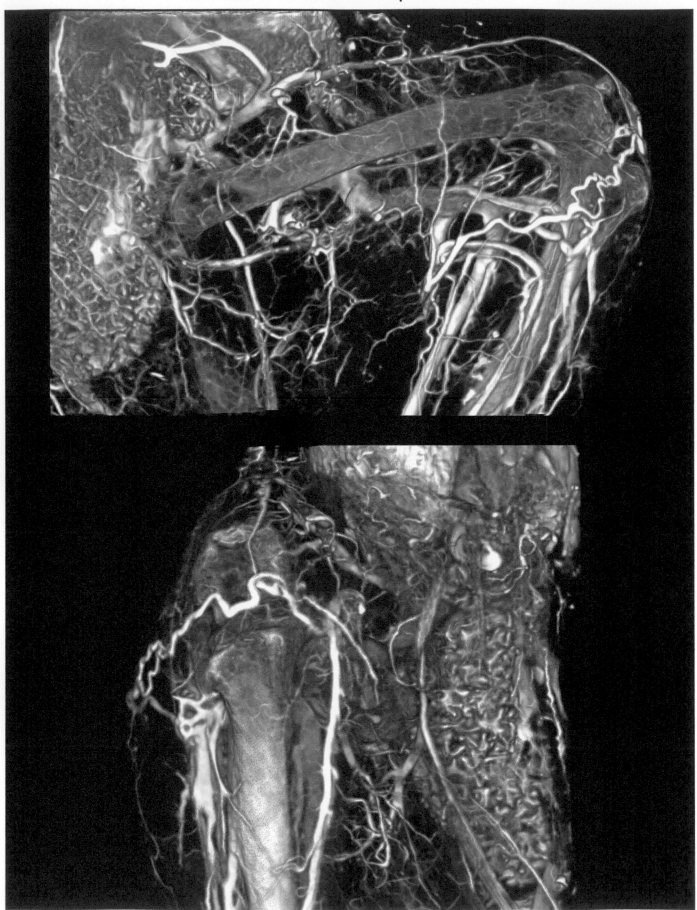

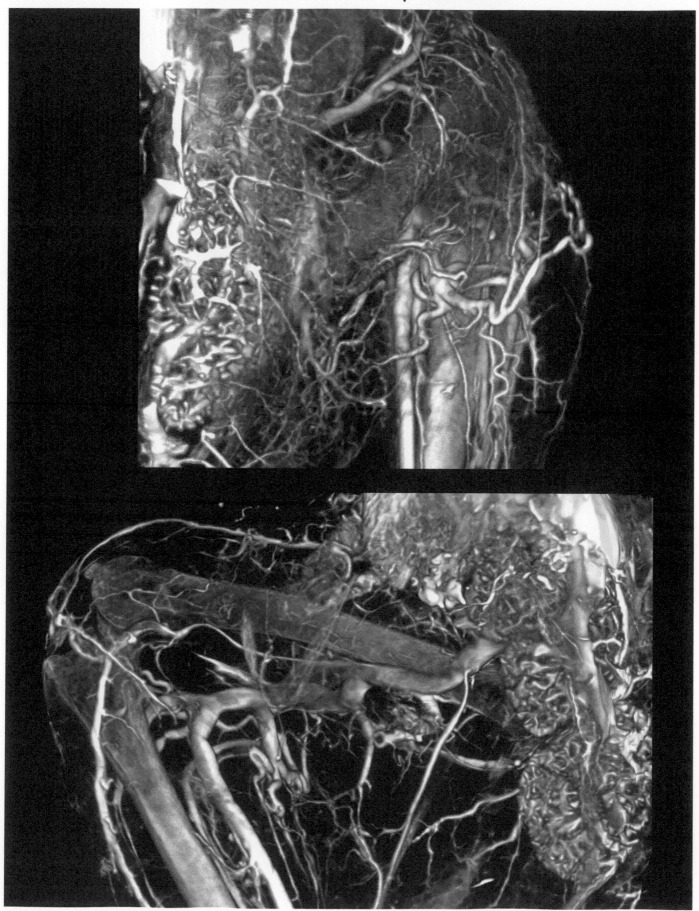

Pigeon (*Columba livia*)
Lateral and Cranial Tibiotarsal-Tarsometatarsal Joint

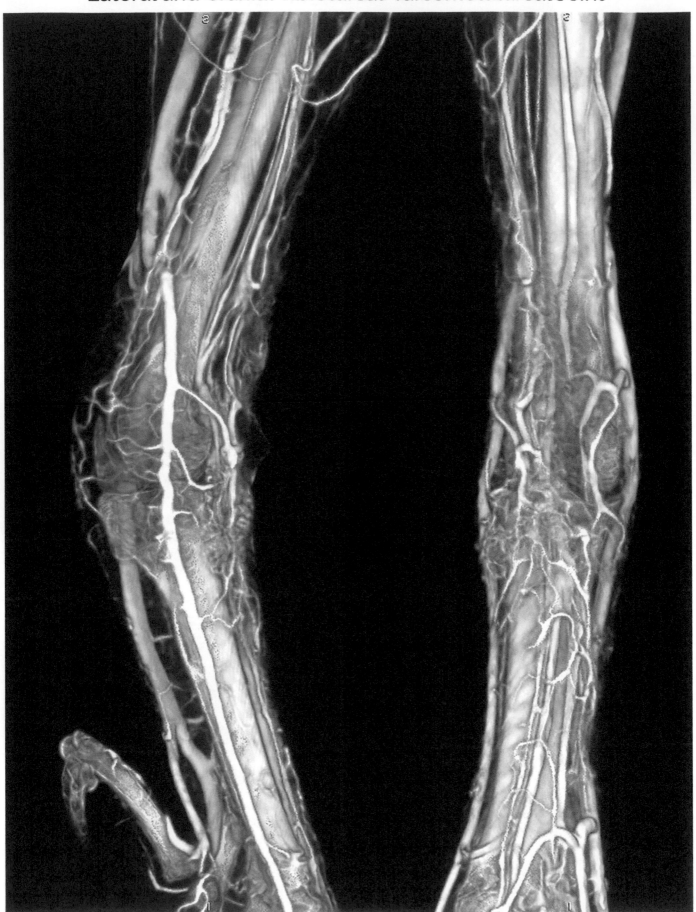

Pigeon (*Columba livia*)
Caudal and Medial Tibiotarsal-Tarsometatarsal Joint

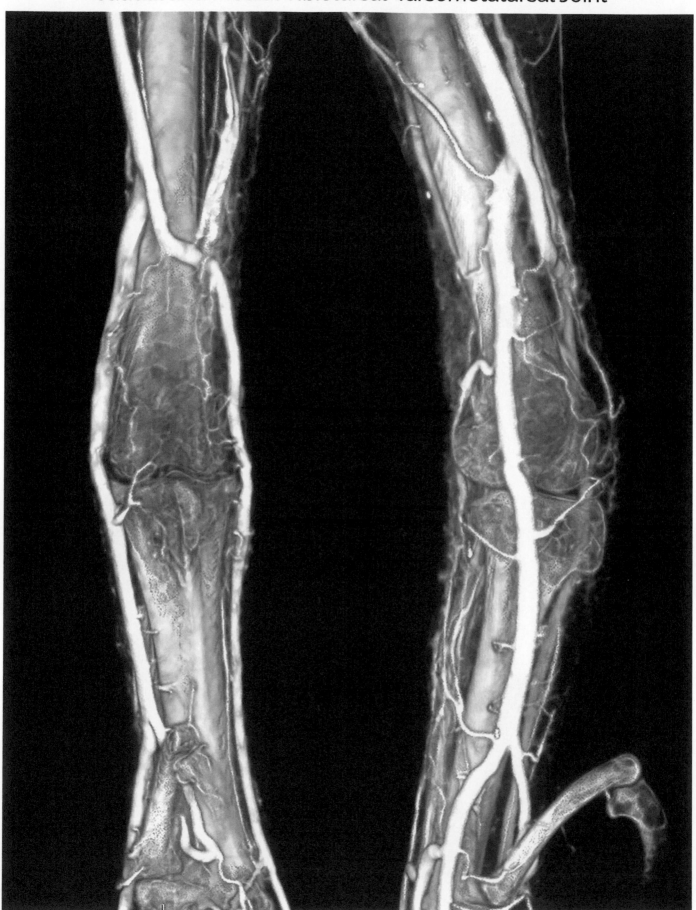

Pigeon (*Columba livia*)
Lateral and Dorsal Foot

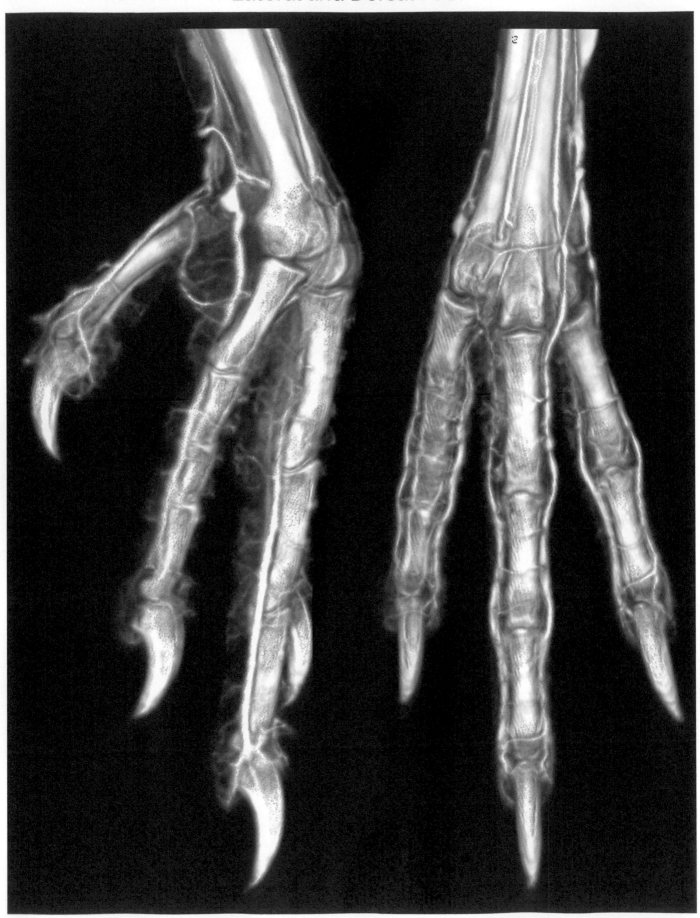

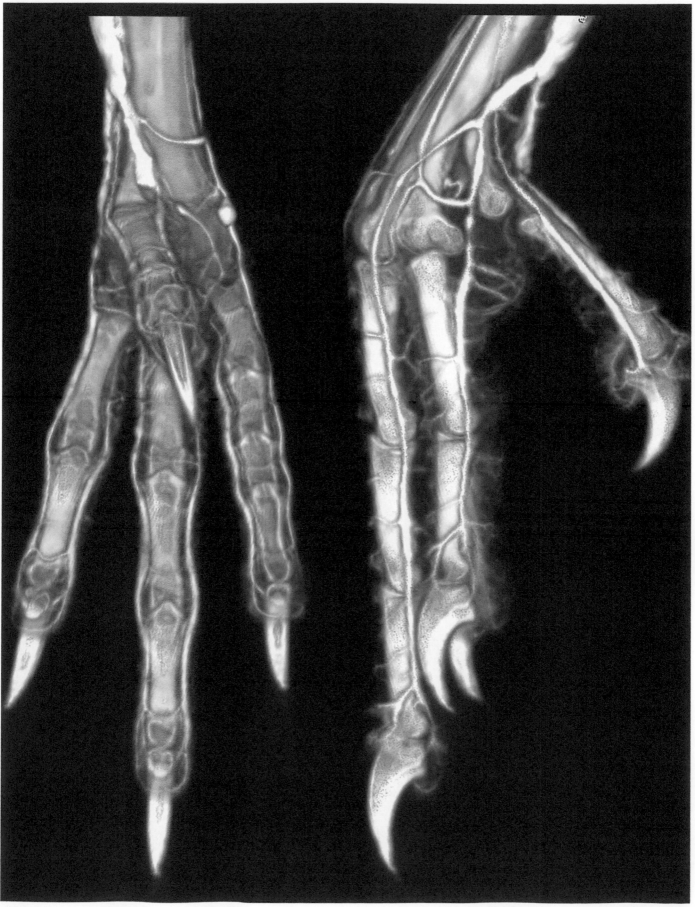

Painted Stork (*Mycteria leucocephala*)
Lateral Hip and Stifle

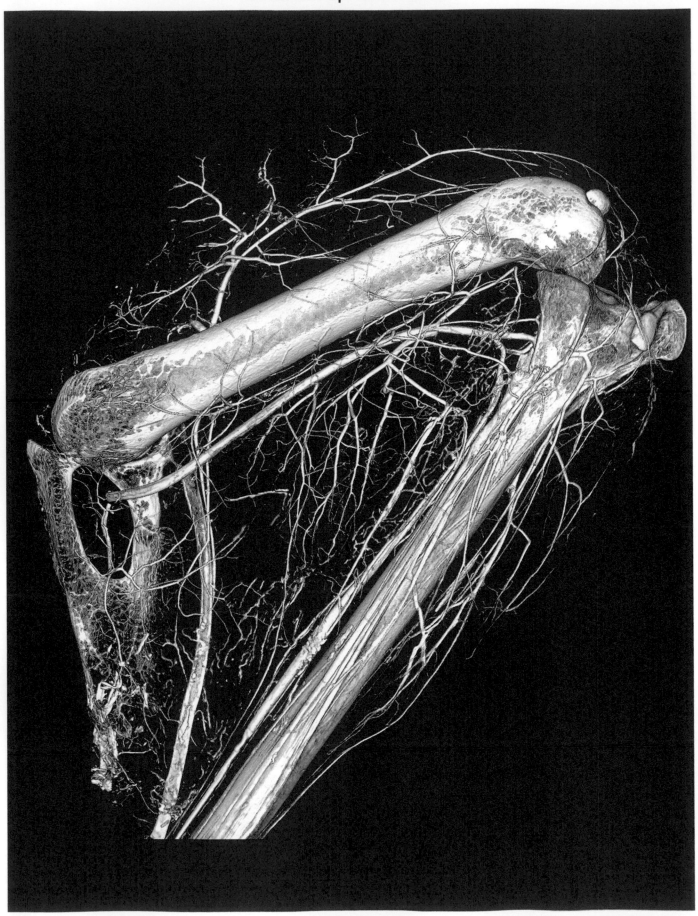

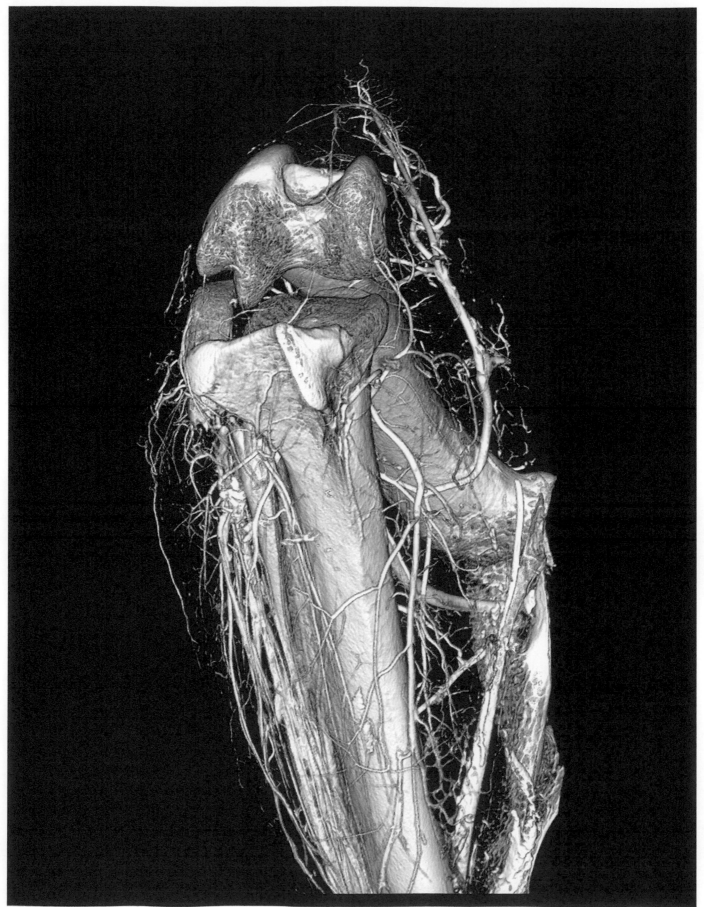

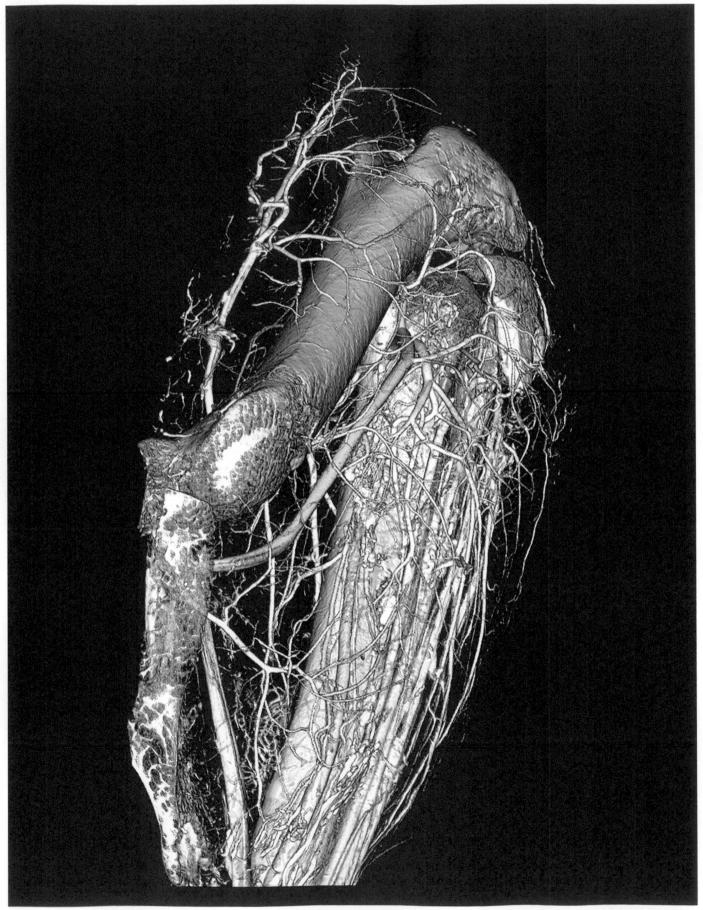

Painted Stork (*Mycteria leucocephala*)
Caudal Hip and Stifle

Painted Stork (*Mycteria leucocephala*)
Medial Hip and Stifle

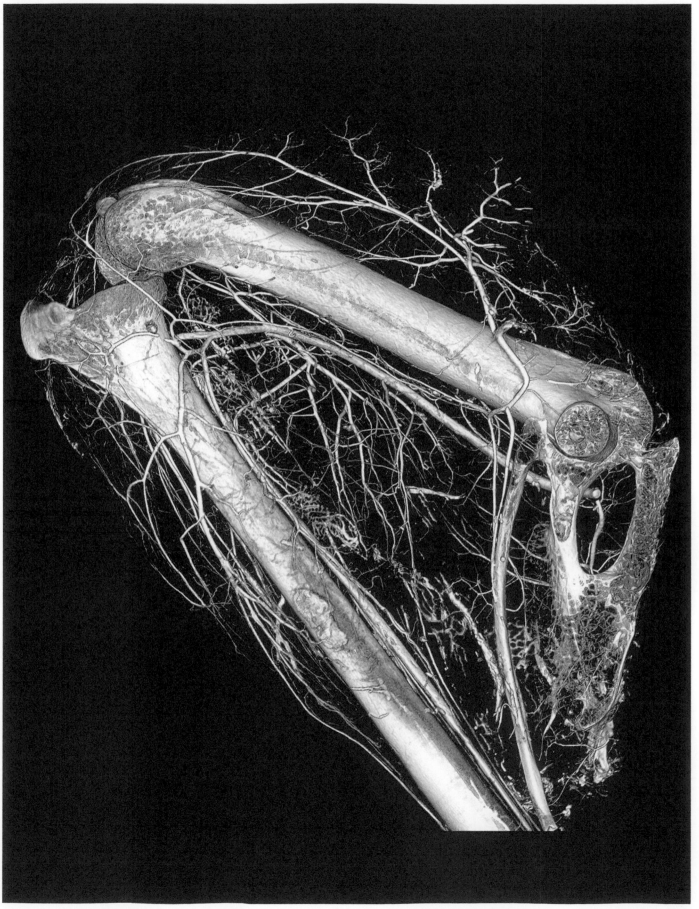

343

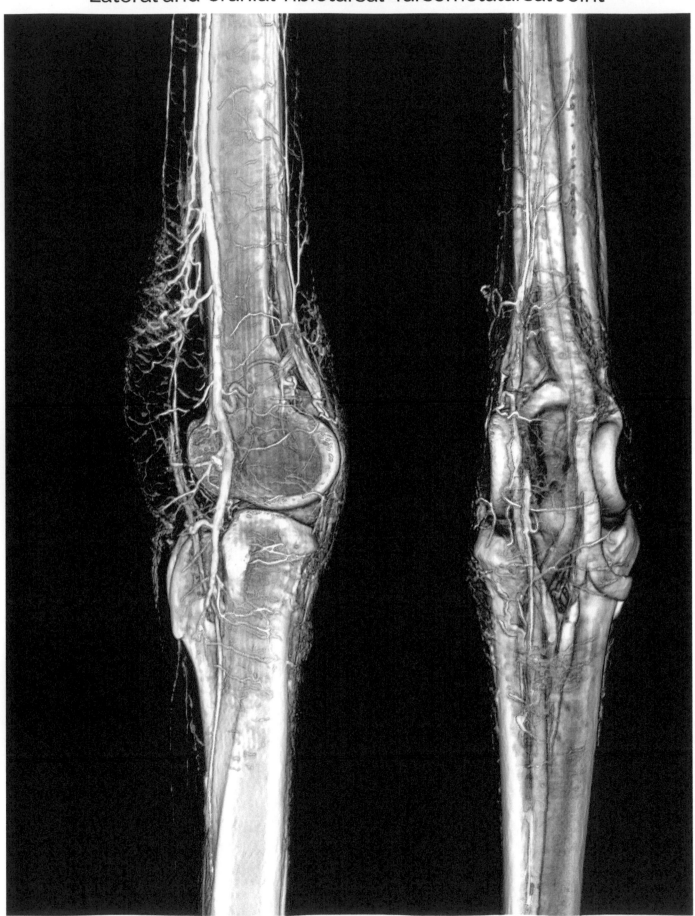

Painted Stork (*Mycteria leucocephala*)
Caudal and Medial Tibiotarsal-Tarsometatarsal Joint

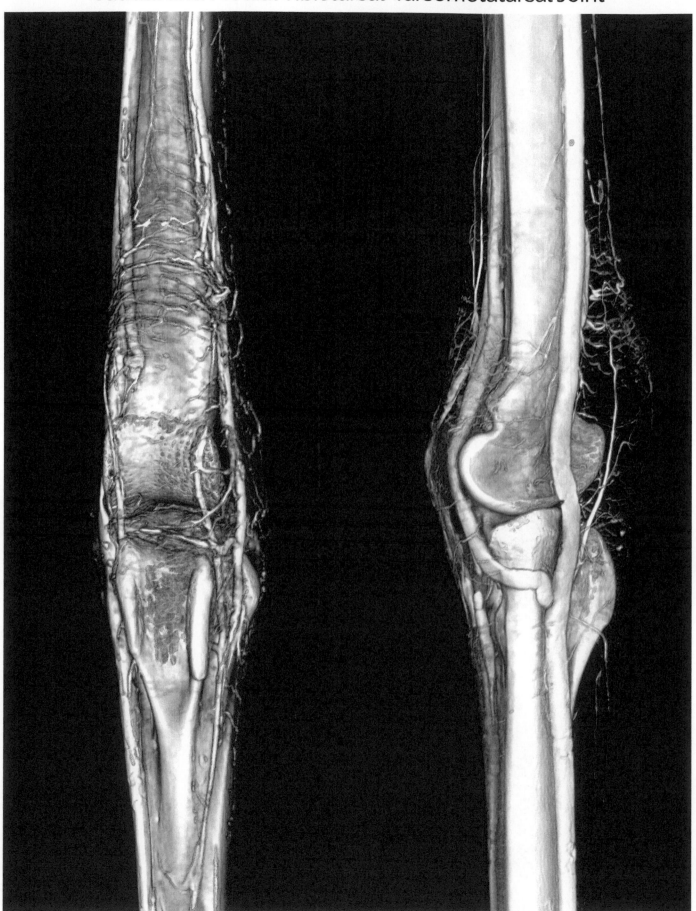

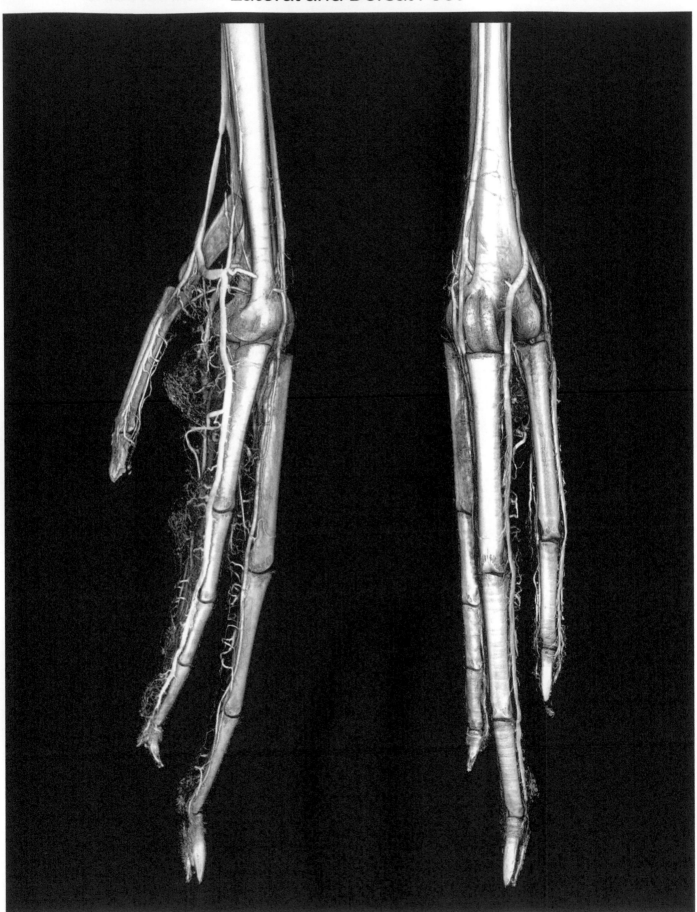

Painted Stork (*Mycteria leucocephala*)
Plantar and Medial Foot

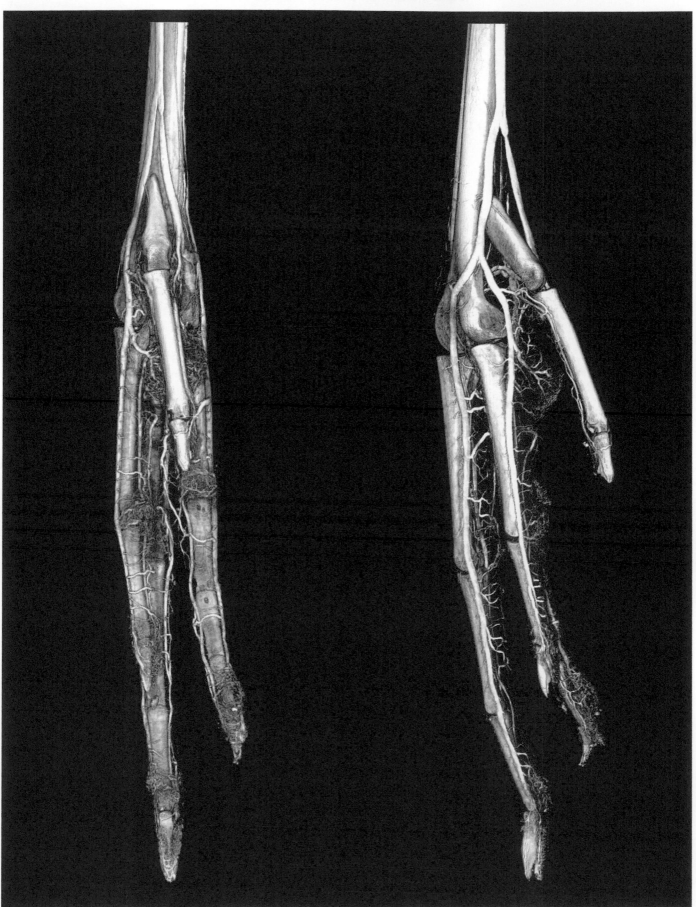

African Goose (*Anser anser domesticus*)
Lateral Hip and Stifle

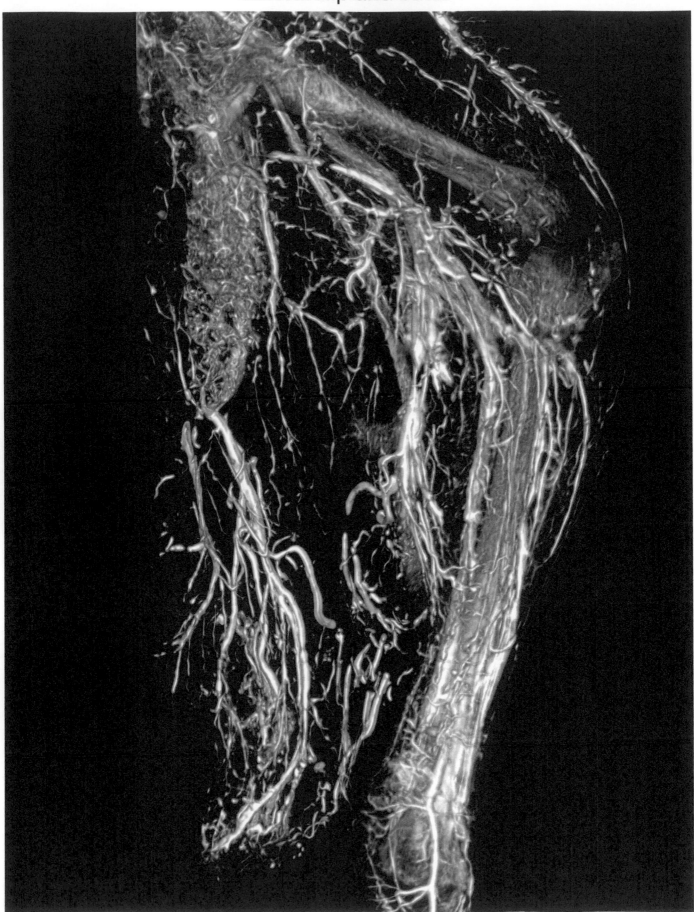

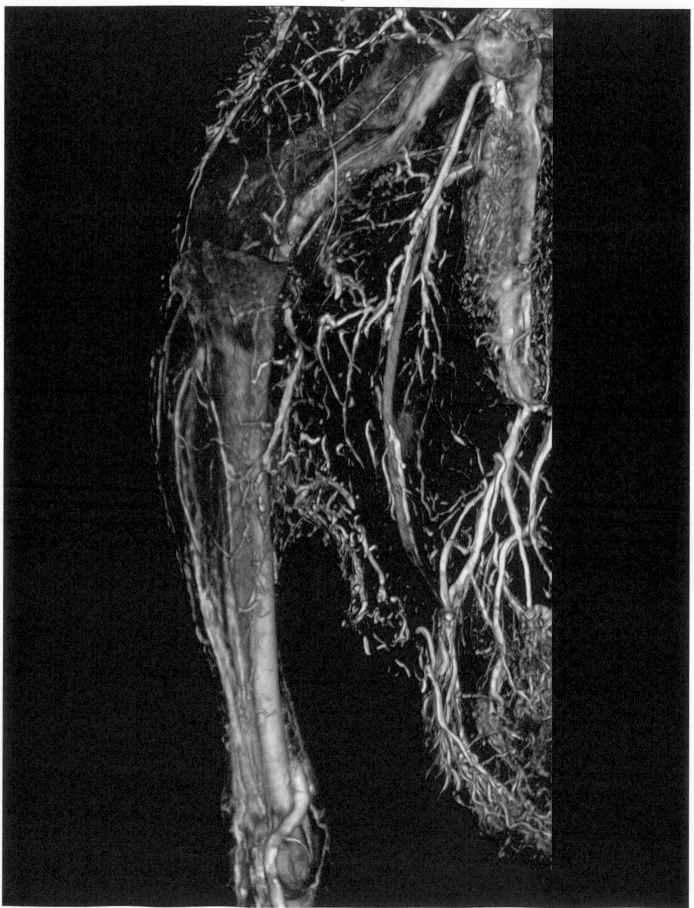

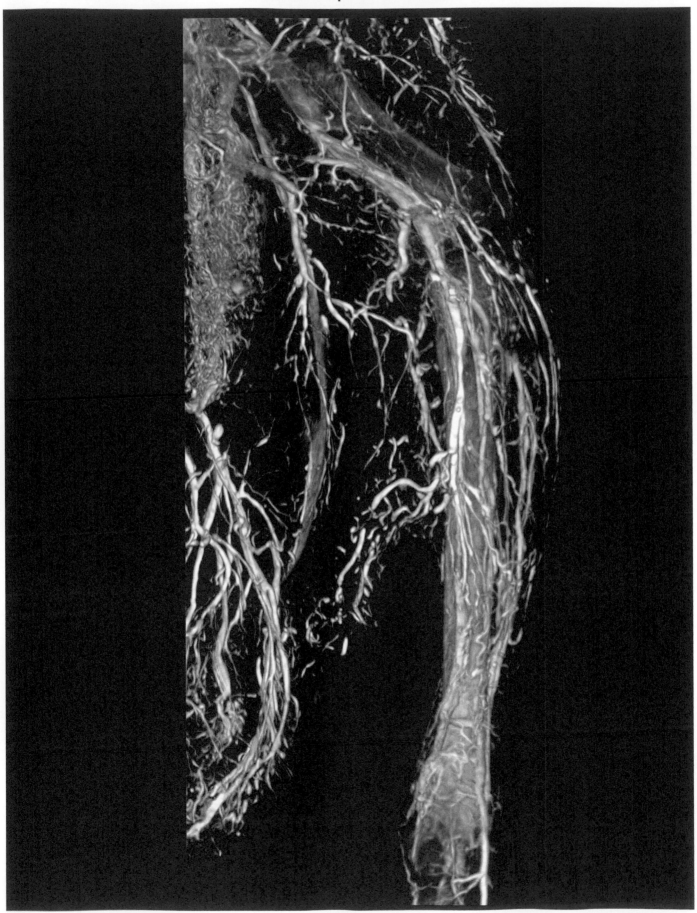

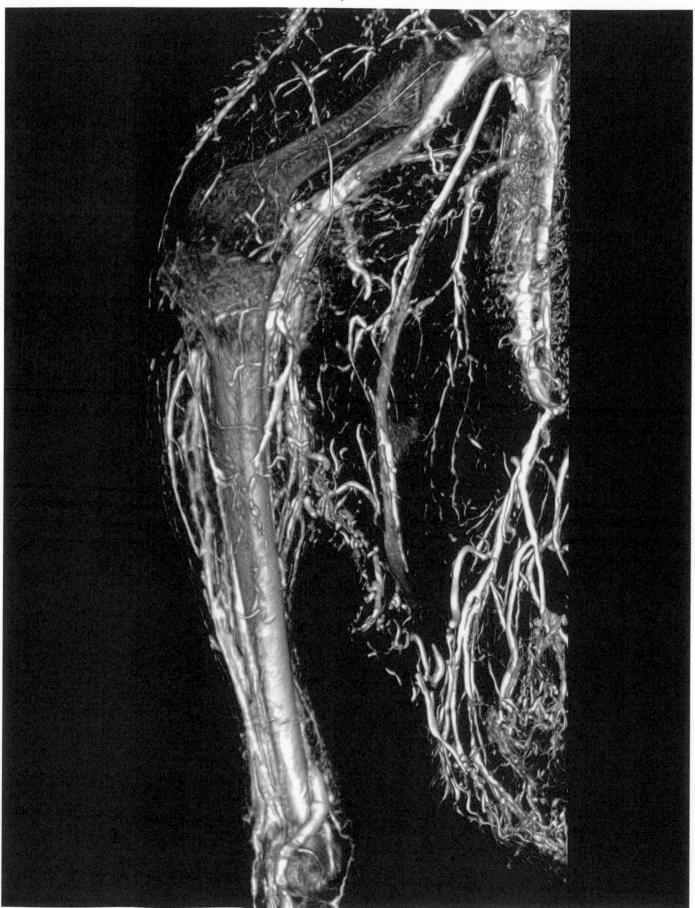

African Goose (*Anser anser domesticus*)
Lateral and Dorsal Foot

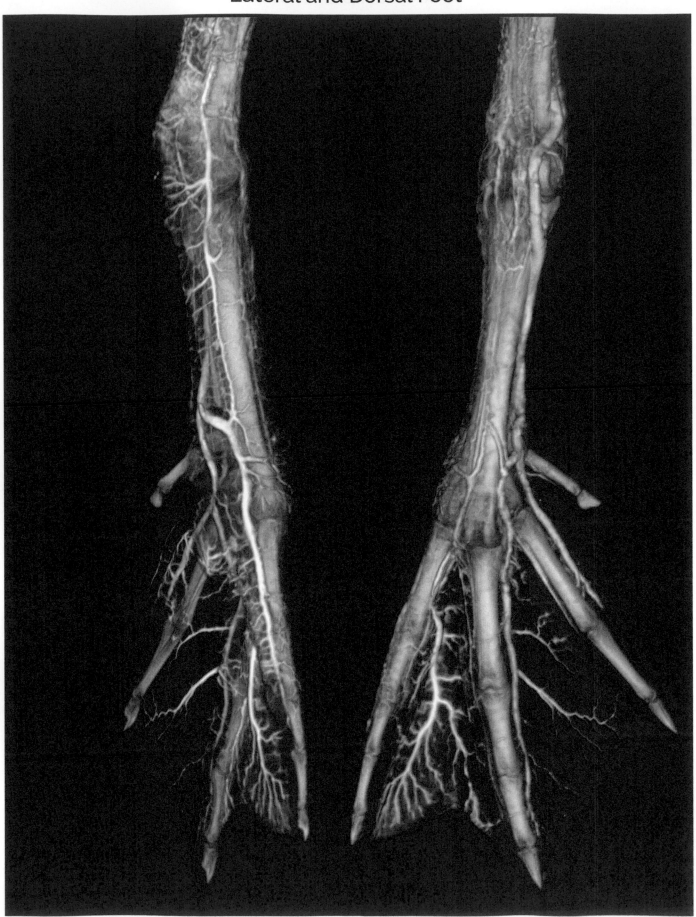

African Goose (*Anser anser domesticus*)
Plantar and Medial Foot

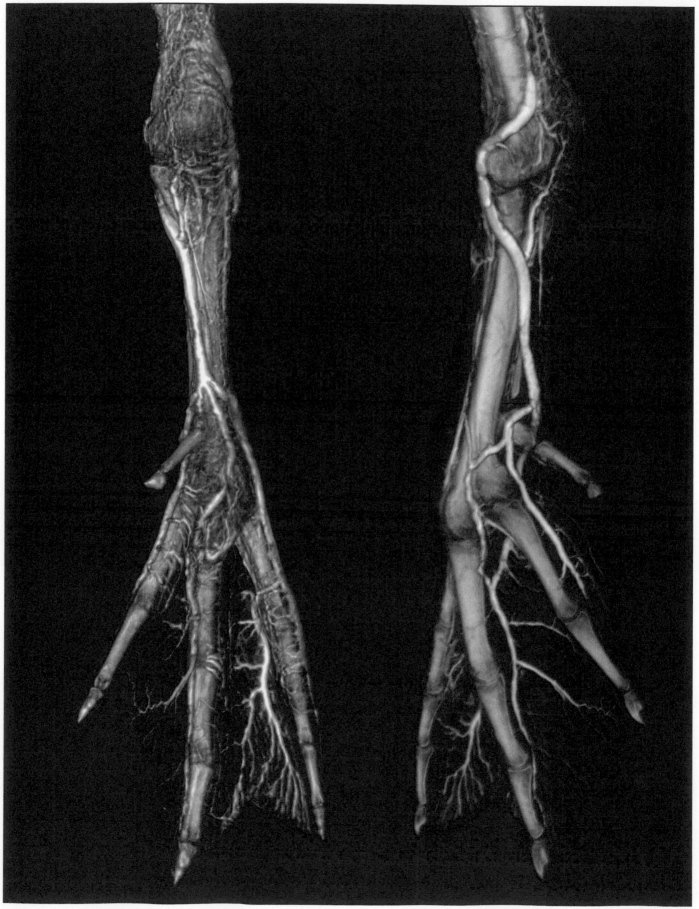

Barn Owl (*Tyto alba*)
Lateral Hip and Stifle

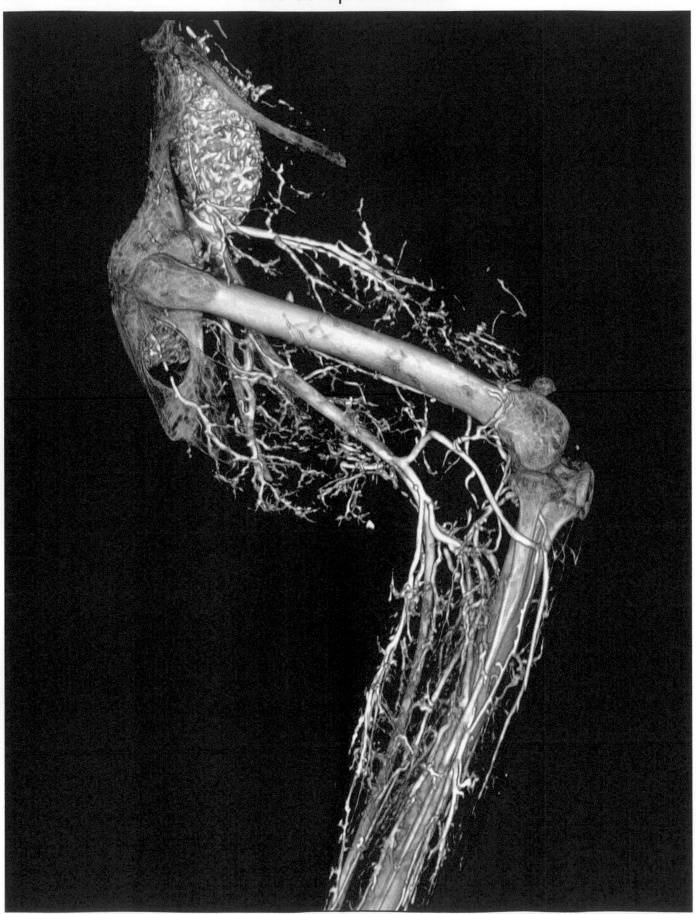

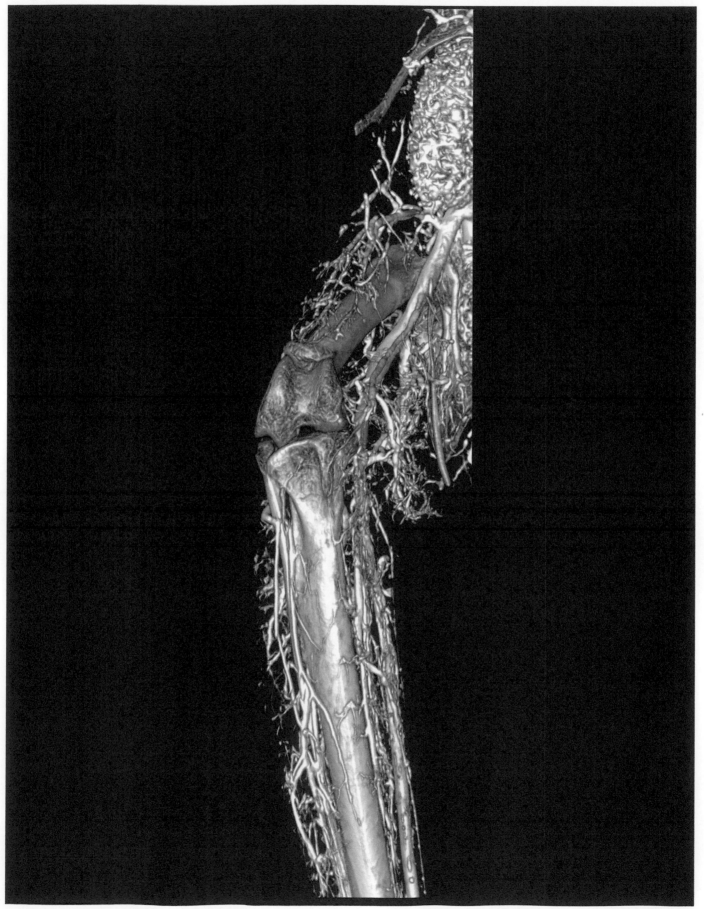

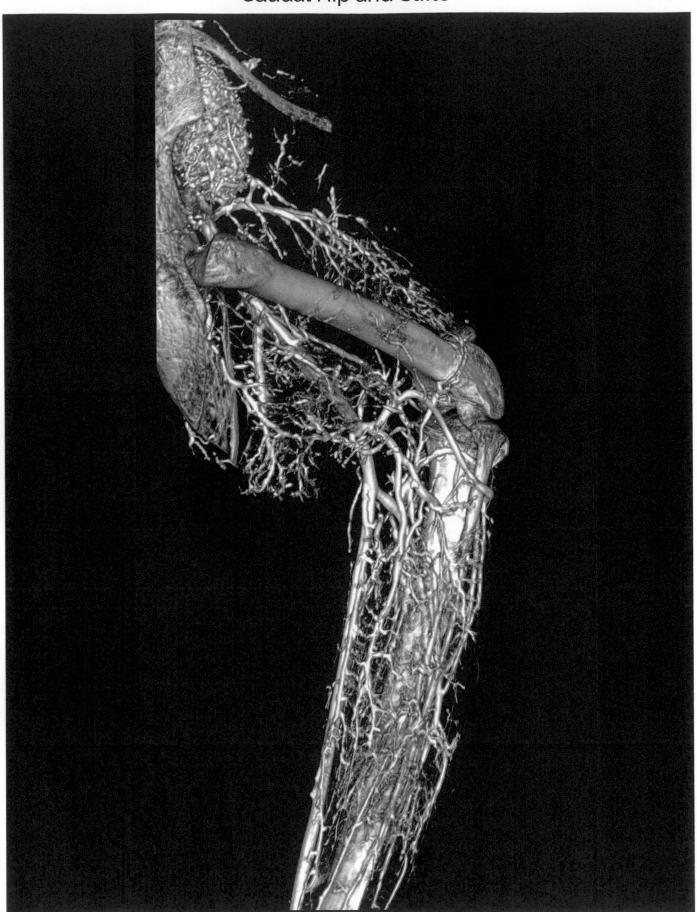

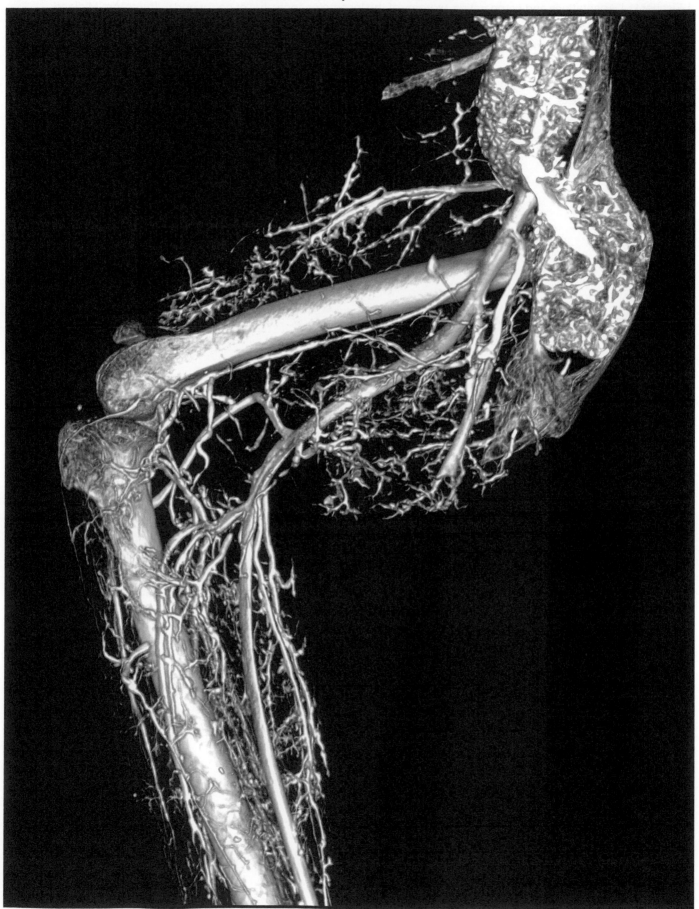

Recommended Reading

1. Baumel J. Functional anatomy of the avian thoracic limb: selected topics. Proc Annu Conf Assoc Avian Vet. 1983;67-70.

2. Fischer H. I. Adaptations and comparative anatomy of the locomotor apparatus of new world vultures. Am Midland Naturalist. 1946; 35:545-727.

3. Getty R. Sisson and Grossman's Anatomy of the Domestic Animals. 5th ed. Vol 2. Porcine, Carnivores, Aves. Philadelphia: WB Saunders; 1975.

4. International Committee on Avian Anatomical Nomenclature. Nomina Anatomica Avium. 1st ed. London: World Association of Veterinary Anatomists; 1979.

CHAPTER 8

Surgical Approaches to the Leg

Application of Tie-in Fixation for Fractures of the Femur
General Considerations

With abundant soft tissue protection afforded by heavy muscle, the femur responds well to most attempts at fixation. The approach to tie-in fixation resembles that of the humerus and the external skeletal fixator-intra-medullary (ESF-IM) pin tie-in works well. Intramedullary pins are most always introduced at the fracture site and driven retrograde at the hip. For insertion of the IM pin, the femur is approached from the lateral aspect. The bird is laid with the contralateral side down. The affected leg is abducted, and the distal portion of the ipsilateral wing placed underneath the leg, between the medial aspect of the leg and the body wall **(Figure 8-1A, B)** with the patient in a semi-ventral recumbency.

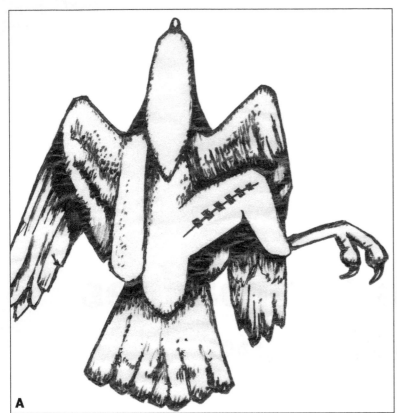

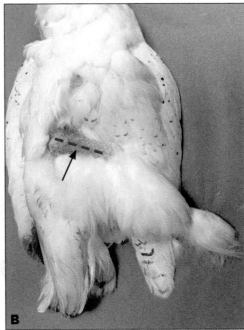

Figure 8-1A, B. Incision line extending from proximal end of the femur to the lateral femoral condyle on the caudal-lateral border of the femur. Species is a snowy owl *(Bubo scandiaca).*

The incision is made at about the 4 o'clock position on the femoral shaft as viewed from the distal end on, extending from the condyles at the distal end to the proximal end. Blunt dissection is used to separate the *iliotibialis lateralis* from the ventral flexor muscle group. Specifically, beginning at the stifle, identify the iliofibularis muscle near its insertion by visualizing the retinaculum that suspends it. Immediately cranial to it is the quadriceps group of muscles (femorotibialis muscles) and with it, the overlying iliotibialis lateralis muscle **(Figure 8-2A, B)**. After incising the fascia overlying these muscles, beginning near the stifle, begin a line of dissection that separates the iliotibialis lateralis muscle cranially and the iliofibularis muscle caudally. Periosteally elevate these muscles from the surface of the femur as necessary to gain access to the fracture site **(Figure 8-2C)**. Closure is accomplished by lightly suturing the muscle bellies together, then closing the overlying fascia. Cutaneous absorbable sutures are used to close the skin with simple interrupted sutures.

The ischiatic nerve divides into the fibular nerve (cranially) and the tibial nerve (caudally) near the distal end of the femur, as shown in Figure 8-2C. The ischiatic artery, vein and nerve lie deep and caudal to the femur; they may be visualized, but do not present a serious hazard during repair of the bone. At this point, additional dissection may be undertaken to elevate bone fragments as needed.

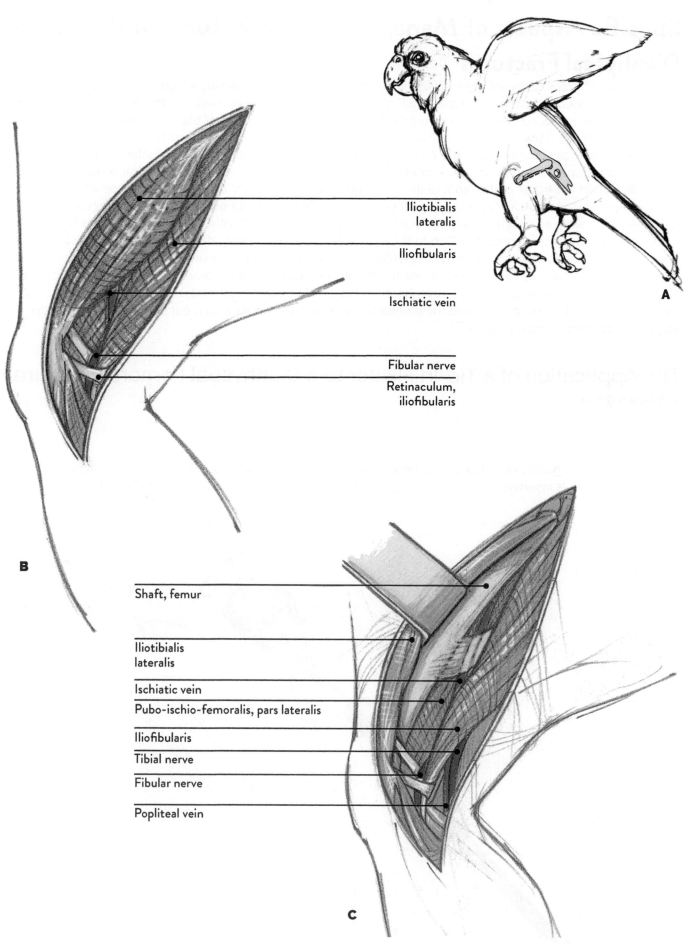

B

Iliotibialis
lateralis

Iliofibularis

Ischiatic vein

Fibular nerve

Retinaculum,
iliofibularis

A

C

Shaft, femur

Iliotibialis
lateralis

Ischiatic vein

Pubo-ischio-femoralis, pars lateralis

Iliofibularis

Tibial nerve

Fibular nerve

Popliteal vein

Figure 8-2A, B, C. Orientation drawing for approach to the lateral femur **(A)**. Anatomical features of the femur for a lateral surgical approach **(B, C)**.

Specific Aspects of Management of Fractures of the Femur:
Diaphyseal Fractures

For diaphyseal fractures, the intramedullary pin for the hybrid fixator is typically introduced at the fracture site and retrograded proximally. The distal ESF pin is placed from lateral to medial in the distal condyles. The proximal ESF pin is placed from lateral to medial by palpating the dorsal rim of the acetabulum and selecting a point on the femur 1-2 bone diameters distad. A smaller pin than that used distally is typically selected as it must share the marrow cavity with the IM pin. As the medial side of the femur cannot be palpated, determination of proper drilling depth for the pin must be done by "feel". Characteristically, resistance to rotation of the pin chuck can be felt when the trocar of the pin is drilling through bone. Accordingly, one feels resistance when passing through the first cortex, lack of resistance as the pin passes through the pneumatized medullary cavity, and increased resistance again when the trocar strikes the opposite cortex. Gentle downward pressure is applied to the pin while threading continues. Two to three full rotations of the chuck after an increase in resistance has been felt is enough to seat the pin in the opposite cortex. Angular deflections of the pin chuck parallel to the long axis should now result in the entire bone fragment moving in concert. If gross movement of the bone is not detected, it means that only one cortex has been engaged. After placement of the ESF pins, the exteriorized portion of the IM pin is bent at 90° and the elements are bonded together with a bar and clamps or with an acrylic bar as in other applications.

The Application of a Tie-In Fixator to a Diaphyseal Femoral Fracture
(Figures 8-3A-D)

Step 1

After exposure and gentle elevation of the proximal fragment, the IM pin, selected to fill approximately 70% of the marrow cavity, is inserted at the fracture site **(Figure 8-3A)**. (Images 8-3A-D by Frank Taylor).

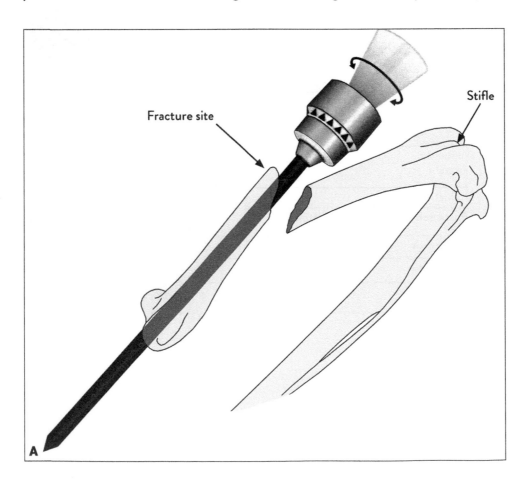

Step 2

The fracture is reduced, and the pin driven and seated in the distal fragment. Locations for placing the two K-wires are indicated (arrows) **(Figure 8-3B)**.

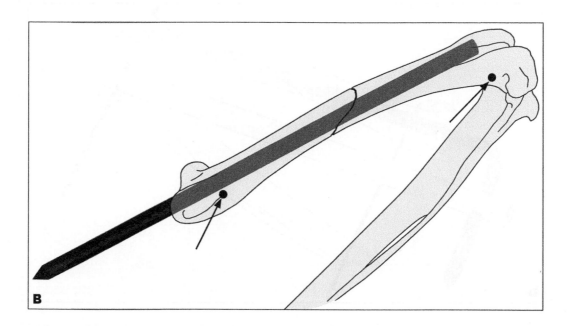

Step 3

The most distal pin is placed first and is driven through the condyles. Since it does not share the bone marrow space with the IM pin, it can be a stout pin (e.g., 0.062 inch [1.6 mm]) in a 1-kg patient. The proximal pin is placed parallel to the distal one and, because it shares the bone marrow space with the IM pin, it must be smaller than the first **(Figure 8-3C)**.

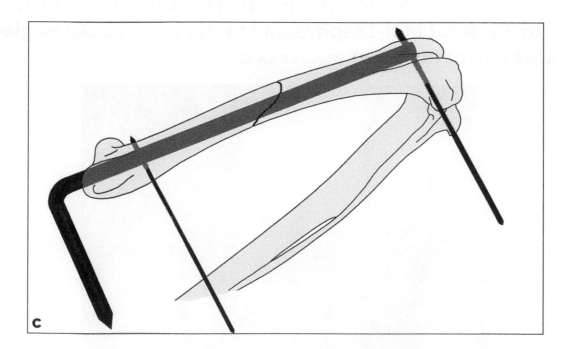

Step 4:

The IM pin is bent 90°, rotated to be in alignment with the ESF pins and an acrylic connecting bar is attached **(Figure 8-3D)**. The protruding pins are trimmed flush with the acrylic bar upon completion.

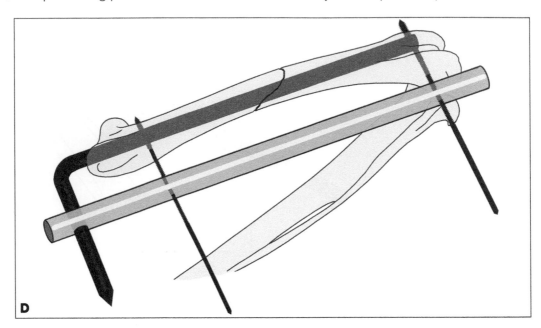

Fractures occurring in the very proximal femur or the femoral neck, where there is insufficient bone length to anchor an ESF pin may be amenable to femoral head ostectomy as a salvage procedure (Burgdorf-Moisuk et al 2011, Ackermann and Redig 1995). The long-term efficacy of this procedure, especially in animals intended for release to the wild, has not been determined. Distal fractures of the femur may be managed with cross-pin tie-in fixators using a procedure similar to the one used for the distal humerus.

Case 1. Radiographic Series Illustrating the Application of Tie-In Fixators to Bilateral Mid-Diaphyseal Fractures in a Bald Eagle (*Haliaeetus leucocephalus*): (Figures 8-4A-E).

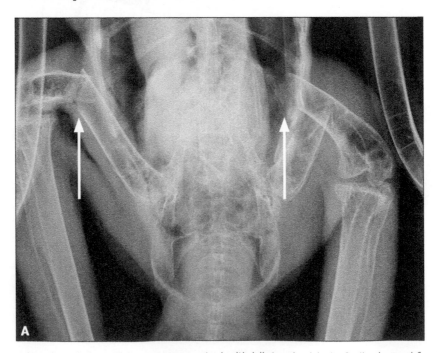

Figure 8-4A. Admission ventro-dorsal view. This case presented with bilateral mid-shaft diaphyseal fractures. *Arrows* indicate locations of the fractures.

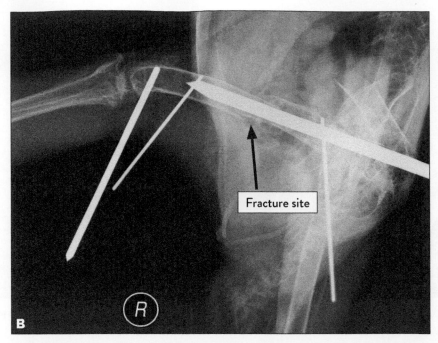

Figure 8-4B. Intra-operative radiograph showing pin placement in the left femur. A 3/16-inch (4.8-mm) diameter IM pin was introduced at the fracture site and driven retrograde; after reduction of the fracture, it was driven partway into the distal fragment. A transcondylar 1/8-inch (3.2-mm) diameter ESF pin was placed followed by two 3/32-inch (2.4-mm) diameter ESF pins on either side of the fracture *(arrow)*. Following placement of the ESF pins, the IM pin was driven further into the distal fragment and the opposite end was bent at 90 degrees. An acrylic bar of 0.75-inch (18-mm) diameter (not yet placed when this radiograph was taken) was used to bond the pins together.

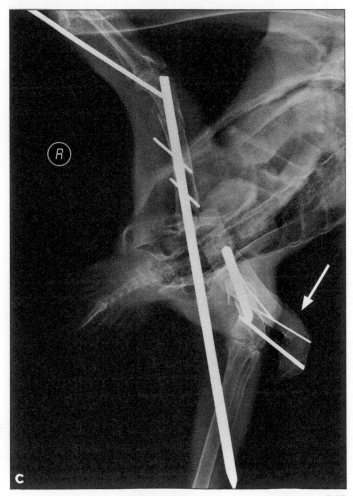

Figure 8-4C. Intra-operative image of the right leg. The placement of the IM pin and the ESF pins proceeded as for the left leg. Note that the distal end of the IM pin was blunted to allow deeper seating of the full pin without risk of penetrating the end of the femur with a sharp trocar. Acrylic bar *(arrow)* has been attached to fixator pins on the left leg.

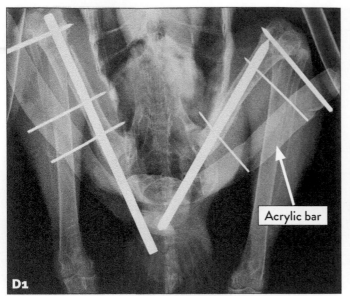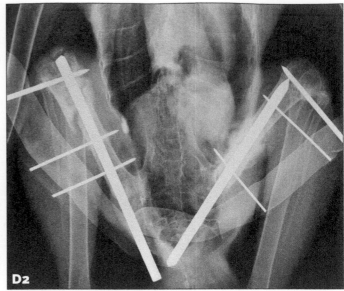

Acrylic bar

Figure 8-4D1, 2. These VD radiographs were taken at days 10 **(D1)** and 25 **(D2)**. Note the large increase in callus formation between the two dates. The fixation hardware was removed from both legs on day 32.

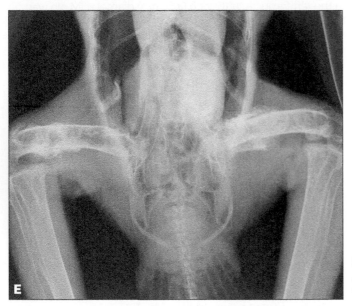

Figure 8-4E. This ventro-dorsal radiograph was taken on day 48 post-operatively. Fracture healing is complete; patient had full use of both limbs and was subsequently released.

Case 2. A Proximal Femoral Fracture in a Broad-winged Hawk (*Buteo platypterus*) with a Short Proximal Fragment:
(Figures 8-5A-E).

Owing to a short proximal fragment, no ESF pin was placed proximally. The Tie-in did not provide rotational stabilization, and the distal ESF pin served as a retainer for the IM pin. Careful post-operative management and the relatively quiet disposition of the patient aided the healing process given the instability of the fixation.

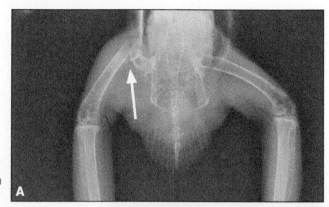

Figure 8-5A. This was the ventro-dorsal radiograph taken at admission. The *arrow* indicates the site of the fracture.

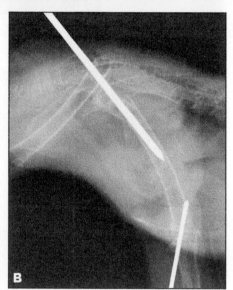

Figure 8-5B. This is an intra-operative radiograph showing the placement of the distal 0.045-inch (1.1-mm) diameter ESF pin proximal to the condyles and partial insertion of the 0.062-inch (1.6-mm) diameter IM pin that was inserted at the fracture site and retrograded at the hip. Following fracture reduction, the IM pin was driven distad into the distal fragment. After this radiograph was taken, it was further driven to a point where it lodged against the ESF pin. Owing to the shortness of the proximal fragment, an ESF pin was not placed in that fragment. Rotational stability was not well attained, necessitating restricted movement of the bird in the immediate post-operative period.

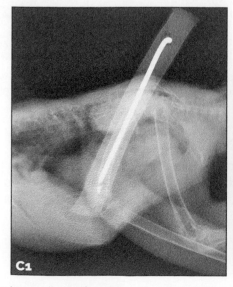

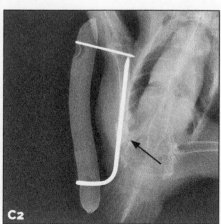

Figure 8-5C1,2. These two radiographs were taken at 7 days post-operatively. Lateral view **(C1)** and a ventro-dorsal view with extended leg **(C2)**. Callus formation is evident in the latter *(arrow)*.

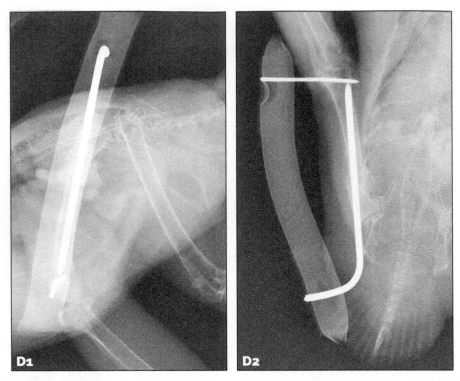

Figure 8-5D1, 2. 27 days post-operatively. Lateral **(D1)** and ventro-dorsal views with extended leg **(D2)**. Bridging callus is evident. Its size is indicative of instability.

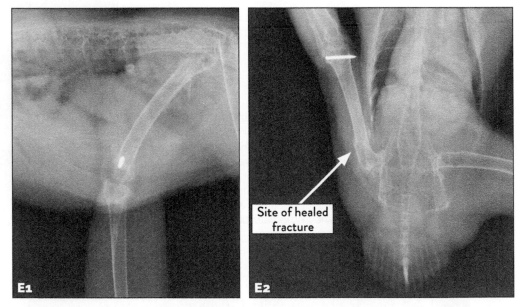

Figure 8-5E1, 2. These radiographs were taken at 37 days post-operatively. Lateral **(E1)** and ventro-dorsal with extended leg **(E2)** views. The fracture is healed, and the fixation hardware removed. The ESF pin had broken and was irretrievable. The patient had normal use of its leg.

Distal (Subcondylar) Femoral Fractures

In these fractures, the distal fragment is within two bone diameters of the joint and too short to gain purchase with an intramedullary pin. The cross-pinning method detailed in the following series of radiographs is an effective modification to the hybrid fixator for this type of fracture. It is similar to the method presented previously for such fractures of the humerus.

Case 3. Radiographic Series in a Golden Eagle (*Aquila chrysaetos*):
(Figures 8-6A-F)

The patient sustained a fracture of the distal femur as well as the ipsilateral ulna in a car collision. Owing to the location of the fracture, conventional tie-in fixation was unsuitable. A cross-pin method was used instead.

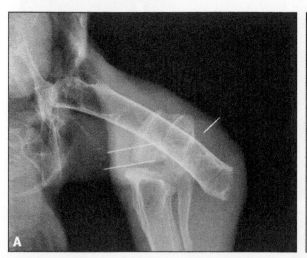
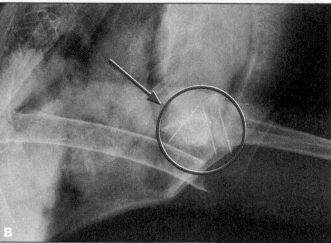

Figure 8-6A. Admission: Ventro-dorsal view of a golden eagle (*Aquila chrysaetos*) with a distal, subcondylar, transverse fracture of the femur. There was severe displacement of the bone fragments. There was insufficient length to the distal fragment to gain purchase with an IM pin. Cross-pinning provided a means of satisfactory fixation.

Figure 8-6B. Pre-operative lateral view – small needles were placed in the skin as external markers for locating sites on bone for insertion of ESF pins. Landmark needles (3 in number, indicated by *yellow arrow*) can be seen.

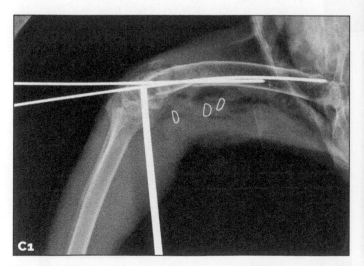
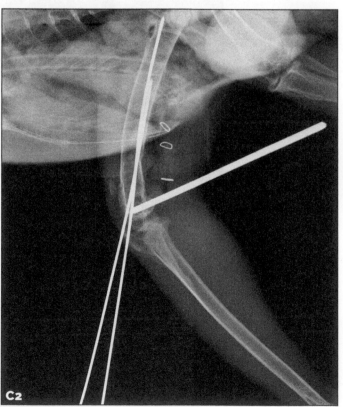

Figure 8-6C1, 2. Intra-operative dorso-ventral **(C1)** and lateral **(C2)** views. These images were taken at a point where a 1/8-inch (3.2-mm) diameter threaded ESF pins had been driven transversely through the condyles, lateral to medial and the two 0.062-inch (1.6-mm) diameter K-wire intramedullary pins had been retrograded in a crossing-fashion in the distal fragment. The fracture was reduced using the transverse ESF pin as a lever to manipulate the overriding distal fragment, at which point, the K-wires were advanced partially into the proximal fragment. Radiographically, alignment and pin placement were deemed satisfactory and the K-wires were subsequently advanced fully into the proximal fragment. Skin staples were used to close the incision made for insertion of the IM pins. Two 3/32-inch (2.4-mm) diameter Steinman pins were used as ESF pins and placed in the proximal fragment **(D1)**.

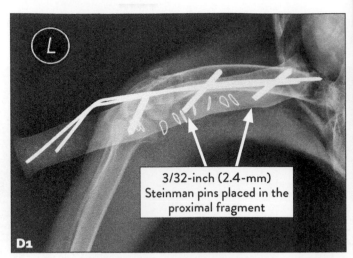

3/32-inch (2.4-mm) Steinman pins placed in the proximal fragment

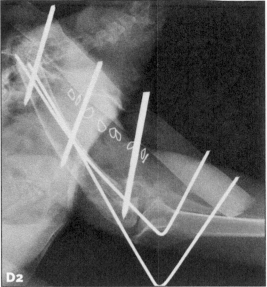

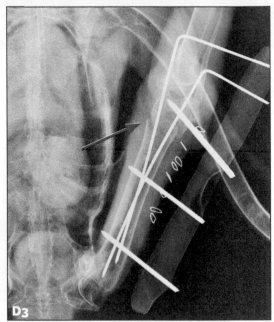

Figure 8-6D1-3. Post-operative views: ventro-dorsal (top), lateral (middle), and ventro-dorsal with extended leg (lower). In these views, two 3/32-inch (2.4-mm) diameter threaded ESF pins can be seen in the proximal fragment. The K-wires have been bent at 90 degrees and incorporated into the acrylic bar that ties the elements of the hybrid fixator together.

Figure 8-6D2. Post-operative lateral radiograph of the distal femoral fracture.

Figure 8-6D3. Post-operative ventro-dorsal view with extended leg. Note location of pins relative to the fracture site *(arrow)*.

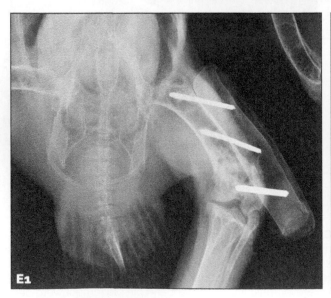

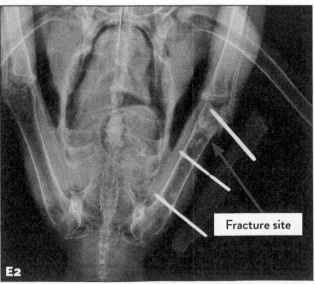

Fracture site

Figure 8-6E1, 2. Cranio-caudal-oblique view **(E1)** and ventro-dorsal view with extended leg **(E2)** taken 46 days post-operatively. The fracture is well healed and stable. The IM pin was removed. The external fixator components were left in place to provide support for another two weeks.

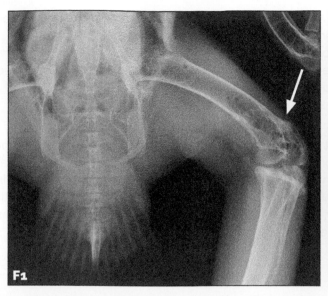
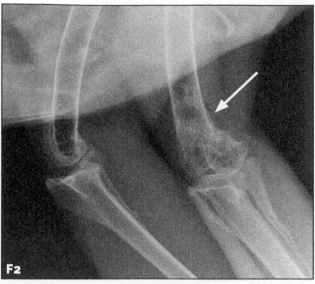

Figure 8-6F1, 2. These radiographs were taken a year post-operatively after the eagle had molted a new set of feathers and was ready for release. Ventro-dorsal **(F1)** and lateral **(F2)** views both show complete remodeling at the fracture *(arrows)*.

Stifle Dislocations and Luxations

Management Methods

Acute stifle dislocations may be repaired conservatively or surgically. With either, there is a high degree of ultimate failure owing to degenerative joint disease. Mild luxations may have reasonable expectations for a good outcome with conservative management following reduction. Attempts to reduce the injury should be conducted under anesthesia. Cage rest may be sufficient if the reduction is successful and stable (and the patient is of a mild temperament). Cage rest is facilitated by using a smooth-sided enclosure (e.g., a fish tank or large plastic container) so that the bird cannot climb or fly out for 2-3 weeks. Some authors have suggested the use of a spica-type splint (over the hip); however, there is insufficient case material available to recommend this approach. If at any point during an attempt at conservative management, the stifle continues to dislocate, surgical repair will likely be required.

Surgical Management of Stifle Dislocations

There is limited clinical experience with surgically managing luxations or dislocations of either the stifle or the hock (tibiotarsal-tarsometatarsal) joint (Rosenthal et al 1994; Jaffe et al 2000, Bowles and Zantop 2002) **(Figure 8-7)**.

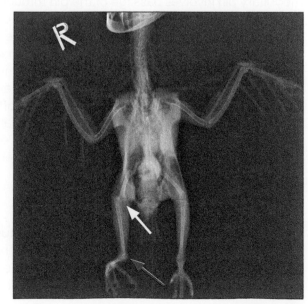

Figure 8-7. Blue-fronted Amazon parrot *(Amazona aestiva)* with a right stifle dislocation. The tibiotarsus commonly dislocates laterally and proximally *(white arrow)*. Note the chronic tibiotarsal-tarsometatarsal joint degeneration *(yellow arrow)*, that may have been related to the stifle dislocation.

A controlled study in pigeons (Villaverde et al 2005) showed that a monofilament polypropylene suture material could be passed caudal to the patellar tendon from lateral to medial, penetrate the proximal tibiotarsus or cnemial crest through a predrilled hole, and anchored to the lateral condyle of the femur using a cortical screw. The procedure is similar to an extracapsular method used in canines. In small birds, a tapered suture needle can be used to penetrate the tibiotarsus or cnemial crest. Non-absorbable braided poly blend suture (FiberWire®, Arthrex Inc, Naples, FL, USA) has also been used as the suture material in this procedure.

An adaptation of the previous method (Chinnadurai et al 2009) eliminates the use of the cortical screw and the suture is passed through a hole drilled in the femoral condyles **(Figure 8-8)**. Recently, experimentation with a hinged transarticular device in a pigeon model has been evaluated (Azmanis et al 2014). In most cases, the aim is stabilization of the joint long enough for scar tissue to form that will provide a modicum of long-term stability. Many factors determine the ultimate outcome; however, degenerative joint disease is not unexpected. No case material is presently available to further demonstrate the utility of this method.

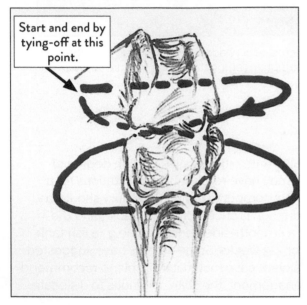

Start and end by tying-off at this point.

Figure 8-8. Illustration of the Chinnadurai method for stabilization of stifle luxations. Stout, nonabsorbable braided or monofilament suture is used. A small hole is drilled through the condyles from lateral to medial. The end of the suture is placed through this hole and brought back through the stifle joint passing caudal to the patellar tendon and exteriorized on the lateral side. Another hole is drilled in the proximal tibiotarsus and the suture passed through that hole exiting on the medial side. It is then passed back through the joint caudal to the patellar tendon, exiting laterally, where it is tied to the free end at the beginning of the suture

Methods of Fixation for Fractures of the Tibiotarsus
General Considerations
The tibiotarsus is a very straight bone with a narrow marrow cavity that tapers from proximal to distal, a crucial factor in selecting an intramedullary pin. The tibiotarsus is covered by joints at both ends and insertion of an intramedullary pin involves passage of the pin through the stifle joint. This joint is in acute flexion in a perched bird **(Figure 8-9)**. This, along with careful placement of the IM pin and restriction of movement of the patient post-operatively, mitigates the potential for joint damage. The proximal portion of the tibiotarsus is well protected by soft tissue, and the primary loads borne during normal use are compressive. Satisfactory orthopedic management of fractures of this limb mandates rotational alignment of the stifle and hock joints which is established when the fixation device is applied. In order to preserve integrity of the contralateral foot, immediate post-operative weight bearing is desirable, although injury to soft tissue often results in impaired use even though the fixation is capable of load bearing. Fractures in the proximal one third are most often transverse, thereby offering opportunities for load sharing. A tie-in fixator has proven effective in managing most fractures of this bone regardless of their location; however, other modes may be effective or required in selected cases.

Fractures of the Tibiotarsus
Among raptors held for falconry purposes, fractures of the tibiotarsus in the proximal one-third arising from bating (jumping at the end of their leash) accidents are seen frequently (Harcourt-Brown 1996), especially if the bird has been tethered with an elastic bungee cord in its leash. These are typically low-energy, transverse fractures. However, wild casualty birds most often have complicated and comminuted, high-energy fractures

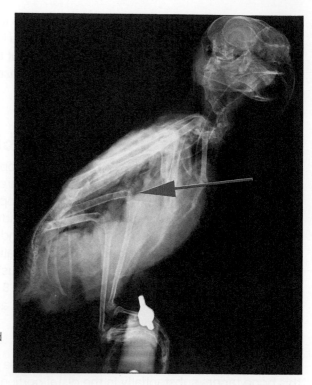

Figure 8-9. The joint of the perching bird, in this case an orange-winged Amazon *(Amazona amazonica)*, is in flexion (yellow arrow), helping to minimize joint damage that might result after insertion of an IM pin.

involving the tibiotarsus. Owing to the large muscle masses, especially in the proximal region, tibiotarsal fractures are seldom open and prognosis is good. Two caveats exist for wild casualty birds: 1) nerve damage often accompanies their fractures of the tibiotarsus resulting in a slow return to use of the lower limb, and 2) spinal injury often accompanies these fractures, but may be hard to detect at admission owing to the analgia in the broken limb. Failure to recognize this condition may lead to an unnecessary and unproductive fixation procedure. With any tibiotarsal fracture it is important to avoid using only an IM pin, as this cannot provide adequate rotational stability. A Type I ESF applied only to the lateral side has proven insufficiently robust.

Midshaft fractures of the tibiotarsus are not uncommon in companion birds. Many such fractures are due to leg entrapment involving toys, leg bands and/or cage material and the relatively low energy fractures are often transverse. Many small birds (< 100 g) and some juveniles of mid-sized species (< 300 g) with closed tibiotarsal fractures can be successfully tape splinted. Mal-union or non-union healing is a common complication with splints **(Figure 8-10)**. Improperly healed tibiotarsal fractures can lead to rotational deformities of the ipsilateral foot, uneven weight loading on the contralateral limb, ambulation abnormalities and ultimately, the lament that surgical repair was not undertaken in the first place.

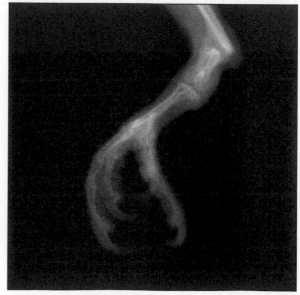

Figure 8-10. This is a radiograph of a Timneh grey parrot *(Psittacus timneh)* with a healed distal tibiotarsal malunion fracture resulting from attempted tape splint stabilization. For repair, the malunion was surgically broken down and bone ends rongeured back to fresh tissue. The new fracture was stabilized with a tie in fixator. It healed successfully; however, there was modest shortening of the leg.

While a Type II ESF has been reported by some to yield satisfactory results (Hess 1994, Bennett 1997, Harcourt-Brown 1996, Redig 2004), we have found, over a large number of cases, that the Tie-in fixator produces exceptional results. It is the method of choice in all but those cases involving severe comminution, wherein a Type II fixator may be an appropriate choice. In the case of very distal fractures, cross-pinning is recommended (Harcourt-Brown 1996).

Surgical Approach to the Tibiotarsus

Where exposure to guide IM pin placement or open reduction is necessary, the diaphysis of the tibiotarsus is approached from the medial aspect. Feathers are removed from the cranial, medial, and caudal aspect of the leg between the hock and the stifle and tape applied as necessary to control the remaining feathers. The skin is incised from a point proximal to the distal condyles and as far proximally as necessary to approach the area of the fracture **(Figure 8-11A)**. Near the distal end of the bone, the gastrocnemius separates from the cranial muscle groups, the fibularis longus and the tibialis cranialis **(Figure 8-11B)**. Incise the overlying fascia. Blunt dissection is used to separate the gastrocnemius from the cranial muscles, and extended proximally, periosteally elevating muscles from the bone **(Figure 8-11C)**. Closure is accomplished by loosely suturing the muscle bellies together along the length of the incision and closing the overlying fascia. Staples or cutaneous sutures are used to close the skin.

When selecting the IM pin, use the internal bone diameter measured at the distal end as a reference because this bone tapers substantially in the distal portion (Harcourt-Brown 1996). For closed application of the Tie-in to the tibiotarsus, in all cases, the IM pin is introduced to the tibial plateau. The approach is from the medial aspect of the femorotibial joint and the pin is driven normograde into the proximal fragment **(Figure 8-12A, B)** in the following manner. The pin is introduced under the skin along the medial edge of the patellar tendon. The trocar of the pin is worked underneath the tendon pushing the tendon laterally. The pin is aligned with the long axis of the tibiotarsus and advanced distally. The fracture is reduced and the pin advanced into the distal fragment.

If open reduction is necessary for reduction and alignment of fragments, after the IM pin is normograded to the level of the fracture, the tibiotarsus is approached from the medial side to allow visualization and manipulation of the fragments for alignment. Following reduction, the IM pin is advanced into the distal fragment to a point immediately proximal to the area of the supratendinal ridge. Threaded ESF pins are placed transversely, distally and proximally. The distal pin must be placed one to two bone diameters proximal to the tibiotarsal-tarsometatarsal joint in order to avoid injury to vessels and tendons at the end of the bone and should not be positioned distal to the supratendinal ridge. The proximal pin should be introduced on the cranio-lateral aspect of the tibiotarsus just distad to the tibial plateau and craniad to the fibula. It should be directed slightly caudo-medially to avoid neurovascular bundles on the medial side of the proximal tibiotarsus (Harcourt-Brown 2000). The IM pin is again bent at 90 degrees and directed laterally so that it can be joined to the ESF pins with an acrylic bar or conventional fixator clamps and a bar **(Figure 8-12C, D)**. *Figures 8-12 A-D used with permission from Samour J, ed. Avian Medicine. 3rd ed. St. Louis: Elsevier; 2016. Figure 12-24(A-D).*

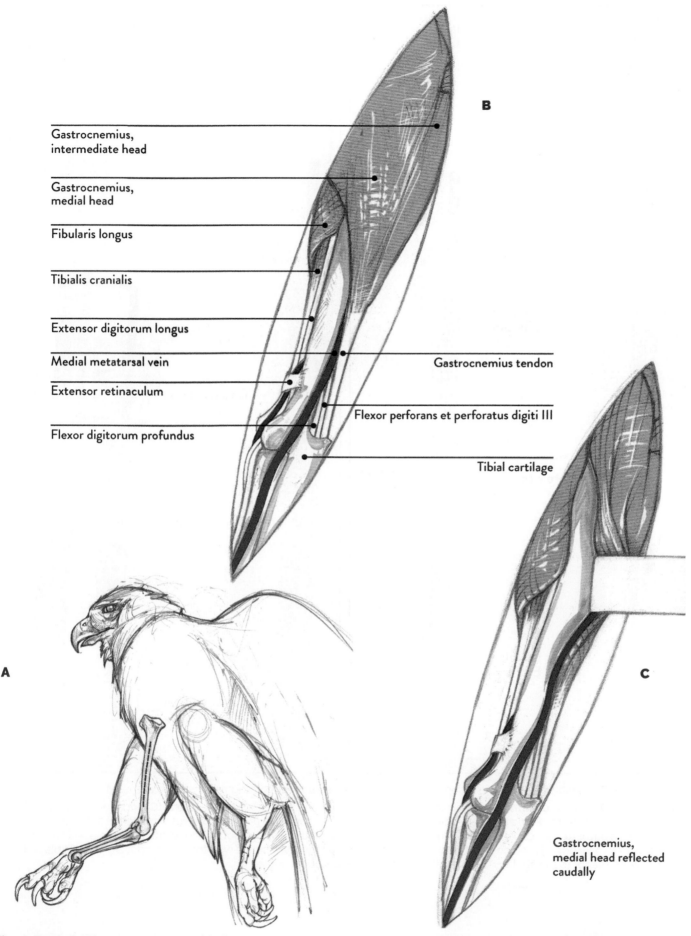

Gastrocnemius, intermediate head

Gastrocnemius, medial head

Fibularis longus

Tibialis cranialis

Extensor digitorum longus

Medial metatarsal vein

Extensor retinaculum

Flexor digitorum profundus

B

Gastrocnemius tendon

Flexor perforans et perforatus digiti III

Tibial cartilage

A

C

Gastrocnemius, medial head reflected caudally

Figure 8-11A-C. Where exposure to guide IM pin placement or open reduction is necessary, the diaphysis of the tibiotarsus is approached from the medial aspect.

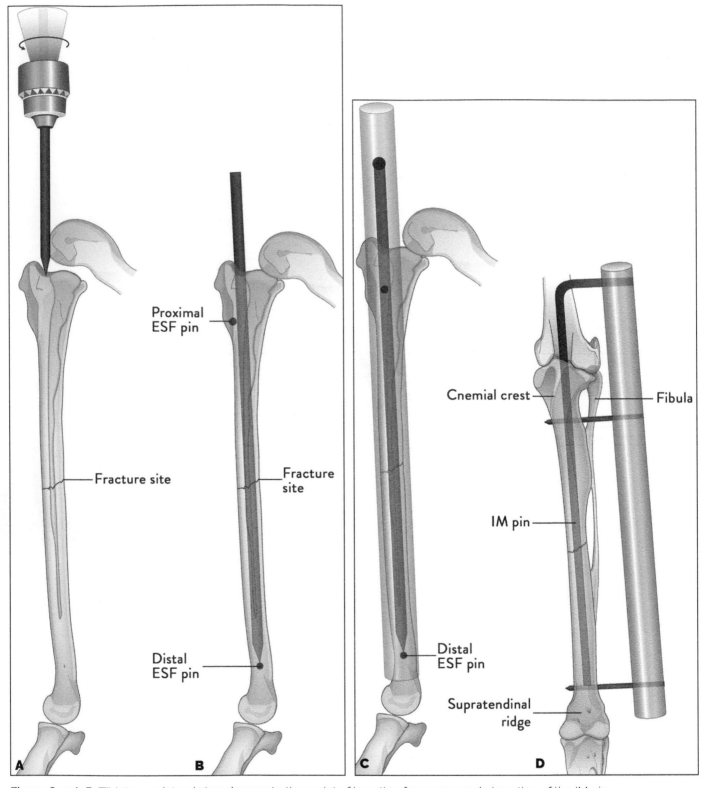

Figure 8-12A, B. Tibiotarsus: lateral view demonstrating point of insertion for normograde insertion of the IM pin.

Figure 8-12C, D. Method of normograde placement of an IM pin into the tibiotarsus bone. Lateral **(C)** and cranial-caudal **(D)** views of the hybrid fixator. Place the distal ESF pin either through the condyles of the tibiotarsus or proximal to the the supratendinal ridge and extensor canal. The proximal ESF pin must engage the diaphysis of the bone and not be placed too far anteriorly as to only engage the cnemial crest. It must share medullary cavity space with the intramedullary pin. It is placed immediately anterior to the fibula and driven at a slightly cranial to caudal angle.

Radiographic Presentation of Tibiotarsal Cases
Case 4. Bald Eagle *(Haliaeetus leucocephalus)*:
(Figures 8-13A-E)

This eagle sustained a mid-shaft fracture of the right tibiotarsal bone that was managed with a tie-in fixator.

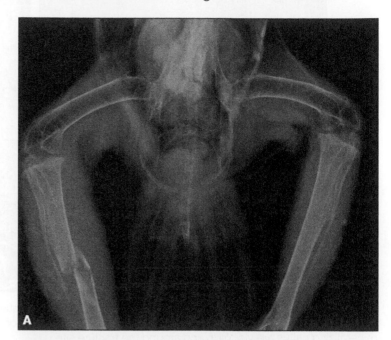

Figure 8-13A. This ventro-dorsal radiograph was taken at admission revealing the midshaft tibiotarsal fracture, partially misaligned and slightly comminuted.

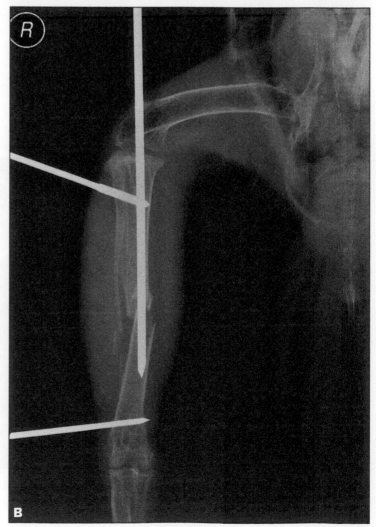

Figure 8-13B. Intra-operative radiograph taken to check alignment and pin locations. The IM pin was driven distally until it rested against the distal ESF pin. It was bent at 90 degrees to form the link for the hybrid fixator. In this case, 1/8-inch (3.2-mm) diameter positive profile pins were used for the ESF components and a 3/16- inch (4.8-mm) diameter Steinman pin was used for the intramedullary pin.

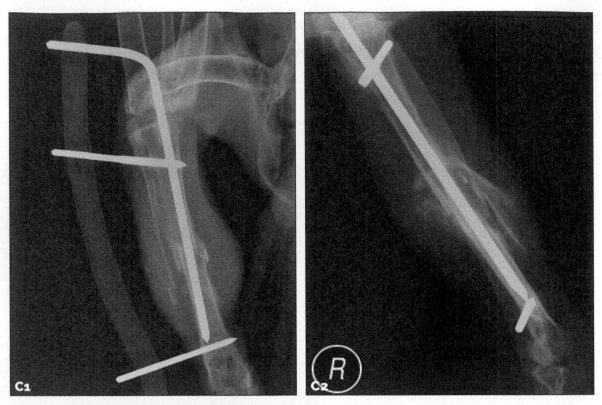

Figure 8-13C1, 2. These radiographs were taken 10 days post-operatively (cranial-caudal view **[C1]**) and 21 days post-operatively (lateral view **[C2)]**) to monitor healing status and integrity of the fixator. The fixator components are holding and both soft and mineralizing callus are visible in and around the fracture site.

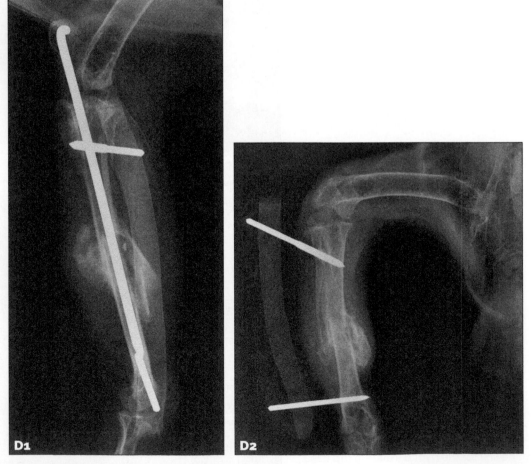

Figure 8-13D1, 2. These radiographs were taken 30 days post-operatively. The fixator was holding well and abundant, remodeling callus was present **(D1)**. The IM pin was removed to minimize potential for joint damage at the stifle **(D2)** The ESF pins were left in place for another 2 weeks to provide continuing support.

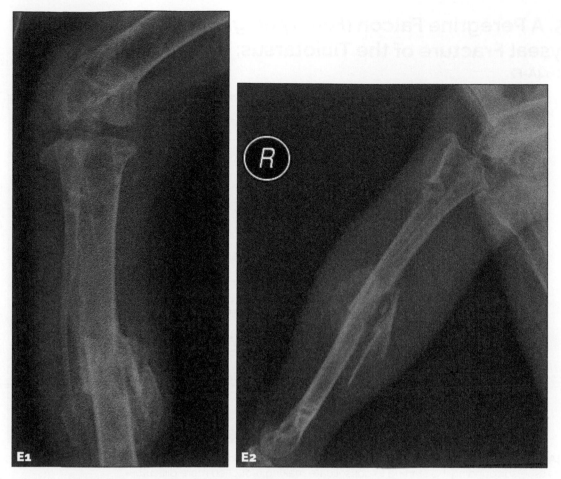

Figure 8-13E1, 2. These radiographs cranial-caudal oblique **(E1)** and medial-lateral **(E2)** were taken 47 days post-operatively. The fracture was well healed, and the comminuted fragments were incorporating into the callus. The eagle was full weight bearing and had normal use of the leg. Note the normal condition of stifle joint elements.

Case 5. A Peregrine Falcon *(Falco peregrinus)* with a Mid-Shaft Diaphyseal Fracture of the Tibiotarsus:

(Figures 8-14A-F)

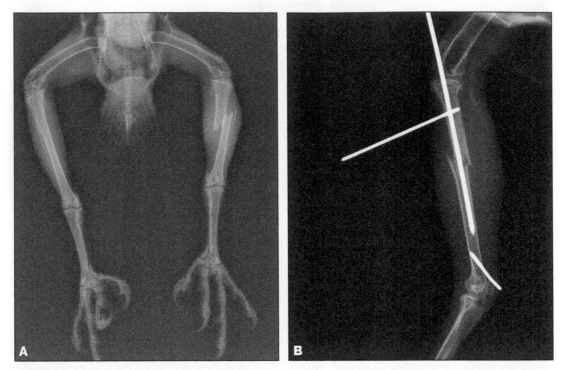

Figure 8-14A. The admission radiograph for the peregrine falcon *(Falco peregrinus)*. The fracture is nearly transverse, overriding, and the soft tissue surrounding it is starting to consolidate making reduction more difficult.

Figure 8-14B. Intra-operative x-ray. The 5/64-inch (2-mm) diameter IM pin was introduced at the stifle and normograded into the proximal fragment. The leg was bent back nearly 180 degrees at the fracture site and the bone ends were brought flush. The leg was straightened, leveraging one end against the other and forcing it to lengthen until longitudinally aligned. The IM pin was advanced into the distal fragment. The 0.062-inch (1.6-mm) diameter ESF pins were inserted, the IM pin advanced until seated, and the acrylic bar attached.

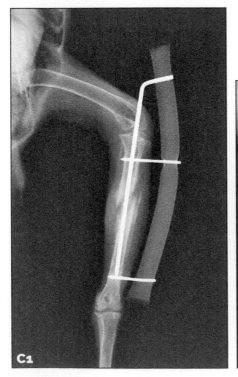
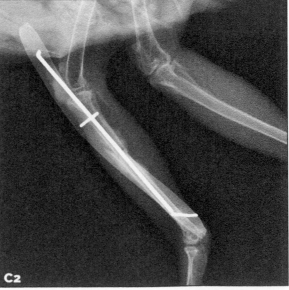

Figure 8-14C1, 2. These radiographs were taken 11-days post-operatively, and they include a cranial-caudal view **(C1)** and a medial-lateral view **(C2)**. The fixator is stable and there is cortical reaction but no bridging callus apparent at the fracture site.

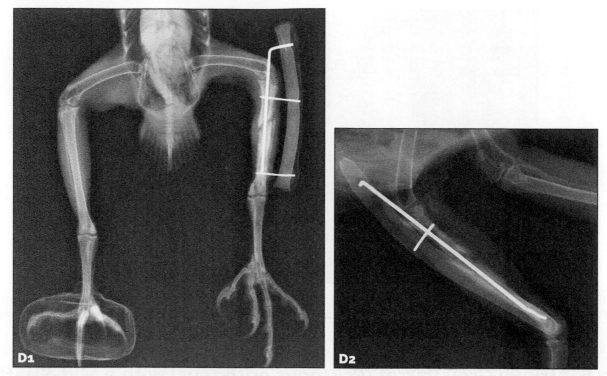

Figure 8-14D1, 2. These cranial-caudal **(D1)** and medial-lateral **(D2)** radiographs were taken 18 days post-operatively. There is a delayed union in process at this point. The fixator is holding well. Note the protective foam shoe on the opposite foot. All else is normal, there are no signs of infection, the foot is warm, so the best course of action was to give it more time.

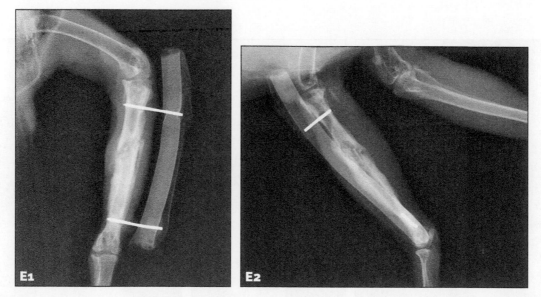

Figure 8-14E1, 2. At 28 days post-operatively, the IM pin has been removed. The external fixator was left in place for support for another week.

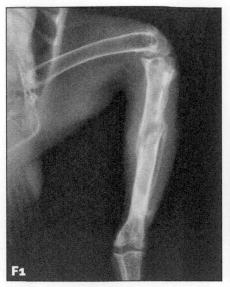
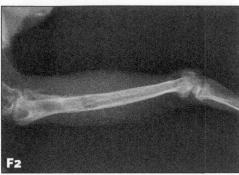

Figure 8-14F1, 2. These radiographs were taken 61 days post-operatively **(F1)** and just prior to release at 214 days post-operatively **(F2)**. The external skeletal fixator was removed at 34 days. The bird had full use of its leg by 42 days post-operatively. Release delayed owing to onset of molt.

Case 6. African Grey Parrot *(Psittacus erithacus)* with a Mid-Shaft Tibiotarsal Repair:

(Figures 8-5A-C)

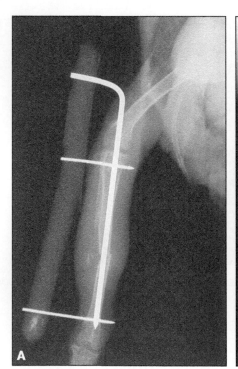
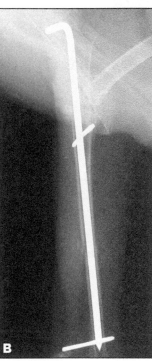
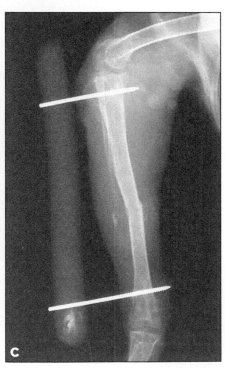

Figure 8-15A-C. These radiographs depict the repair of a midshaft tibiotarsal fracture in an African grey parrot *(Psittacus erithacus)* at post-operative periods of 1 week **(A)**, 2 weeks **(B)**, and 4 weeks **(C)**. A 5/64-inch (2.0-mm) diameter pin was used as the intramedullary pin and 0.045-inch (1.1-mm) diameter pins were used for the ESF components. A 3/8-inch (10-mm) diameter latex tube (Penrose drain) was used as the mold for the acrylic bar. The IM pin was removed at 18 days post-operatively. The remaining ESF elements were removed after the radiograph was taken at four weeks.

Case 7. Placement of a Tie-In Fixator in a Cockatiel *(Nymphicus hollandicus)*:

(Figures 8-16A-C)

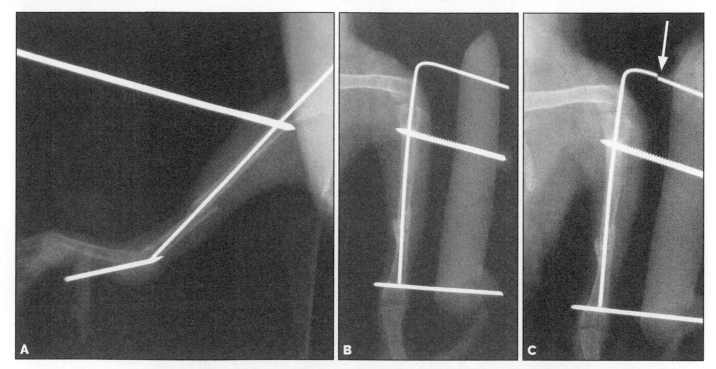

Figure 8-16A-C. This partial radiographic series displays the placement of a tie-in fixator on the tibiotarsus of a cockatiel *(Nymphicus hollandicus)*. The intra-operative image **(A)** shows the placement of the 1/6-inch (1.6-mm) diameter IM pin placed by closed reduction and normograde (from the tibiotarsal plateau) insertion and ESF pins (0.028-inch [0.7-mm] distally and 0.035-inch [0.9-mm] proximally) in place. The next image **(B)** was taken at 6 weeks post-operatively and shows modest callus formation. The acrylic bar was excessively large in this case. At 9 weeks post-operatively **(C)**, the callus was remodeling and the link between the IM pin and the ESF pins had been cut *(arrow)* to transfer more load to the leg. The entire apparatus was removed one week later. This fracture appeared to take an exceptionally long time to heal; however, in retrospect, the fracture was healed some time before the fixation was removed.

Case 8. Transarticular Fixator Applied to a Proximal Tibiotarsal Fracture in a Cooper's Hawk *(Accipiter cooperii)*:
(Figures 8-17A-C)

Proximal fractures of the tibiotarsus are not uncommon, but unlike fractures of the humerus and femur near a joint, these fractures are not amenable to cross-pinning and the proximal fragment is too short to accept a tie-in fixator. Transarticular fixators have been useful in managing these fractures.

This patient was a bird trained for and flown in falconry. It fractured its tibiotarsus in a tussle with a much larger pheasant that it had pursued, caught, and wrestled to the ground. *(Figures used with permission from Samour J, ed. Avian Medicine. 3rd ed. St. Louis: Elsevier; 2016. Figure 12-27 A, B, C)*

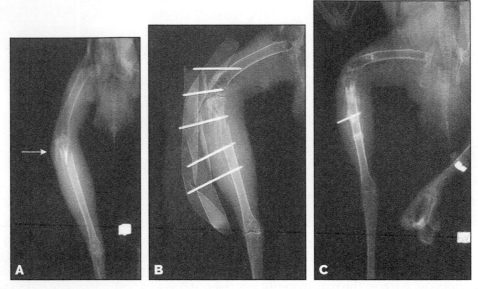

Figure 8-17A. Admission radiograph cranial-caudal view. The proximal fracture of the tibiotarsus and fibula is evident *(arrow)* in a Cooper's hawk *(Accipiter cooperii)*.

Figure 8-17B. A post-operative radiograph anterior-posterior oblique view. Two 0.045-inch (1.1-mm) diameter threaded pins were placed in the femur and three in the tibiotarsus, including one in the short proximal fragment: this created a Type I transarticular configuration. The stifle was partially flexed and an acrylic bar that followed the contour of that flexure was formed using a latex tube. The Cooper's hawk is relatively small (350 g), and the bar was not reinforced. Had it been a larger bird, a bar connecting the most proximal pin in the femur to the most distal pin in the tibiotarsus would have been needed (i.e., complete the triangle as shown in the metatarsal case involving the bald eagle (Case 12 below).

Figure 8-17C. A cranial-caudal-oblique radiograph taken 27 days post-operatively shows a fully healed fracture. One ESF pin was broken below the skin line and was irretrievable; 4 months was required for full return to function.

Alternate Approach with a Proximal Tibiotarsal Fracture in a Very Tractable Patient – Hybrid Falcon
Case 9. Cage Rest
(Figure 8-18A-C)

Cage rest is another management modality that may be useful. The patient was a young (12-week-old) imprinted hybrid falcon (gyrfalcon x peregrine falcon cross) that sustained a proximal transverse fracture of its tibiotarsus and fibula that was reasonably well-aligned. Surgical options in the form of a transarticular Type I Fixator were considered. However, consideration was given to the very calm demeanor of this bird, accustomed as it was to perch quietly with its head covered by a hood. It was placed in a large, front-opening cardboard box on a transverse perch covered with sisal rope. The hood was removed once a day for hand feeding. Within 3 weeks, the fracture was healed, and the bird was able to perch. It eventually acquired full use of the leg. Cage rest is another option for consideration when the nature of the fracture, the temperament of the patient, and the handling skills of the owner combine.

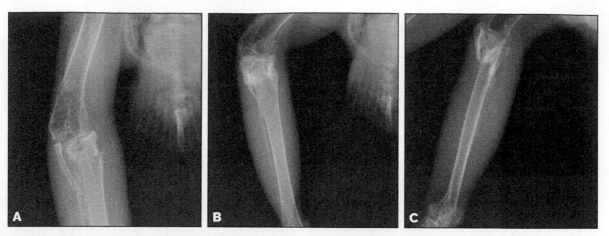

Figure 8-18A-C. These radiographs were taken of a 12-week-old imprinted hybrid falcon with a well-aligned proximal fracture of the proximal tibiotarsus and fibula **(15A)**. After 3 weeks of confinement and careful management, the fracture was healed and the bird had use of the leg (**B & C**, cranial-caudal and lateral, respectively).

Use of Coaptation to Manage a Distal Tibiotarsal Fracture in a Blue and Gold Macaw *(Ara ararauna)*

Distal, subcondylar tibiotarsal fractures are challenging to manage surgically. Owing to the blood vessels and tendons that traverse the area, placement of pins runs a high risk of iatrogenic injury. This is one of the few instances where coaptation with a modified Schroeder-Thomas splint is useful.

Case 10. Blue and Gold Macaw *(Ara ararauna)*:
(Figures 8-19A-E)

This case involved a blue and gold macaw *(Ara ararauna)* whose leg had been entangled and fractured in the ensuing struggle to free itself. The parrot was presented for treatment within hours of the injury.

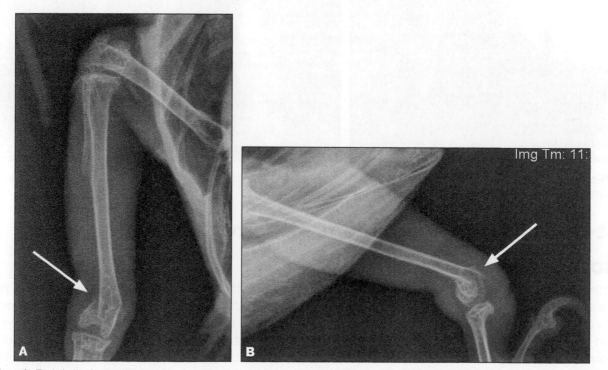

Figure 8-19A, B. Admission radiographs: cranial-caudal **(A)** and lateral **(B)**. *Arrows* indicate the location of the moderately displaced fracture in a blue and gold macaw *(Ara ararauna)*.

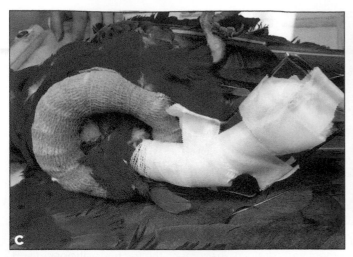
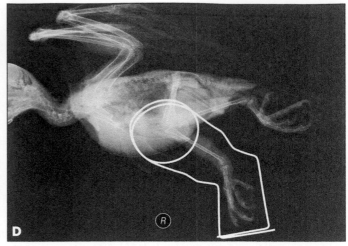

Figure 8-19C, D. The fracture was manually reduced **(C)**. For stabilization, a modified Schroeder-Thomas splint made from 3/32-inch (2.4-mm) soft wire was shaped and affixed to the leg such that it held it in a position compatible with perching on a flat surface. After radiographs to check positioning **(D)**, it was overwrapped with a layer of conforming adherent tape (Vetrap™, 3M, Maplewood, MN, USA).

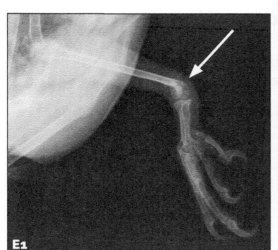
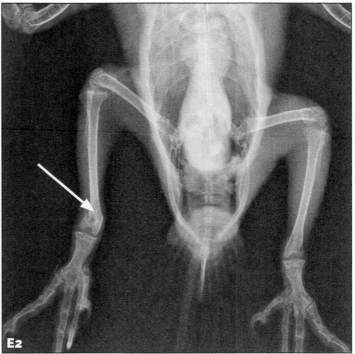

Figure 8-19E1, 2. Lateral **(E1)** and ventro-dorsal **(E2)** x-rays 4 weeks after application of the splint. The fracture has healed in normal anatomical alignment and the bird had full use of the leg.

Post-operative Management of Femoral and Tibiotarsal Fractures

Post-operatively, one should expect little or no weight-bearing on the affected leg for 3-5 days. General pain and transitory neuroparalysis arising either from the injury itself or the surgical procedure; "knuckling over" is common. It is important to wrap the digits of the affected limb with protective materials (e.g., Vetrap™) to prevent abrasion of the dorsal surfaces. Concurrently, the asymmetric weight bearing predisposes bumblefoot formation in the contralateral foot, so it too should be given protective bandaging. This may be as little as an interdigitating bandage or may require a polypropylene shoe. Other management methods may include keeping patients in smooth sided containers, so they can't attempt to climb (e.g., cardboard box, aquarium, animal incubator, fiberglass pet carrier), maintaining them in the dark to reduce activity, and bedding them in a deep layer of shredded paper that encourages them to rest in sternal recumbency. Physical therapy is of lesser concern than for wings; however, occasional passive range of motion movements should be applied during the healing period.

Methods of Stabilization and Fixation for Tarsometatarsal Fractures

General Considerations

Like the metacarpus, the tarsometatarsus has a paucity of soft tissue coverage and therefore many of the same management problems. Anatomically, it is quite different in that it has no marrow cavity in the proximal one-third in hawks and owls, while in falcons a marrow cavity runs the full length (Harcourt-Brown 2000). In cross-section, it is a "U"-shaped bone formed embryonically from the fusion of elements of the metatarsal and tarsal bones. The flexor tendons run in a channel on the plantar side of the bone **(Figure 20A)**; veins are present on the lateral and medial aspects and arterial blood supply along with nerves are found on the cranial aspect. The bone is protected by articular surfaces at both ends. In addition, the tarsometatarsal bone has an inconsistent internal structure that makes placing longitudinal pins impossible **(Figure 20B)**. These factors combine to render intra-medullary pinning a poor fixation choice. Additionally, when a bird is perching at rest, the bone is positioned at an angle to the perching surface, so load bearing applies bending forces as well as rotational forces to the bone.

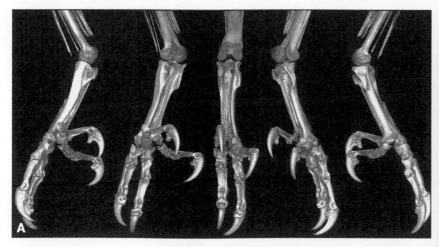

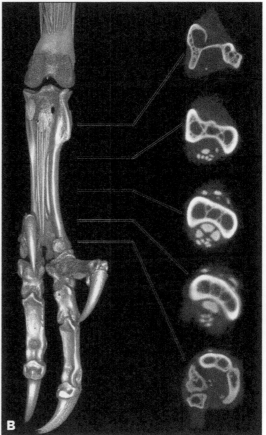

Figure 8-20A, B. Lower leg CT (100 μm) of the Great Horned Owl *(Bubo virginianus)*. The focus is placed on the plantar aspect of the tarsometatarsus **(A)**. The lower leg is rotated at 45° angles. From left to right: medial, medial-plantar, plantar, lateral-plantar and lateral **(B)**. Cross-sectional images of the tarsometatarsus *(right)* and their respective position on the plantar view *(left)*. The unusual and inconsistent shape of the tarsometatarsal bone makes placing longitudinal pins impossible.

Fixation Choices

Fixation choices for tarsometatarsal fractures range from limited use of coaptation (tape splints, Schroeder-Thomas), Type II ESF and variations on that theme, and transarticular-reinforced Type II constructs.

Tape Splint

This splint has limited use in very small birds - < 50 grams. It has long been included in the list of recommendations and was originally referred to as the Altman Tape Splint – a call back to the 1960s. While useful in some cases, it fails to meet the essential requirement of coaptation – that of immobilizing the joints proximal and distal to the fracture site *(See Chapter 4)*.

The Type II ESF is applicable in a wide variety of situations and is the method of choice in any situation where there is comminution or there are open wounds that require management; Type I ESFs are not sufficiently strong and will often fail before a fracture heals. Owing to the bending loads applied to this bone, it is recommended to place, if possible, three pins rather than only two on either side of the fracture site. One author was successful in the use of a locking compression plate in a Bald Eagle *(Haliaeetus leucocephalus)* (Montgomery et al 2011) demonstrating a novel method of fixation in larger birds. Regardless of what is used, care must be taken not to pass the pins through the flexor channel on the plantar side of the tarsometatarsal bone.

Radiographic Series of Cases for Tarsometatarsal Fractures
Case 11. Type II Fixation of an Oblique Fracture of the Tarsometatarsal Bone in a Broad-winged Hawk *(Buteo platypterus)*:
(Figures 8-21A-D)

Such a fracture is unstable and has no potential for load sharing during healing. Experience in treating such fractures with coaptation has been unrewarding, leaving surgical fixation as the next best option. As the tarsometatarsus had no medullary cavity in which an IM pin can be placed, a Type II fixator was the best option. Use of at least one center-threaded pin in the construct greatly increased the strength and durability of the fixator.

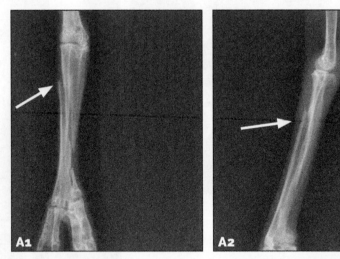

Figure 8-21A1, 2. These cranial-caudal **(A1)** and lateral **(A2)** radiographs taken at admission reveal a long oblique fracture of the tarsometatarsus that was minimally displaced *(arrow)* in a broad-winged Hawk *(Buteo platypterus)*.

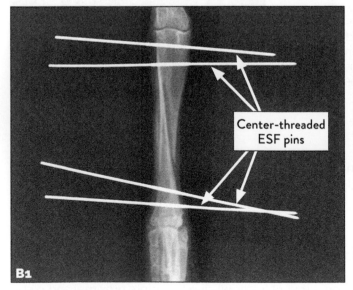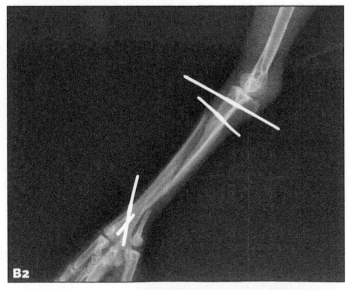

Figure 8-21B1, 2. Radiographs cranial-caudal view **(B1)** and lateral **(B2)** taken intra-operatively. The ESF pins (0.045-inch [1.1-mm] diameter) were placed at sites most proximal and distal owing to the long oblique nature of the fracture. Center-threaded pins were used to improve the purchase with the bone.

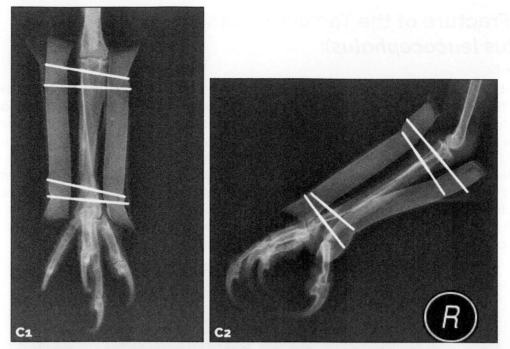

Figure 8-21C1, 2. Cranial-caudal view **(C1)** and medial-lateral **(C2)** radiographs taken 37 days post-operatively. Note acrylic connecting bars placed laterally and medially. Fracture healing was nearly complete with little evidence of excess callus formation.

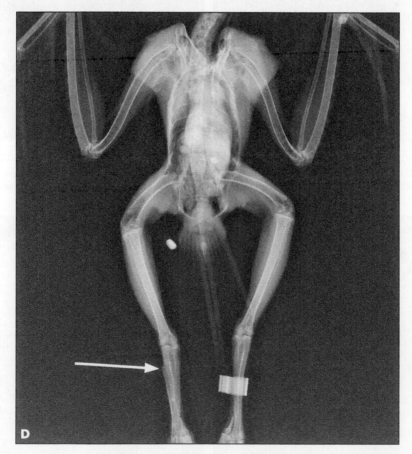

Figure 8-21D. This pre-release radiograph was taken 7 months post-operatively; the arrow indicates the site of the original fracture. The patient was retained for the winter as this species migrates to South America returning to Minnesota in April of each year. A U.S. Fish and Wildlife Bird Banding Laboratory band was attached to the left leg.

Case 12. Fracture of the Tarsometatarsus in a Bald Eagle (*Haliaeetus leucocephalus*):

(Figures 8-22A-F)

A second-year bald eagle *(Haliaeetus leucocephalus)* sustained a fracture of the proximal tarsometatarsus in a collision with a moving vehicle. The significant factors in fixation selection for this case included: 1) no medullary cavity in which to insert an IM pin, 2) short proximal fragment that limited fixation device attachment, 3) weight of the patient (> 5 kg), 4) closed, transverse, well-aligned fracture, with no capacity for load-sharing giving the angular relationship of the hock joint, and, 5) an anticipated prolonged healing time. A type II fixator, transarticular fixator, using center-threaded 1/8-inch (3.2-mm) diameter IM pins, along with conventional Steinmann pins was applied. The hock was flexed to approximate the normal perching position. One-half inch (15-mm) diameter acrylic bars were placed on the medial and lateral sides of the leg. In addition, another bar, extending from the most proximal to the most distal pins on the lateral side, constituting the base of a triangle, was applied in order to establish structural strength to the construct.

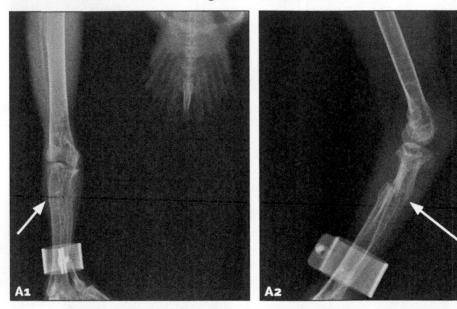

Figure 8-22A1, 2. These cranial-caudal oblique **(A1)** and medial-lateral **(A2)** radiographs were taken at admission. Evident in both projections is a well-aligned, unstable, transverse fracture of the proximal tarsometatarsal bone *(arrows)* in a bald eagle *(Haliaeetus leucocephalus)*. Figures used with permission from Samour J, ed. *Avian Medicine.* 3rd ed. St. Louis: Elsevier; 2016. Figure 12-31.

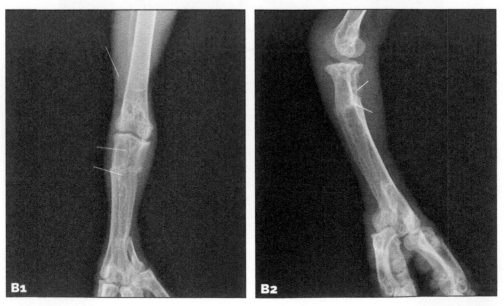

Figure 8-22B1, 2. Pre-operative radiographs: cranial-caudal oblique **(B1)** and lateral **(B2)**. 25-gauge hypodermic needles were placed in the skin as landmarks to aid accurate placement of the ESF pins, particularly in the proximal fragment where precise placement of the ESF pin was critical.

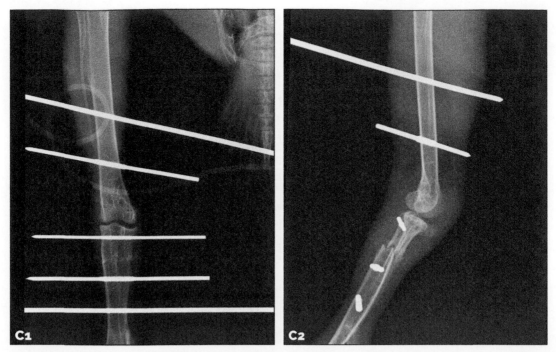

Figure 8-22C1, 2. This intra-operative radiograph (cranial-caudal **[C1]**) and medial-lateral **[C2]**) shows placement of the ESF pins in a transarticular arrangement to impart enough strength to the overall construct. Note the center threaded pins in the tibiotarsus and the tarsometatarsus. Pin sizes ranged between 3/32-inch (2.4-mm) diameter and 1/8-inch (3.2-mm) diameter. The alignment of the fracture fragments has been maintained. These pins were placed with a hand chuck and there was no pre-drilling of holes.

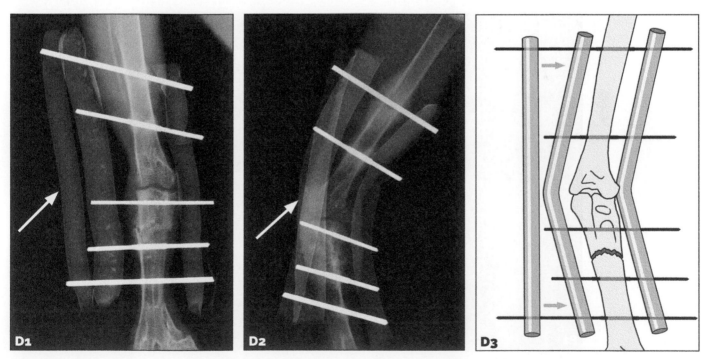

Figure 8-22D1-3. These cranial-caudal **(D1)** and lateral **(D2)** radiographs were taken 11 and 21 days post-operatively and show locations of fixator bars. Note the extra connector bar *(arrows)* attached on the lateral side between the most proximal and most distal ESF pins to add configurational strength (i.e., triangle) to the construct. The arrangement of the acrylic fixator bars is shown in **8-22D3**. Line drawing by Frank Taylor.

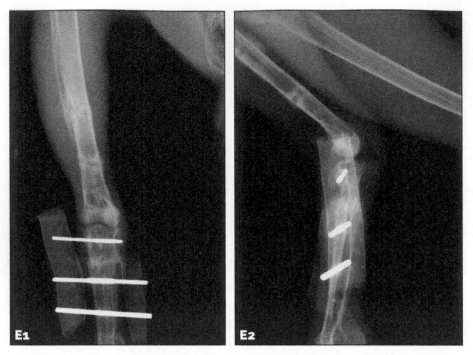

Figure 8-22E1, 2. Cranial-caudal **(E1)** and lateral **(E2)** x-rays 47 days post-operatively. The fracture has healed, and the fixator deconstructed in stages, beginning at day 28, as the patient began to show signs of weight-bearing on the limb.

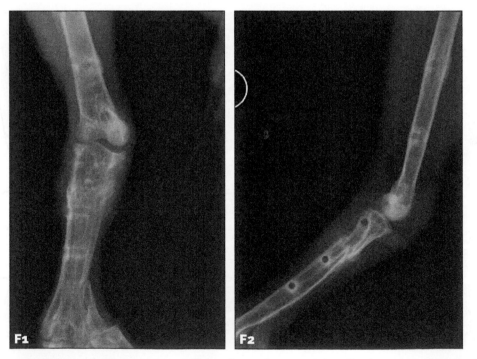

Figure 8-22F1, 2. These cranial-caudal **(F1)** and lateral **(F2)** radiographs were taken 60 days post-operatively. All fixation was removed, the fracture was healed and remodeled. The eagle was full weight bearing. It was released to the wild with a radio transmitter that allowed tracking. It ranged throughout Minnesota and Southern Ontario and back to its natal site in Oklahoma over a two-and-a half-year period before being struck by a car and killed in Iowa.

Recommended Reading

1. Ackermann J, Redig PT. Surgical repair of elbow luxation in raptors. *J Avian Med Surg.* 1997;11(4):247-254.

2. Azmanis PN, Voss K, Hatt J-M. Evaluation of short-term outcomes of experimental stifle luxation in feral pigeons *(Columba livia domestica)* treated with a hinged transarticular external skeletal fixator and physical therapy. *Int J Appl Res Vet Med J Applied Res Vet Med.* 2014;12(2):160-167.

3. Bennett RA. Orthopedic surgery. In: Altman RB, Clubb SL, Dorrestein GM, Quesenberry K, eds. *Avian Medicine and Surgery.* Philadelphia: WB Saunders; 1997:733-766.

4. Bowles HL, Zantop DW. A novel surgical technique for luxation repair of the femorotibial joint in a monk parakeet *(Myiopsitta monachus). J Avian Med Surg.* 2002; 16:34–38.

5. Burgdorf-Moisuk A, Whittington JK, Bennett RA, et al. Successful management of simple fractures of the femoral neck with femoral head and neck excision arthroplasty in two free-living avian species. *J Avian Med Surg.* 2011;25(3):210-215.

6. Chinnadurai SK, Spodnick G, Degernes L, et al. Use of an extracapsular stabilization technique to repair cruciate ligament ruptures in two avian species. *J Avian Med Surg.* 2009;23(4):307-313.

7. Harcourt-Brown NH. Foot and leg problems. In: Benyon PH, Forbes NA, Harcourt-Brown NH, eds. *Manual of Raptors, Pigeons and Waterfowl.* Cheltenham: BSAVA; 1996:163-167.

8. Harcourt-Brown NH: Birds of Prey: Anatomy, Radiology, and Clinical Conditions of the Pelvic Limb (CD-ROM). Lake Worth, FL, Zoological Education Network, 2000

9. Hess R. Management of orthopedic problems of the avian pelvic limb. *Semin Avian Exotic Pet Med.* 1994;3(2):63-72.

10. Jaffe MH, Fitch R, Tully T. Medial release and extracapsular stabilization in a 7-month old blue and gold macaw *(Ara ararauna)* with a grade IV medial patella luxation. *Proc Annu Conf Assoc Avian Vet.* 2000;101-104.

11. Montgomery RD, Crandall E, Bellah JR. Use of a locking compression plate as an external fixator for repair of a tarsometatarsal fracture in a bald eagle *(Haliaeetus leucocephalus). J Avian Med Surg.* 2011;25(2):119+.

12. Ponder JB, Redig P. Orthopedics. In: Speer BL, ed. Current Therapy in Avian Medicine and Surgery. St Louis: Elsevier; 2016: 657-667.

13. Redig P. Fractures. In: Samour J. ed. *Avian Medicine.* St. Louis; Mosby; 2000:131-169.

14. Rosenthal K, Hillyer E, Mathiessen D. Stifle luxation repair in a moluccan cockatoo and a barn owl. *J Assoc Avian Vet.* 1994;8(4):173-178.

15. Villaverde S, de la Vibora B, Gonzales R, et al. Management of the femorotibial luxation by coaptation splinting, intramedullary pins, external skeletal fixator and tension bands; a pilot study in domestic pigeons *(Columba livia domestica).* In: Proc 8th Eur Assoc Avian Vet/6th Scientific ECAMS meeting Arles, France. 2005;196-202.

16. Zsivanovits P. Repair techniques in case of intertarsal joint luxation: two case reports. *EAAV Proceedings.* 2011;58.

Post-operative Management of the Orthopedic Patient

Introduction

The success of the orthopedic procedure is ultimately determined by care in the ensuing post-operative period. There are six factors that require attention:

- Surgical wound management
- Active promotion of joint and limb movement
- Active management of soft tissue integrity and healing
- Alertness to and management of damage arising from post-op bandaging; minimize length of time such bandaging is used
- Prevention of collateral injury to other limb components, especially contralateral bumblefoot when dealing with leg fractures
- Monitoring and actively ensuring fixator integrity

General Considerations with Emphasis on the Pectoral Limb

Pain management through proper use of medications such as NSAIDS and the various opioids commonly used in avian medicine (tramadol, torbugesic, and buprenorphine), and dynamization of the fixator as bone healing progresses are important adjuncts to promote patient comfort, health and optimization of the recovery process. Wound management and bandage changes in the immediate post-operative period, allowing sufficient time for the patient to stabilize following prolonged anesthesia and sedation periods, and hospitalization for 48 hours are highly recommended.

The Immediate Post-operative Period; 24-48 Hours

Within the first 12 – 24 hours post-operatively, the patient should be anesthetized, bandages removed, and the surgical wound attended to. The pin tracts will have encrusted plasma and blood that seals the wound and prevents drainage. These should be gently loosened and removed with a cotton-tipped applicator soaked in chlorhexidine. Apply a small amount of triple antibiotic at these sites and replace the bandages, ensuring that there is non-adherent, absorbent dressing material in proximity to the wounds. The limb, especially if the procedure has involved the humerus or the radius/ulna, should be subjected to very gentle passive range of motion (PROM) movement. This can be painful, hence the need for anesthesia and pain management. A few small excursions to the limits of what the combined skeletal and soft tissue elements permit is sufficient.

In the second 24-hour post-operative period, check the bandages for strike-through, the appearance of blood or fluids on the outer surface, and change them if necessary. Fractious patients will require anesthesia or sedation to prevent uncontrolled limb movements that would endanger the fixation. Wing injuries involving the humerus and radius/ulna with adequate, robust fixation, will not need additional coaptation to stabilize the wing beyond this point. Metacarpal fracture patients will require additional coaptation for most of the healing period to prevent wing-flapping from dislodging the fixator. In the case of humerus and radius/ulna injuries, bandaging is restricted to that necessary to contain wound dressing materials. Assess the patient's weight, hydration and overall condition and consider discharge with appropriate instructions to the owner or care staff.

Passive Range of Motion Exercises – the Wing

Limb and soft tissue manipulation involve passive-range-of-motion (PROM) and stretch-and-hold procedures. In the former, the elbow and carpal joints are extended and flexed multiple times within the range of motion that the current soft tissue conditions permit. It is desirable to press the extension a slight amount each time to stretch the tissues. Stretch-and-hold involves extending the limb to slightly beyond the retarding pull of the soft tissues and holding it for 10-15 seconds, then releasing it. In practice, PROM and stretch-and-hold are alternated with each other **(Figure 9-1A-C)**. In the beginning, there may only be 20-30 degrees of extension of the humerus – this will loosen with time and the elbow should ultimately extend to approximately 120 degrees. Beyond that, further passive manipulation is not usually necessary. Similarly, the carpo-metacarpal joint will extend to near 180 degrees at completion. A further test of the functionality of the combined wing elements is obtained by grasping the elbow in moderate extension between the fingers and thumb of one hand and pushing outward on the leading edge of the carpus. This should result in the primary feathers extending into near full flight position with a slight bounce or recoil in their extension owing to the rebound of the ligaments and tendons. Such a reaction will not be apparent until well into the healing and post-recovery process but should be evident at the time of full recovery **(Figure 9-2A, B)**.

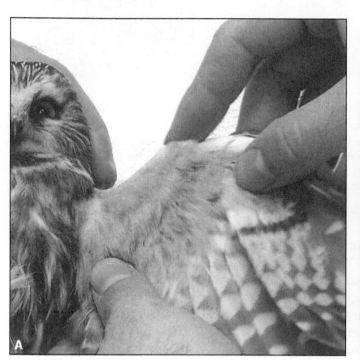

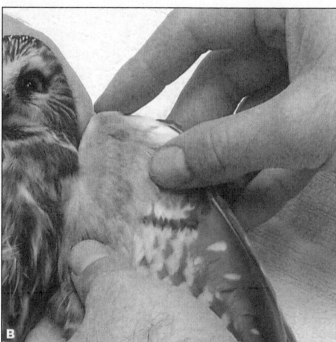

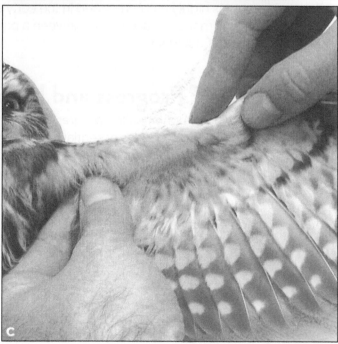

Figure 9-1A-C. These three images show the basic elements in passive-range-of-motion (PROM) **(A and B)** and Stretch-and-hold **(C)** post-operative management of an orthopedic patient (saw whet owl, *Aegolius acadicus*). In the Stretch-and-hold, the elbow is stabilized by the thumb and fingers while the carpus is extended by applying pressure to the leading edge, resulting in the reflex extension of the primary flight feathers (Figures are from Speer, Current Veterinary Therapy – with permission).

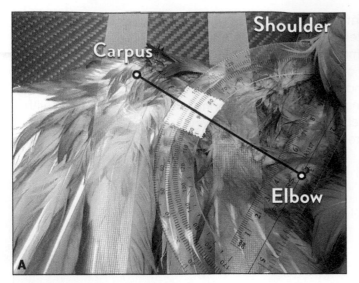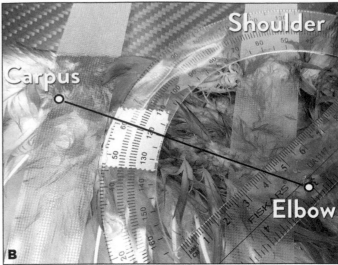

Figure 9-2A, B. When performing passive-range-of-motion (PROM) and stretch-and-hold procedures, it is helpful to measure the degree of contracture of affected joints. This gives caretakers a means to measure progress during post-operative care. A domestic duck *(Anas platyrhynchos)* serves as a model. A common protractor or goniometer can be used to measure the angle of the elbow on the ventral side of the wing. In this example, the elbow rests at approximately 90 degrees **(A)**. With PROM the wing is extended, and the angle of the elbow fully extends to 120 degrees **(B)**.

Longer Term Considerations

Over the ensuing 3-4 weeks, the forelimb fracture patient will be favored by having twice weekly sessions where there is attendant wound cleaning and PROM exercises. The latter should be gradually increased in intensity, always pushing the limits of extension of the joints and soft tissues, and increased numbers of repetitions. The soft tissues of the propatagial are inclined to contract, which if left unchecked, will result in deformity of the leading edge and limitations on extension *(see figure 9-2B)*. Therefore, in addition to PROM, massage and kneading of the propatagium and the propatagial ligament along the leading edge of the wing, breaking down fibrous knots that appear in the latter, is essential to ensuring wing function. Use of anesthesia is at the discretion of the clinician but is highly recommended in the early stages of this process. Attention to this intensive period of management will make the difference between a patient that flies again and one that has a significantly reduced likelihood of doing so.

Monitoring of Progress and Interdiction of Problems

Optimally, monitoring of bone healing progress is done radiographically at 7-10 day intervals post-operatively. Frequent radiographic evaluation is essential to detect problems such as pin loosening, sequestrum formation, or evidence of delayed union. Uncomplicated humeral fractures can be expected to heal in as little as 21 days, forearm fractures (radius or ulna) in approximately 4 weeks, and metacarpal fractures in five to six weeks. Femoral fractures, like the humerus heal in 3-4 weeks, tibiotarsal fractures in 4-5 weeks and metatarsal fractures in 5-6 weeks. Given the pace of healing, frequent radiographic evaluation provides information necessary to interdict any problems that may occur within the window of opportunity that exists for proper bone healing. Failure to recognize and mitigate problems, not only increases the amount of time required for healing but may result in ultimate failure because beyond certain time frames, the healing process often stagnates or ceases altogether. Such an event will require a repeat operation with lessened chances for success.

Concurrent with radiographic evaluation, blood sampling in the form of a simple CBC (hematocrit, total and differential white cell counts) is a valuable tool for overall assessment of patient health, recovery from bodily insult due to original and surgical trauma, and presence of infection. In the case of infection, increased white cell counts and total protein will wax and ultimately wane with adequate antibiosis.

Sequestrum formation is important to recognize and manage. A sequestrum is a piece of dead bone, usually sterile and interposed between healthy bone that has evident callus formation. The sequestrum itself is non-reactive and often is surrounded by a ring of radioluscency. Sequestra typically become evident at approximately half-way through the expected bone-healing time. Its continued presence, if it is left in place and becomes incorporated into the callus, will delay healing and constitute a weak point that is highly subject to refracture. Management requires surgical intervention, removal of the dead bone, culture, irrigation, and wound closure. If removal of the sequestrum leaves a large defect, the options for adequate bone healing are limited. The application of a bone graft in such situations is warranted, however, the state of development of that procedure in avians is not adequately developed – limited in no small part because of the dearth of cancellous bone in the avian skeleton.

Osteomyelitis (*See Figure 6-16D2*) is an infrequent occurrence and is detected radiographically. It is managed in the usual way with antibiotics. It may be possible to obtain a culture and sensitivity through sampling of exudates present along a pin tract. In some cases, the intramedullary pin is removed and its surface cultured. Infected bone will heal, but the infection needs to be controlled for adequate bone healing. Absent material from which to obtain antibiotic sensitivity, clindamycin has proven useful in treating osteomyelitis.

Loosening of the ESF pins and occasionally, their breakage is a possible event in the recovery period. The former is typically detected radiographically as an area of lucency around the pin-bone interface. Such pins are no longer contributing to the strength of the fixator construct, and in fact, are causing damage to the bone and serving as a site of introduction of infection. They should be removed at the first indication that they are failing. Depending on the state of healing and the adequacy of the remaining construct, remedies may include placing another ESF pin through the acrylic bar and attaching it to the bone in near proximity to the removed pin or employing coaptation for a short period of time while healing continues.

PROM goals – elbow to extend 120 degrees and carpal-metacarpal joint to nearly 180 degrees.

Post-operative Issues of the Pelvic Limb

Most of the preceding discussion, particularly regarding PROM, has pertained to the wing. Fractures of the pelvic limb require much less active management. There are areas of concern. Since the pelvic limb is weight-bearing, the fixation must be sufficiently robust to withstand forces applied to it. It is also expected that for the first two weeks of healing, owing to pain and perhaps nerve damage associated with the injury, there will be limited weight-bearing and the other leg will be carrying the brunt of the weight. The greatest resulting concern is the development of plantar ischemia, epithelial breakdown, infection, and formation of bumblefoot or pododermatitis. The remaining points made above regarding monitoring of the fracture and patient apply.

Management approaches and strategies for leg fractures include 1) limiting opportunities for movement by housing in solid sided containers (no climbing), 2) reduced lighting to discourage movement, 3) removal of perches to encourage the patient to rest in the prone position, 3) bedding the holding container with several inches of shredded newspaper that again encourages them to rest without putting pressure on their legs, and 4) protection of the contralateral foot. Other considerations include, in the case of tibiotarsal fractures, removal of the IM pin at approximately the mid-point of healing between two and three weeks when there is radiographic evidence of callus formation. This will reduce the likelihood of stifle injury from the protruding pin. The remaining ESF elements are left in place until healing is complete. While not essential, the practice of removing the IM pin when able is recommended.

Protection of the contralateral foot is an essential consideration and must be undertaken immediately in the post-operative period. It is recommended that a protective interdigital wrap of conforming gauze overlayed with Vetrap be applied to the foot at the conclusion of the surgical procedure on the opposite limb and that that the foot be examined every time the patient is examined. Waiting until there is evidence of loss of epithelial integrity on the plantar surface, or worse yet, breakdown and infection because of lack of protection, is to invite a difficult management situation and possibly loss of the patient. Readers are encouraged to consult materials in other avian texts on bumblefoot prevention and treatment.

Beyond Recovery

For wild birds, especially raptors, that are intended for release to the wild, but also including any others where practical, attainment of bone healing and fixation removal is not the endpoint. These patients will require another 2-3 months of quiet recovery in appropriate flight cages or facilities during which time healed bones acquire adequate strength (full bone strength may take close to a year) and body condition is regained. At that point, usually marked by the ability to reach high perches in their enclosure, they can be entered into an active exercise program. The goal is to give them athletic ability and endurance comparable to that of an uninjured wild bird. This will necessitate several weeks on a 2-3 times a week basis of active, controlled exercise. An excellent method of providing this is the "creance flying" method (Arent 2000). Briefly, this consists of attaching leather straps (jesses) to each leg, tethering these to a length of parachute cord or other appropriate light-weight line (50-100 meters long) with a length of wood at the other end for a drag, and taking the bird to an open area and encouraging it to fly the length of the cord. Over a period of 3-4 weeks, a remarkable improvement in flight ability will be observed that will prepare it for ultimate release. There is much more to this method than can be addressed here and readers are encouraged to pursue this in the referenced text or the many on-line videos available.

Recommended Reading

Arent, L. 2000. Reconditioning Raptors: A Training Manual for the Creance Technique. The Raptor Center, University of Minnesota, St. Paul, MN.

CHAPTER 10

Digital Radiographs of the Limbs

Radiograph Plate: I

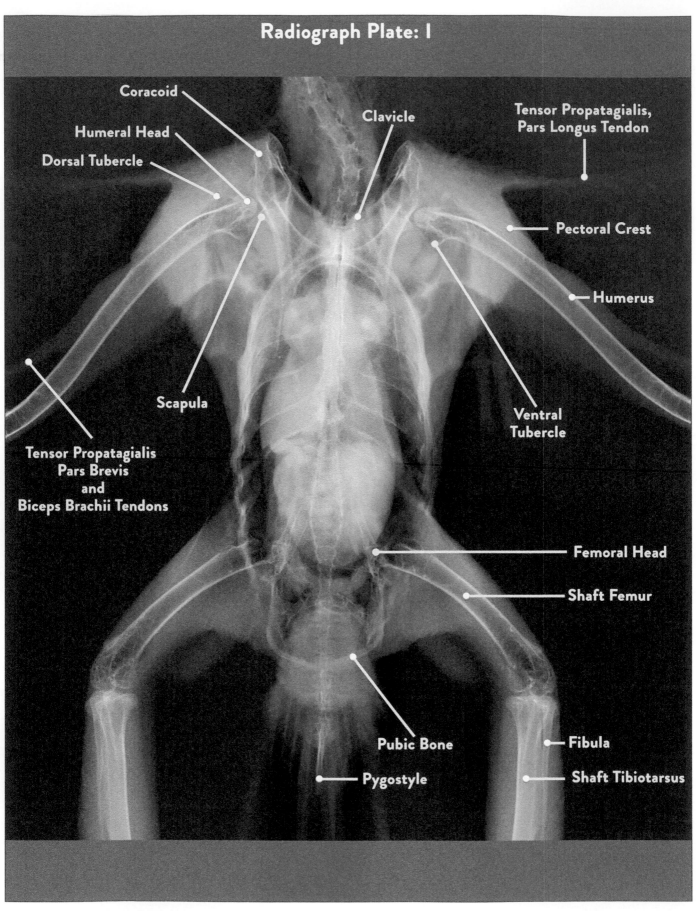

Radiograph Plate I: Ventro-dorsal view of the body and proximal limbs. Swainson's hawk (*Buteo swainsoni*).

Radiograph Plate: II

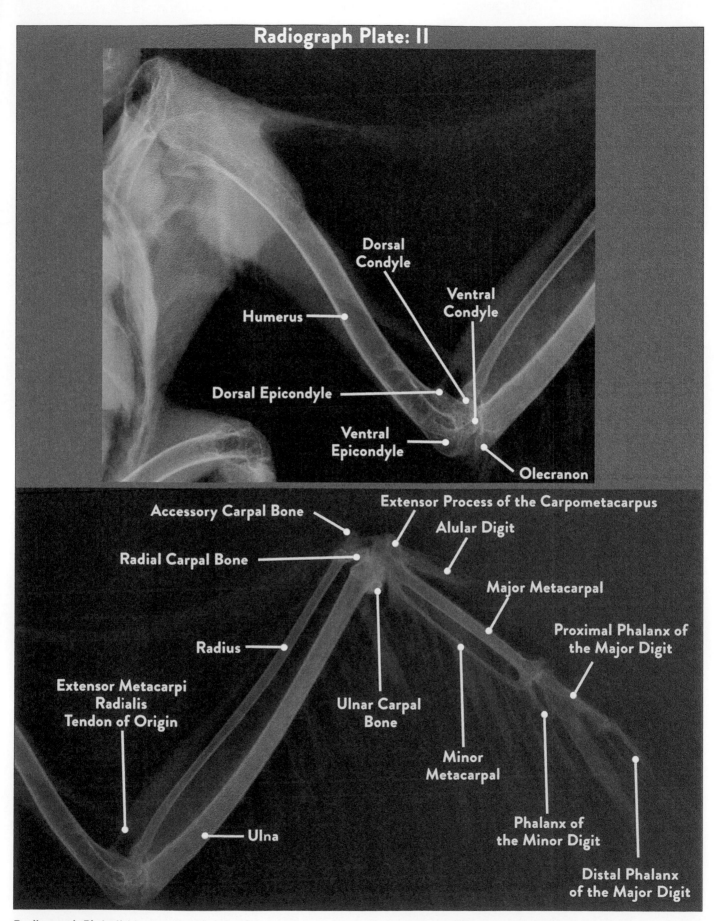

Radiograph Plate II: Ventro-dorsal view of the partially extended wing—proximal *(top)* and distal *(bottom)*. Swainson's hawk *(Buteo swainsoni)*

Radiograph Plate: III

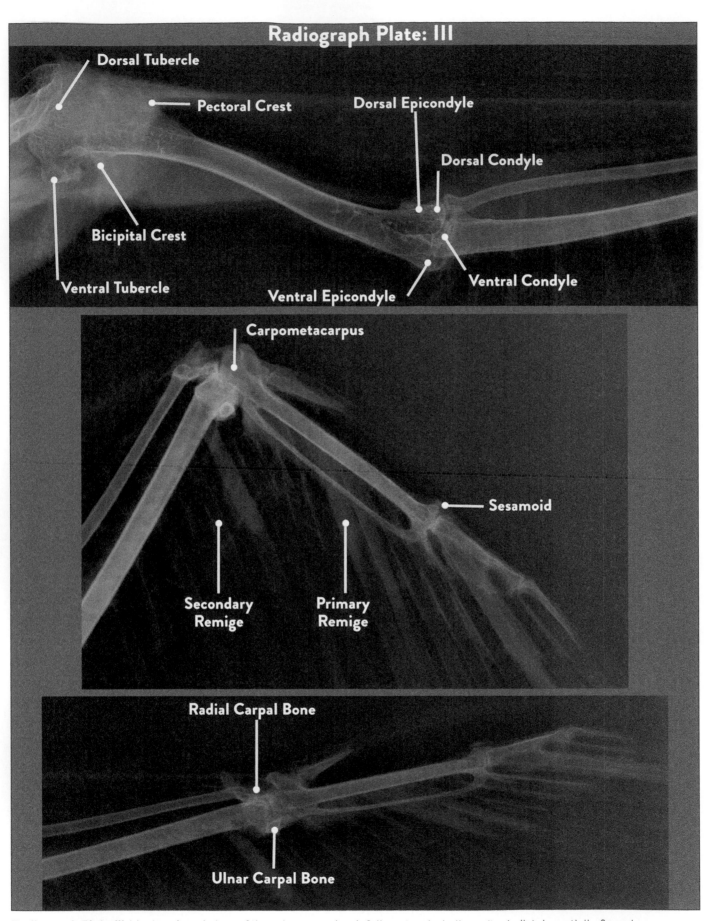

Radiograph Plate III: Ventro-dorsal view of the wing—proximal, fully extended elbow *(top)*; distal, partially flexed carpus *(middle)*; and distal, fully extended carpus *(bottom)*. Swainson's hawk *(Buteo swainsoni)*.

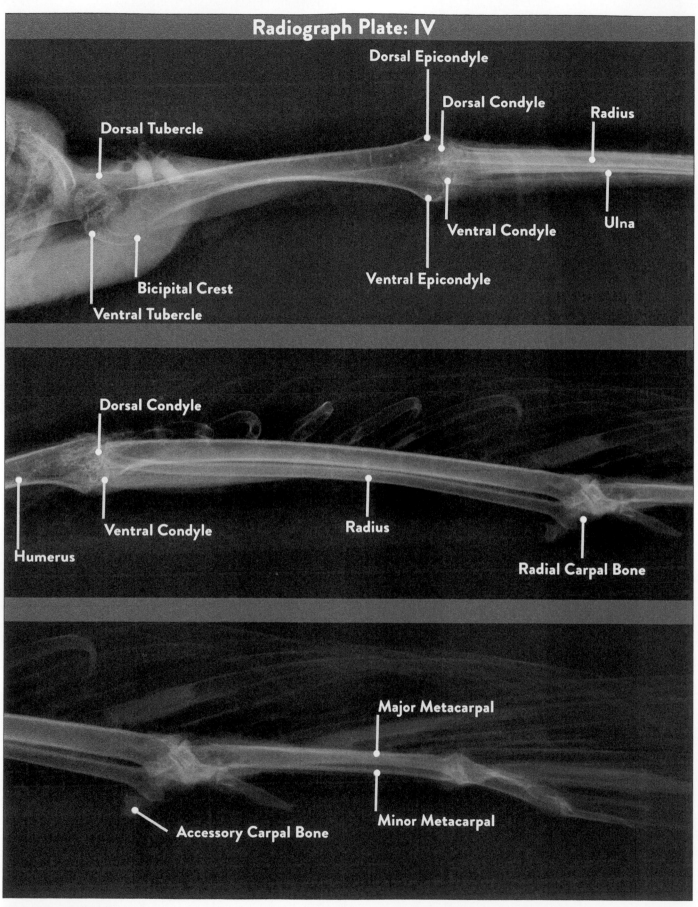

Radiograph Plate: IV

Dorsal Epicondyle

Dorsal Condyle

Radius

Dorsal Tubercle

Ventral Condyle

Ulna

Bicipital Crest

Ventral Epicondyle

Ventral Tubercle

Dorsal Condyle

Ventral Condyle

Radius

Humerus

Radial Carpal Bone

Major Metacarpal

Minor Metacarpal

Accessory Carpal Bone

Radiograph Plate IV: Caudo-cranial view of the fully extended wing—proximal *(top)*; mid *(middle)*; and distal *(bottom)*. Swainson's hawk *(Buteo swainsoni)*.

Radiograph Plate: V

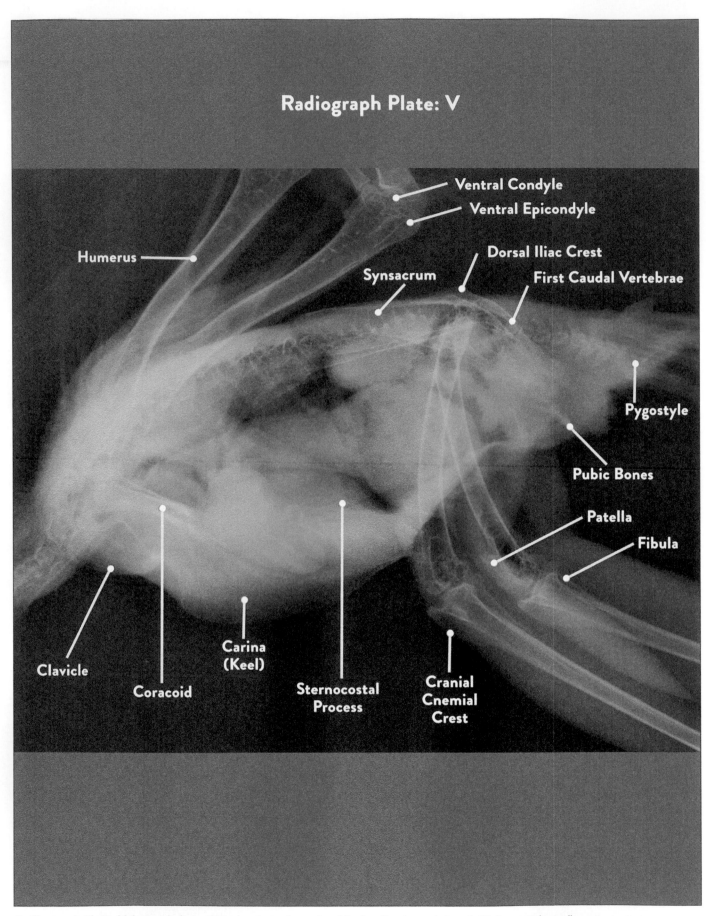

Ventral Condyle

Ventral Epicondyle

Humerus

Dorsal Iliac Crest

Synsacrum

First Caudal Vertebrae

Pygostyle

Pubic Bones

Patella

Fibula

Clavicle

Coracoid

Carina (Keel)

Sternocostal Process

Cranial Cnemial Crest

Radiograph Plate V: Lateral view of the body and proximal limbs. Swainson's hawk (*Buteo swainsoni*).

Radiograph Plate: VI

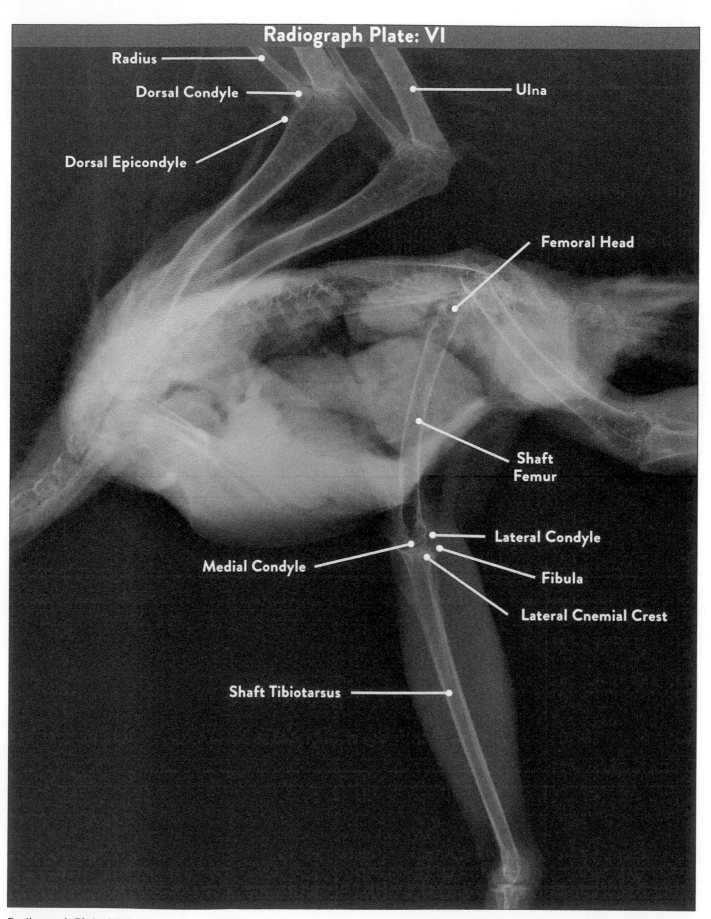

Radius

Dorsal Condyle

Dorsal Epicondyle

Ulna

Femoral Head

Shaft
Femur

Lateral Condyle

Medial Condyle

Fibula

Lateral Cnemial Crest

Shaft Tibiotarsus

Radiograph Plate VI: Partially rotated lateral view of the body and proximal limbs with one leg in extension and the other in flexion. Swainson's hawk *(Buteo swainsoni)*.

Radiograph Plate: VII

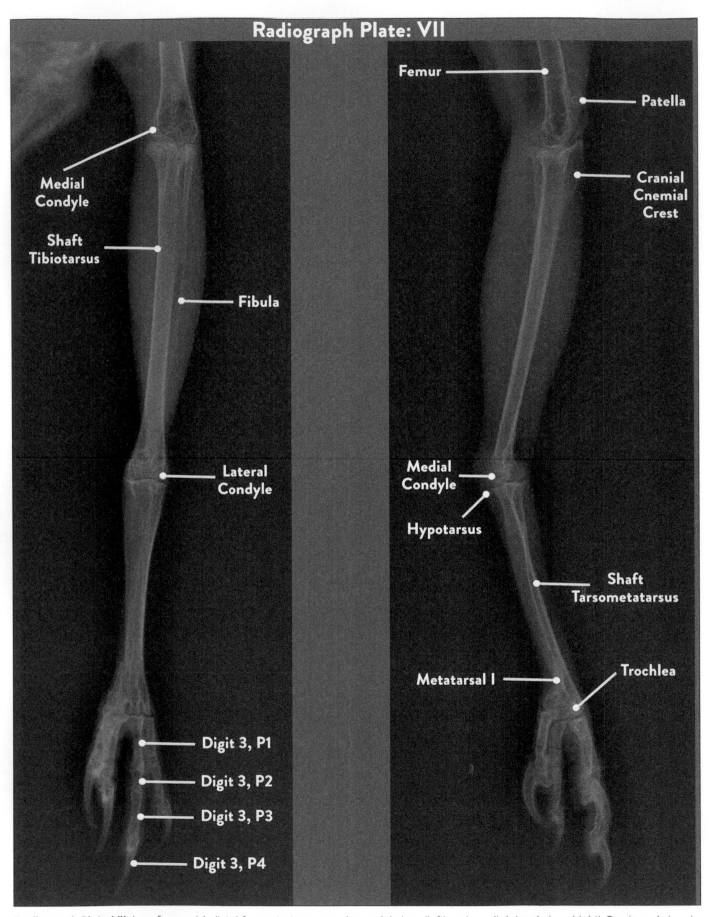

Radiograph Plate VII: Leg from mid-distal femur to toes- craniocaudal view *(left)* and mediolateral view *(right)*. Swainson's hawk *(Buteo swainsoni)*.

Appendices

TABLE OF GUIDELINES OF PIN SIZES FOR LONG BONES OF VARIOUS SPECIES

Species	Humerus	Radius	Ulna	Femur	Tibiotarsus	ESF Pin	Finished Bar Diameter
Bald & Golden Eagle	3/16	1/8	3/16	3/16	5/32-3/16	3/32-1/8	0.75-1.0 (3/4-1)
Gyrfalcon	5/32	5/64	1/8-5/32	1/8-5/32	1/8	0.078	0.625 (5/8)
Peregrine & Prairie Falcon	3/32	0.062			5/64	0.062	0.5 (1/2)
Merlin	0.062	0.035-0.045	0.062	0.062	0.045	.035-.045	0.25-0.375 (3/8)
Kestrel	0.045	NA	0.035	0.045	.035	.035	0.375 (3/8)
Red-Tail & Ferruginous	9/64	0.062	5/64-3/32	1/8-5/32		0.062	0.5 (1/2)
Rough Leg, Swainson's, Red Shouldered	7/64	0.062	3/32/-7/64	7/64	3/32	.062	0.5 (1/2)
Broad-Wing	3/32	0.045	5/64	5/64	0.062	0.045	0.375-0.5 (3/8-½)
Goshawk	1/8	0.062	5/32-7/64	1/8	7/64-3/32	0.062	0.5 (1/2)
Cooper's Hawk	5/64	0.045	5/64	5/64	1/16	0.045	0.375 (3/8)
Sharpshinned Hawk	0.062	NA	0.045	0.045-.062	0.035	0.035	0.25 (¼)
Great Horned & Snowy Owl	1/8	0.062	7/64	9/64	1/8	0.062-0.078	0.5-0.75 (1/2-¾)
Great Grey Owl	7/64	.045-.062	7/64	1/8	1/8	0.062	0.5 (1/2)
Barred Owl	3/32	0.062	5/64	3/32	5/64	0.062	0.5 (1/2)
Long & Short Eared Owl	5/64	0.045	5/64	5/64-3/32	5/64	0.045	0.375-0.5 (3/8-½)
Screech Owl	1/16	0.035	.035	0.062	0.045-0.062	0.035	0.25 (1/4)
Saw-Whet Owl	0.045	NA	0.035	0.045	0.035-0.045	0.028	0.25 (1/4)
African Grey Parrot	5/64	0.045	1/16-5/64	5/64-3/32	1/16-5/64	0.045	0.5 (1/2)
Cockatiel	0.045-0.062	NA	0.035	0.035	0.045	0.028	0.25 (1/4)
Blue & Gold Macaw	1/8	0.062	5/32	1/8	5/32/-7/64	0.062	0.5

All dimensions are provided in inches. Pin sizes less than 1/16" (0.062") are given as decimals while larger sizes are expressed fractionally. Where a range of sizes is provided, this reflects variation known to exist within that species or reflects gender size difference (female raptors are larger than males). In all instances, this is a guide. Pin sizes should be checked against radiographic measurements and intra-operatively to ensure that the pin moves freely in the medullary cavity. Impingement of the endothelial surface by a too large pin will result in ischemic bone necrosis. Ideally, the pin would be sized to 60-70% of the medullary cavity – a slightly larger pin is useful in holding an oblique fracture in alignment. NA refers to situations in which the medullary cavity is generally too small to accept conventionally available pin sizes. In general, external fixator bar size should be at least as large or slightly larger than the bone being repaired.

3/16 = 4.8mm	3/32 = 2.4 mm	1/16 = 0.062 = 1.6mm
1/8 = 3.2 mm	5/64 = 2mm	0.028 = 0.7mm

Table of Homologous Terms

Thoracic Limb

Easy Reference Terms	Fisher[1]	NAA[2]	Getty[3]
Abductor alulae	Abductor pollicis	Abductor alulae	Abductor alulae
Abductor digiti majoris	Abductor indicis majoris	Abductor digiti majoris	Abductor· digiti majoris
Adductor alulae	Adductor pollicis	Adductor alulae	Adductor alulae
Anconeus	Anconeus	Ectepicondylo-ulnaris	Ectepicondylo-ulnaris
Biceps brachii	Biceps	Biceps	Biceps brachii
Brachialis	Brachialis	Brachialis	Brachialis
Common digital extensor	Extensor digitorum communis	Extensor digitorum communis	Extensor digitorum communis
Coracobrachialis caudalis	Coracobrachialis caudalis	Coracobrachialis caudalis	Coracobrachialis
Coracobrachialis dorsalis	Coracobrachialis anterior	Coracobrachialis cranialis	Coracobrachialis cranialis
Deep pectoral	Pectoralis superficialis, deep layer	--	--
Deltoideus major	Deltoideus major	Deltoideus major	Deltoideus major
Deltoideus minor	Deltoideus minor	Deltoideus minor	Deltoideus minor
Dermotensor patagii	Dermotensor patagii	Dermotensor patagii	Dermotensor patagii
Extensor brevis alulae	Extensor pollicus alula	Extensor brevis alulae	Extensor brevis alulae
Extensor brevis digiti majoris	Flexor metacarpi brevis	Extensor brevis digiti majoris	Extensor brevis digiti majoris
Extensor longus digiti majoris	Extensor indicis longus	Extensor longus digiti majoris	Extensor longus digiti majoris
Extensor longus alulae	Extensor pollieus longus	Extensor longus alulae	Extensor longus alulae
Extensor metacarpi radialis	Extensor metacarpi radialis	Extensor metacarpi radialis	Extensor metacarpi radialis
Flexor alulae	Flexor pollicis	Flexor alulae	Flexor alulae

Easy Reference Terms	Fisher[1]	NAA[2]	Getty[3]
Flexor carpi ulnaris	Flexor carpi ulnaris, posterior part	Flexor carpi ulnaris	Flexor carpi ulnaris
Flexor digiti minoris	Flexor digiti Ill	Flexor digiti minoris	Flexor digiti minoris
Flexor digitorum profundus	Flexor digitorum profundus	Flexor digitorum profundus	Flexor digitorum profundus
Flexor digitorum superficialis	Flexor carpi ulnaris, anterior part	Flexor digitorum superficialis	Flexor digitorum superficialis
Flexor metacarpi caudalis	Flexor metacarpi pollicus	Ulnometacarpalis dorsalis	Ulnometacarpalis dorsalis
Interosseous dorsalis	Interosseous dorsalis	Interosseous dorsalis	Interosseous dorsalis
Interosseous ventralis	Interosseous palmaris	Interosseous ventralis	Interosseous ventralis
Latissimus dorsi, pars cranialis; pars caudalis	Latissimus dorsi, pars anterior and pars posterior	Latissimus dorsi; pars cranialis; pars caudalis	Latissimus dorsi cranialis and caudalis
Pronator brevis	Pronator brevis	Pronator superficialis	Pronator superficialis
Pronator longus	Pronator longus	Pronator profundus	Pronator profundus
Superficial pectoral	Pectoralis superficialis, superficial layer	Pectoralis	Pectoralis, pars thoracicus
Supinator	Supinator brevis	Supinator	Supinator
Supracoracoideus	Supracoracoideus	Supracoracoideus	Supracoracoideus
Tensor propatagialis pars brevis and longus	Tensor patagii brevis and longus	Tensor propatagialis pars brevis and longus	Tensor propatagialis pars brevis and longus
Triceps brachii	Triceps	Triceps brachii	Triceps brachii
Ulnaris lateralis	Flexor metacarpi radialis	Extensor metacarpi ulnaris	Extensor metacarpi ulnaris
Ulnometacarpalis ventralis	Flexor metacarpi posterior	Ulnometacarpalis ventralis	Ulnimetacarpalis ventralis

Thigh and Leg

Easy Reference Terms	Fisher[1]	NAA[2]	Getty[3]
Abductor digiti II	Abductor digiti II	Abductor digiti II	Abductor digiti II
Abductor digiti IV	Abductor digiti IV	Abductor digiti IV	Abductor digiti IV
Adductor	Adductor superficialis	Pubo-ischio-femoralis pars lateralis	Pubischiofemoralis, pars lateralis
Adductor digiti II	Adductor digiti II	Adductor digiti II	Adductor digiti II
Adductor magnus et brevis	Adductor profundus	Pubo-ischio-femoralis, pars medialis	Pubischiofemoralis, pars medialis
Biceps femoris, cranial head	Extensor iliotibialis lateralis	Illiotibialis lateralis	Illiotibialis lateralis
Biceps femoris, caudal head	Extensor iliofibularis	Illiofibularis	Illiofibularis
Caudofemoralis	Caudofemoralis	Caudo-ilio-femoralis, caudofemoralis	Caudo-ilio-femoralis, caudofemoralis
Extensor brevis digiti III	Extensor brevis digiti III	Extensor brevis digiti III	Extensor brevis digiti III
Extensor brevis digiti IV	Extensor brevis digiti IV	Extensor brevis digiti IV	Extensor brevis digiti IV
Extensor digitorum longus	Extensor digitorum longus	Extensor digitorum longus	Extensor digitorum longus
Extensor hallucis longus	Extensor hallucis longus	Extensor hallucis longus	Extensor hallucis longus
Flexor digitorum longus	Flexor digitorum longus	Flexor digitorum longus	Flexor digitorum longus
Flexor hallucis brevis	Flexor hallucis brevis	Flexor hallucis brevis	Flexor hallucis brevis
Flexor hallucis longus	Flexor hallucis longus	Flexor hallucis longus	Flexor hallucis longus
Flexor perforans et perforatus digiti II	Flexor perforans et perforatus digiti II	Flexor perforans et perforatus digiti II	Flexor perforans et perforatus digiti II
Flexor perforans et perforatus digiti III	Flexor perforans et perforatus digiti III	Flexor perforans et perforatas digiti III	Flexor perforans et perforatus digiti III
Flexor perforatus digiti II	Flexor perforatus digiti II	Flexor perforatus digiti II	Flexor perforatus digiti II
Flexor perforatus digiti III	Flexor perforatus digiti III	Flexor perforatus digiti III	Flexor perforatus digiti III

Easy Reference Terms	Fisher[1]	NAA[2]	Getty[3]
Flexor perforatus digiti IV	Flexor perforatus digiti IV	Flexor perforatus digiti IV	Flexor perforatus digiti IV
Gastrocnemius lateral head	Gastrocnemius pars externa	Gastrocnemius pars lateralis [externa]	Gastrocnemius pars externa
intermediate head	pars media	pars intermedia	pars media
medial head	pars interna	pars medialis [interna]	pars interna
Gluteus medius	Gluteus profundus	Iliotrochantericus caudalis	Illiotrochantericus caudalis
Gluteus profundus	Illiacus	Iliotrochantericus cranialis	Iliotrochantericus cranialis
Obturator externus	Flexor ischiofemoralis	Ischiofemoralis	Ischiofemoralis
Obturator internus	Obturator internus	Obturatorius medialis	--
Peroneus brevis	Peroneus brevis	Fibularis brevis	Fibularis (peroneus) brevis
Peroneus longus	Peroneus longus	Fibularis longus	Fibularis (peroneus) longus
Piriformis	Piriformis	Iliofemoralis externus	Iliotrochantericus externus
Sartorius	Extensor iliotibialis anterior	Iliotibialis cranialis	Iliotibialis cranialis
Semimembranosus	Flexor cruris medialis	Flexor cruris medialis	Flexor cruris medialis
Semitendinosus	Flexor cruris lateralis	Flexor cruris lateralis, pars pelvica	Flexor cruris lateralis
Semitendinosus, accessory head	Flexor cruris lateralis accessory head	Flexor cruris lateralis, pars accessoria	Flexor cruris lateralis
Tibialis cranialis	Tibialis anterior	Tibialis cranialis	Tibialis cranialis
Vastus intermedius	Vastus medialis	Femorotibialis medius	Femorotibialis pars medius
Vastus lateralis	Vastus lateralis	Femorotibialis externus	Femorotibialis, pars externus
Vastus medialis	Femorotibialis internus	Femorotibialis internus	Femorotibialis pars internus

References

1. Fisher HI. Adaptations and comparative anatomy of the locomotor apparatus of new world vultures. *Am Midland Naturalist.* 1946;35:54

2. Association *of Veterinary Anatomists. International Committee on Avian Anatomical Nomenclature: Nomina Anatomica Avium.* 1st ed. London: 1979.

3. Getty R. *Sisson and Grossman's Anatomy of the Domestic Animals. Vol. 2. Porcine, Carnivores, Aves.* 5th ed. Philadelphia: WB Saunders; 1975.

Index

Printed and bound by CPI Group (UK) Ltd, Croydon, CR0 4YY

23/10/2024

01777682-0015